The Human Body Made Simple

This book is dedicated to my wife, Netta

For Churchill Livingstone:

Senior Commissioning Editor: Sarena Wolfaard
Project Manager: Gail Wright
Design Direction: Judith Wright
Main illustrator: Eitan Lavon MD

The Human Body Made Simple

A Guide to Anatomy, Physiology and Disease

Eran Tamir MD

SECOND EDITION

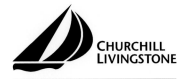
CHURCHILL
LIVINGSTONE

EDINBURGH LONDON NEW YORK OXFORD PHILADELPHIA ST LOUIS SYDNEY TORONTO 2002

CHURCHILL LIVINGSTONE
An imprint of Elsevier Science Limited

First edition 1999
Second edition 2002
  Reprinted 2003

ISBN 0 443 07161 6

British Library Cataloguing in Publication Data
A catalogue record for this book is available from the British Library

Library of Congress Cataloging in Publication Data
A catalog record for this book is available from the Library of Congress

Note
Medical knowledge is constantly changing. As new information
becomes available, changes in treatment, procedures, equipment and
the use of drugs become necessary. The author and the publishers have
taken care to ensure that the information given in this text is accurate
and up to date. However, readers are strongly advised to confirm that
the information, especially with regard to drug usage, complies with
the latest legislation and standards of practice.

 **ELSEVIER
SCIENCE** your source for books,
journals and multimedia
in the health sciences
www.elsevierhealth.com

The
publisher's
policy is to use
**paper manufactured
from sustainable forests**

Printed in China
C/02

Contents

Preface

The book *The Human Body Made Simple* is intended for the student commencing the study of medicine, or complementary or alternative medicine.

Many students encounter difficulty in the early stages of their studies when they start learning about the human body. Part of the difficulty arises because of the lack of suitable texts for the beginner in this field. Most of the texts dealing with the human body are written in technical terms and present the information in excessive detail.

The Human Body Made Simple is written for the reader who has no or little prior knowledge of biology, medicine, or the structure and function of the body. In spite of the simple non-technical language, the book is medically and scientifically accurate and up to date. The reader is gradually and painlessly introduced to the basic technical terminology, yet the inform-ation is presented in a light and highly readable fashion.

The Human Body Made Simple provides a basic overview of the structure and function of the human body, and some common diseases. The explanations are clear and simple, and stress the principles behind the various processes in the body. The text is accompanied by accurate, eye-catching illustrations.

My intention has been to simplify complex topics so that they can be included in this basic text, without sacrificing scientific and medical exactitude. The reader of *The Human Body Made Simple* will acquire a thorough basic understanding of the structure and function of the human body, which can be used as a foundation for more advanced studies.

Ramat Gan 2001   Eran Tamir

Acknowledgement

I wish to thank Felix Klajner for his valuable advice and great contribution in editing the first edition of this book.

From matter to man

MATTER IN THE BODY

Every substance in the world is made up of basic particles called **atoms**. An atom is a tiny particle that cannot be seen with even the most powerful microscope. Each atom consists of a nucleus, which itself is made up of particles called protons and neutrons, and other particles called electrons that revolve around the nucleus. In nature, there are over 100 different types of atoms, which differ one from the other by the number of particles in their nuclei.

An **element** is a substance made up of only one type of atom. For example, oxygen, uranium, iron, zinc, helium and copper are elements. Water is not an element, because it is made up of two different elements – oxygen and hydrogen.

A **molecule** is formed when two or more atoms are joined together. The number of atoms in a molecule can be anything from two to tens of thousands. Very large molecules can even be seen and photographed with an electron microscope (a powerful microscope that enlarges objects by hundreds of thousands of times).

CONSTITUENTS OF THE BODY

The human body is made of water (60% of the

body weight), organic matter (40% of the body weight), and minerals.

The organic matter is made up largely of hydrogen, oxygen, carbon and nitrogen. Organic substances are found only in living things (plants and animals). In the human body, the main organic substances are lipids (fats), carbohydrates (sugars), and proteins.

Lipids (fats) are used mainly as an energy source for the body's activities, and they function as an energy store. The molecules of fat contain oxygen, hydrogen, and carbon. The energy is stored in the form of fatty molecules known as **triglycerides**. Each triglyceride molecule is made up of **glycerol** combined with three **fatty acids**.

Carbohydrates (sugars) are used mainly to provide energy but are also structurally important in certain tissues. They contain carbon, oxygen and hydrogen atoms, which make up molecules called **monosaccharides**, such as **glucose**. When several monosaccharides are joined together they form molecules called **polysaccharides. Starch**, for example, is a polysaccharide made up of many units of the monosaccharide glucose. **Sucrose** (table sugar) is a carbohydrate known as a **disaccharide**, because it is made up of two monosaccharide units (glucose and fructose).

Proteins are the main building blocks of the tissues of the body. They are made up of individual basic units called **amino acids**. Amino acids contain nitrogen in addition to hydrogen, carbon and oxygen. There are 22 different types of amino acid. Proteins are made of chains of amino acids. There are small proteins comprising several tens of amino acids and huge proteins containing hundreds of thousands of amino acids. The chain of amino acids is folded into various shapes (Fig. 1.1). The

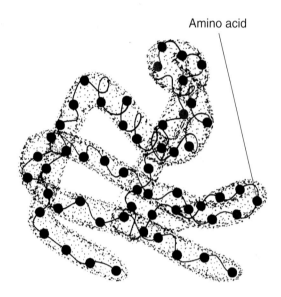

Amino acid

Figure 1.1   The spatial structure of a protein molecule. The protein is made up of a chain of amino acids, and is folded in space to create a three-dimensional structure. The order of the amino acids in the chain determines the spatial structure of the molecule.

average human will contain around 100 000 different proteins, which differ from one another in the number and arrangement of their component amino acids. The body uses information from the genetic material – **DNA** – to help construct the proteins from amino acids. Proteins are used in the construction of the body's tissues, and also serve as enzymes.

An **enzyme** is a protein that carries out a specific function in the body. For example, the digestive system produces digestive enzymes whose function is to break down food into its chemical constituents. Amylase is an enzyme that is involved in the breakdown of the polysaccharide starch into the monosaccharide glucose.

Minerals make up some 4.5% of the body weight. They are mainly made up of elements such as calcium, phosphorus, sodium, potassium, chloride, magnesium, iron, sulfur or copper.

THE CELL

If you examine any tissue of the body under a microscope, you will see that it is made up of many individual cells.

The **cell** is the basic unit from which the body tissues are made. Cells vary in size from 5 thousandths of a millimeter to 150 thousandths of a millimeter.

In nature, there are creatures that can move around and multiply, and which consist of a single cell only; these are called unicellular organisms. Man is a multicellular organism, with billions of different cells in the body.

Each type of cell has a structure that is suited to its specific function in the body. For example, a muscle cell is long and thin, and is capable of contracting and shortening, while a skin cell is flat and waterproof.

In spite of the fact that cells in the body differ from one another, most of them contain the same sorts of organelles (internal components). These components can be seen with the aid of a microscope (Fig. 1.2).

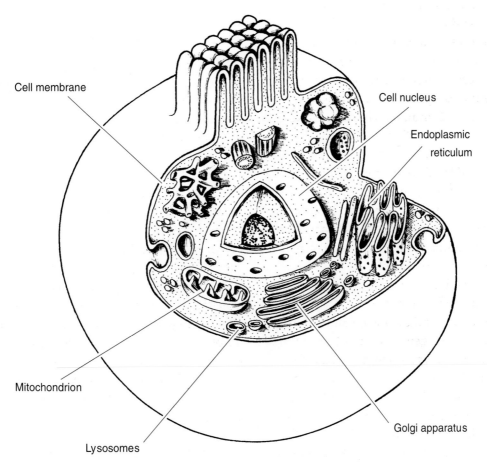

Figure 1.2 Structure of a cell.

Cell organelles

Cell membrane

The cell membrane has two layers, made up of various lipids and proteins. The membrane defines the 'borders' of the cell, and separates it from the surrounding environment. Inside the cell – within the boundaries of the cell membrane – there are various cell organelles, within a watery substance called the **cytoplasm**.

The most important feature of the cell membrane is that it is **selective**. The proteins within the cell membrane act as sentinels that control which substances can get into or out of the cell. Different types of body cells contain different types of protein within their cell membranes. The presence of specific proteins within the cell membrane of certain cells allows the entry of certain substances into that type of cell, depending on its function in the body. For example, substances that can get into liver cells are not the same as substances that can get into skin cells (Fig. 1.3).

Mitochondria

These (the singular is Mitochondrion) are sausage-shaped organelles that function as the 'power stations' of the cell (Fig. 1.4). In the mitochondria, the 'fuel' derived from food is burnt using oxygen, producing energy. The final destination of the oxygen that we breathe is, in fact, the mitochondria, where it takes part in chemical reactions with molecules that are derived from sugars or fats, to produce energy, water and carbon dioxide. The energy pro-

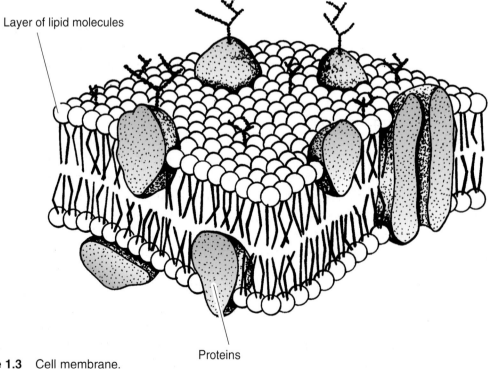

Layer of lipid molecules

Proteins

Figure 1.3 Cell membrane.

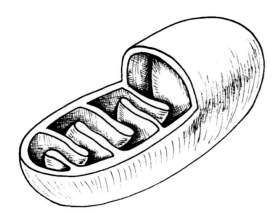

Figure 1.4 Mitochondrion.

duced is stored in a special molecule called **ATP**.

Nearly all processes in the cell that require energy involve ATP molecules, which then break down, releasing energy.

The carbon dioxide produced in the mitochondria is removed from the body via the respiratory system. The water that is produced (some 400 cm^3 a day on average), is used by the body for various purposes.

Lysosome

This is a tiny sac-like structure whose wall is similar in structure to that of the cell itself. Lysosomes are involved in transporting substances within the cell – a sort of delivery van. For example, a substance that is produced in some organelle of the cell, and which is destined to be 'exported' out of the cell, is packed inside a lysosome. The lysosome then moves to the cell membrane, its wall becomes incorporated into the cell membrane, and its contents are discharged out of the cell.

The task of some cells is to engulf and destroy bacteria. To do this, the bacterium is first surrounded by part of the cell wall, which then (with the bacterium inside it) separates off from the rest of the cell wall and becomes a lysosome. The lysosome then joins up with another lysosome that contains enzymes that can digest and destroy the bacterium.

Endoplasmic reticulum

This organelle acts as a 'factory' for the production of proteins. The 'workers' on the protein assembly line are organelles called **ribosomes**. Ribosomes are found inside the endoplasmic reticulum and they join amino acids together into chains, which are called proteins (Fig. 1.5). The 'instructions' that tell the ribosomes how to assemble the proteins come from a special molecule that is derived from the cell nucleus.

Golgi apparatus

This organelle is a processing and packaging station for the proteins formed in the endoplasmic reticulum (Fig. 1.2).

Cell nucleus

The nucleus of the cell (see Fig. 1.2) contains the genetic material, called **DNA**, which holds the information needed to produce proteins.

DNA is made up of a long chain of units called **nucleic acids**, and forms structures called **chromosomes**. In each human cell nucleus, there are 23 chromosomes. The part of a chromosome that contains the information needed for the production of a single protein is called a **gene**. To utilize the information for protein production contained in a gene, another molecule called **RNA** is used. The structure of RNA is similar to that of DNA,

Ribosomes

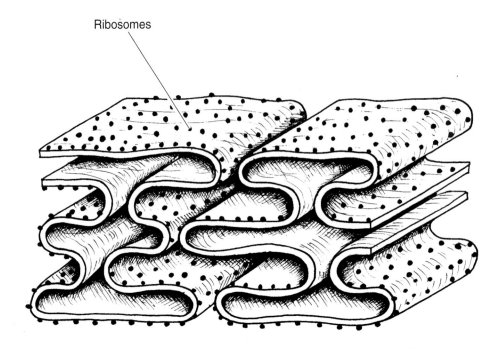

Figure 1.5 Endoplasmic reticulum and ribosomes. Proteins are produced in this organelle. The 'workers' that make the proteins are the ribosomes.

because it is also made up of nucleic acids. The RNA molecule transfers the information stored in the DNA in the cell nucleus to the ribosomes that actually produce the protein.

Every set of 23 chromosomes contains all the information needed to produce every protein in the body. Any single cell in the body obviously makes use of only a small portion of the genes it contains, depending on that cell's tasks and requirements. For example, a cell in a salivary gland will make use of the specific genes that are responsible for the production of the proteins secreted in saliva. Other cells in the body do not use those genes, and so will not make those proteins, but they will make other proteins that are needed for their own particular function.

Adaptation of cell structure to its function

The shape of a cell varies, depending on its function (Fig. 1.6). For example, the task of a skin cell is to cover a surface, and so it is flat; a muscle cell has to contract and shorten, and so it is long and thin; the task of a nerve cell is to transmit changes in electric voltage, and so it has a long filament that extends out of the main cell body.

The make-up of the intracellular organelles also varies from cell to cell, depending on its function. For example, cells that produce large amounts of protein (pancreatic cells that produce digestive enzymes), contain a large amount of endoplasmic reticulum. Cells that use a lot of energy (e.g. skeletal muscle cells)

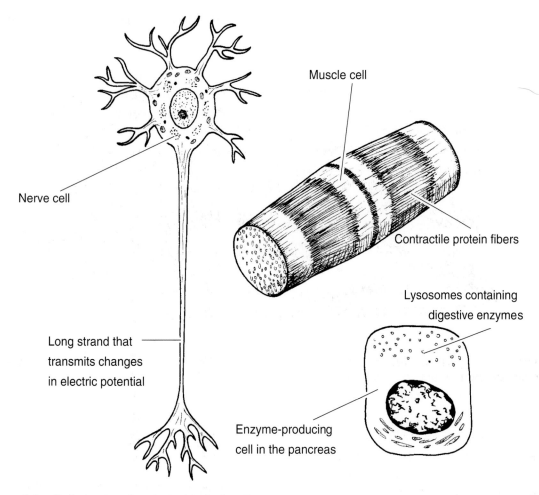

Muscle cell

Nerve cell

Contractile protein fibers

Lysosomes containing
digestive enzymes

Long strand that
transmits changes
in electric potential

Enzyme-producing
cell in the pancreas

Figure 1.6   Cell structure is adapted to its function.

contain a larger number of mitochondria. Mature red blood cells, whose task it is to carry oxygen, contain no organelles, but only a protein called hemoglobin.

TISSUES

A **tissue** is defined as a collection of cells with a common structure and function. There are four types of tissue in the body: epithelial tissue, connective tissue, muscle tissue and nervous tissue. These four types of tissue contain over 200 different types of cells.

Epithelial tissue

This type of tissue serves as a covering tissue and glandular tissue. Epithelium covers all the external surfaces of the body (skin), as well as the internal surfaces of tubes, hollow organs and spaces within the body. The tubular organs for the blood, digestive system, urine, genital organs, respiratory system, biliary system and others are all lined with epithelial tissue on the side facing the lumen (the middle) of the tube.

Epithelial cells can be of various shapes – flat cells, cuboid cells or tall column-like cells.

Some lining tissues contain only one layer of epithelial cells, such as the layer that lines the blood vessels, while others, such as the skin, are made up of several layers of epithelial cells (Figs 1.7 and 1.8).

Glandular epithelium. This makes up the glands in the body. A **gland** comprises a collection of epithelial cells that produce and secrete a certain product. This product might be excreted out of the body (sweat glands), into a tubular space (e.g. the pancreas secretes digestive juices into the digestive tract), or into the bloodstream (e.g. the thyroid gland secretes thyroid hormone into the bloodstream).

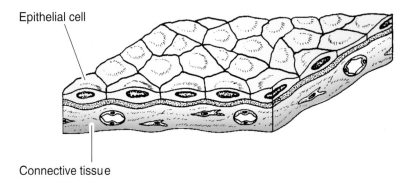

Epithelial cell

Connective tissue

Figure 1.7   Unilayered epithelium.

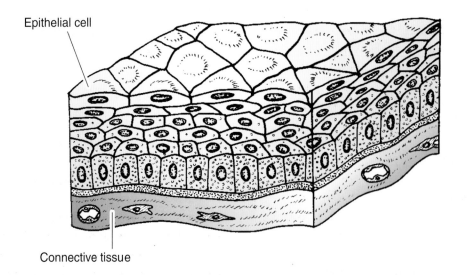

Epithelial cell

Connective tissue

Figure 1.8   Multilayered epithelium.

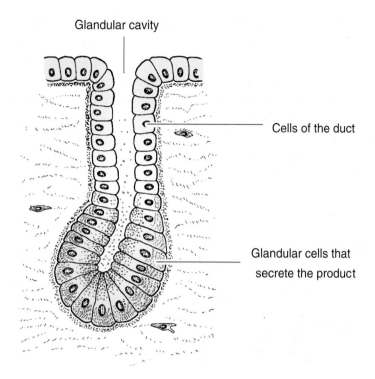

Glandular cavity

Cells of the duct

Glandular cells that
secrete the product

Figure 1.9 A gland.

Glandular tissue is derived during embry-onic development from lining or covering tissue. During the process of formation of the gland, some of the epithelial cells that form the lining or covering move down into the deeper tissues. Those cells that penetrate the most deeply undergo a change, and become cells that produce a certain substance. The cells nearer to the surface become the duct (tube) for the gland. The deep cells secrete their substance into the cavity of the gland, and it then passes along the duct to the external surface (Fig. 1.9).

The process of gland formation can occur in the skin, to form glands that secrete their product onto the skin (sweat glands, sebaceous glands), or in a tube (such as the bowel), result-ing in glands that secrete their product into the cavity of the tube (e.g. mucus glands). Glands whose product is secreted into the bloodstream are not connected by a duct to any surface. Tiny blood vessels pass through the gland and the secretory product of the gland passes directly into the blood in these vessels.

Connective tissue

This type of tissue joins, connects and supports structures in the body. In contrast to epithelial tissue, in which the cells are closely attached to each other, the cells in connective tissue are not joined to each other, and there is a substance called the **extracellular matrix** between them. This substance contains protein fibers (such as collagen fibers) embedded in a gel-like sub-stance. The connective tissue cells are scattered throughout the extracellular matrix (Fig. 1.10).

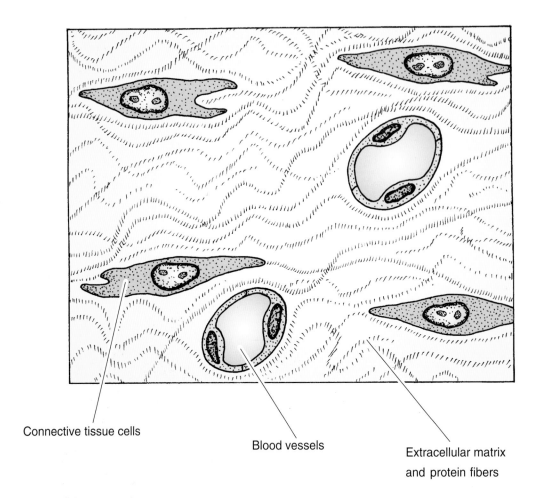

Connective tissue cells

Blood vessels

Extracellular matrix
and protein fibers

Figure 1.10   Connective tissue.

Bone, cartilage, tendons and ligaments, and the subcutaneous (beneath the skin) tissues are all connective tissue. Various types of connective tissue differ in their strength and elasticity, depending on their function. The difference in the characteristics of the various tissues derives mainly from the composition of their extracellular matrix. The type of protein fibers in the matrix, their crowding and the way that they are arranged spatially, vary from one type of connective tissue to another.

Blood and fat are also defined as connective tissues, despite the fact that each has a unique structure.

Nervous tissue and muscle tissue will be discussed in more detail in the chapters dealing with the nervous system and with the motor (movement) system.

ORGANS

Several tissues that are organized into a structure with a specific function form an **organ**.

For example, the heart is made up of three types of tissue. The outer covering of the heart is made of connective tissue, which covers the heart and attaches it firmly to the sternum (breastbone) in front and to the diaphragm below. The wall of the heart is made up of muscle tissue, which can contract. The cavities of the heart are lined with epithelial tissue.

As another example, the hand is an organ that contains epithelial tissue (the skin), connective tissue (subcutaneous tissue, bone and others), muscle tissue and nervous tissue (the peripheral nerves). All these tissues are organized into an organ – the hand. The hand is involved in the motor (movement) system (Fig. 1.11).

SYSTEMS

A number of organs with related functions form a **system**. Each organ in the system has a specific role in the overall function of that system in the body.

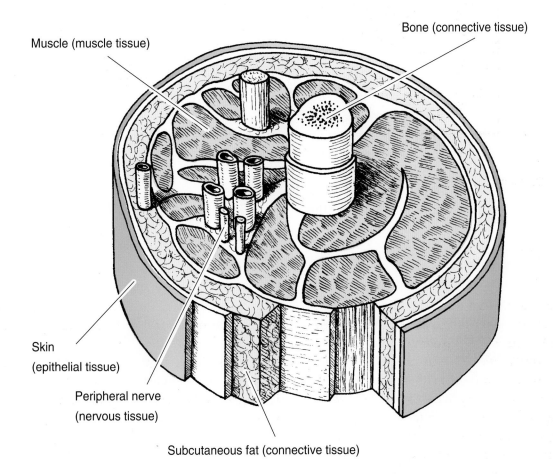

Muscle (muscle tissue)

Bone (connective tissue)

Skin
(epithelial tissue)

Peripheral nerve
(nervous tissue)

Subcutaneous fat (connective tissue)

Figure 1.11   A limb as an example of an organ. A section across a limb demonstrates the layout of the various tissues that comprise it.

For example, the function of the digestive system is to break down and absorb food. Each of the individual organs of the digestive system has a specific task that contributes to the overall function of the system. The mouth breaks down the food mechanically, the esophagus (gullet) then moves the chewed food from the mouth to the stomach, which continues the mechanical breakdown of the food and releases it in a controlled fashion to the small intestine. In the small intestine, the food is broken down chemically and is absorbed into the bloodstream. The large intestine absorbs water and salts, and within it feces are formed. The rectum acts as a reservoir for the feces prior to their expulsion from the body.

Systems of the body

Motor system. Allows movement. Includes the bones, joints, ligaments, tendons and muscles.

Cardiovascular system. Is the body's transport system and includes the heart (the Greek. word *kardia* = heart), blood vessels and the blood itself.

Nervous system. Controls all the body organs. Includes the brain, spinal cord and peripheral nerves.

Respiratory system. Is responsible for supplying oxygen to the blood and for removing carbon dioxide from it. This system includes the respiratory passages, the lungs and some accessory organs used in breathing.

Digestive system. Breaks down food and allows for its absorption into the blood. Comprises the digestive tract and various glands that secrete digestive juices into it.

Endocrine system. Secretes hormones that affect various bodily processes. Comprises a series of glands at various places within the body.

Urinary system. Eliminates waste products from the blood and maintains the correct balance of water and salts within the body. The system comprises the kidneys, ureters, bladder and urethra.

Immune system. Destroys infecting agents that get into the body. Includes the lymphatic vessels and lymph glands, the spleen and an 'army' of cells in the blood and within various tissues.

Reproductive system. In the male, the reproductive system delivers sperm to the woman, while in the woman it allows pregnancy and birth.

All the systems together make up the complete body.

FROM MATTER TO MAN

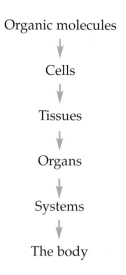

Organic molecules
↓
Cells
↓
Tissues
↓
Organs
↓
Systems
↓
The body

Terms

MEDICAL DISCIPLINES

There are various disciplines dealing with the science of the body. The amount of knowledge that has accumulated is enormous, and today there are tens of thousands of terms to describe structures and processes within the body. Here are the major scientific disciplines dealing with the human body.

Anatomy.   The study of the macroscopic (able to be seen with the naked eye) structures in the body. This is an ancient discipline, going back thousands of years, whose development required only a body, a knife, and a keen eye. Today, the trend in anatomy is to use English terms, rather than Latin or Greek terms, as used to be the case in the past.

Histology.   The study of the microscopic (able to be seen only with a microscope) structures of the body. This is a relatively modern discipline that followed the invention of the microscope in the seventeenth century. The first microscope was a light microscope, which allows magnification of up to 1500 times. In the twentieth century, the invention of the electron microscope, which provides magnification of up to half a million times, revealed a whole new complex world within the body.

Physiology. The study of the function of the various structures in the body. Physiology makes use of anatomic and histologic terms.

Biochemistry. The study of the chemical processes that take place in the body.

Pharmacology. The study of medications and how they affect the body.

Microbiology. The study of microorganisms (infectious agents) and their effect on the body.

Genetics. The study of the arrangement of the hereditary material and the relationship between this hereditary material and the body's structure and diseases.

Psychology. The study of behavior and mental and behavioral processes.

Epidemiology. The study of the incidence and frequency of diseases in various populations.

Immunology. The study of the body's defense system.

Pathology. The study of disease processes within the body. Pathology includes the study of the macroscopic appearance of diseased organs, the microscopic appearance of diseased tissues, and the processes that occur in disease – a field called **pathophysiology**.

MEDICAL SPECIALTIES

Medicine comprises the diagnosis, treatment and prevention of disease. The study of medicine involves acquiring knowledge about each of the disciplines of the biologic sciences. Medicine is broadly divided into those fields related to internal medicine and those related to the surgical specialties. The surgical disciplines involve surgery as part of the treatment of the patient. Below are some of the medical specialties.

Internal medicine specialties

Internal medicine. The general name for all the non-surgical specialties.

Cardiology. Deals with diseases of the heart.

Pulmonology. Deals with diseases of the lungs.

Neurology. Deals with diseases of the nervous system.

Gastroenterology. Deals with diseases of the digestive system and the liver.

Psychiatry. Deals with mental and emotional diseases.

Pediatrics. Deals with diseases of children .

Rheumatology. Deals with autoimmune diseases, in which the body is attacked by its own defense system.

Radiology. Deals with the display of images of the body using various imaging and photographic techniques.

Oncology. Deals with cancer.

Geriatrics. Deals with the diseases and problems of the elderly.

Nephrology. Deals with diseases of the kidney.

Dermatology. Deals with diseases of the skin (and traditionally also with sexual diseases).

Surgical specialties

General surgery. Deals mainly with the diagnosis and surgical treatment of diseases of abdominal organs and the breast.

Anesthesiology. Deals with anesthetizing patients for surgery, and also with resuscitation and intensive care.

Orthopedics. Deals with the diagnosis and treatment of diseases and injuries of the skeletal system.

Ear–nose and throat (otolaryngology). Deals with diseases of the ear, nose, and neck region.

Plastic surgery. Deals with the correction of congenital (present from birth) abnormalities, cosmetic corrections, the reconstruction of organs following accidents or the removal of growths and scars.

Neurosurgery. Deals with surgery of the central nervous system.

Urology. Deals with diseases and surgery of the urinary tract and male genital system.

Gynecology. Deals with diseases of the female genital system, pregnancy, and childbirth.

Thoracic surgery. Deals with surgery of the chest cavity.

Vascular surgery. Deals with surgery of the blood vessels.

Ophthalmology. Deals with diseases of the eye.

BASIC MEDICAL TERMS

In medical textbooks, there is a standardized method of presenting information about diseases, with the information being presented under conventional headings. Below are some of the more commonly used concepts, in the usual order in which they appear in a description of a disease.

Epidemiology. Describes the incidence of diseases among various populations. Epidemiological data includes a description of the occurence of diseases in various populations, the age of the patients, their ethnic origin, socioeconomical status of the patients, and so on – within specific populations.

Etiology. Refers to the causes of the disease. In many instances, the precise etiology is not known and the epidemiologic informa-

tion helps to suggest directions for research that may reveal the causes of the disease.

Pathogenesis. Describes the sequence of events that occur in the patient's organ(s) from the first stages of the disease until its later stages.

Clinical features. Refer to the subjective and objective findings in the patient as a result of the disease. **Symptoms** are subjective feelings that the patient reports (such as pain) and **signs** are objective findings that are revealed upon examining the patient. The **diagnosis** defines those criteria needed to establish the nature of the disease.

Treatment. Includes the accepted methods for dealing with the disease. Any given illness may have several forms of treatment.

Prognosis. Refers to the likelihood of the patient's recovery from the illness, either with or without treatment. The data regarding prognosis are based on statistics derived from large numbers of patients.

THE ANATOMIC POSITION

Is the standard position for drawing the human body in anatomic drawings. In all anatomy books the anatomic position is identical, so as to ensure common reference points (Fig. 2.2).

PLANES

If one looks at a drawing of a body in the anatomic position, one can imagine lines producing 'slices' through the body in various directions. These slices are known as planes, or sections, and they describe the anatomy of the body in the various planes. Certain imaging techniques that are available today, such as CT (computerized tomography) or MRI (magnetic resonance imaging) allow us to actually visualize such sections of the body in detail, and to obtain images of internal organs in various planes without actually cutting open the body. These images can be used to help diagnose various pathologies in the body organs. Below are details of the various sections.

Sagittal plane.   Cuts the body at right angles to the ground from front to back. The mid-sagittal plane cuts the body exactly in its midline.

Coronal plane.   Cuts the body at right angles to the ground, from side to side.

Transverse plane.   Cuts the body parallel to the ground.

Oblique plane.   Cuts the body at an angle (Fig. 2.1).

RELATIVE DIRECTIONAL TERMS

These terms describe directions and relations among different parts of the body, again referring to the body as depicted in the anatomic position (Fig. 2.2).

Cranial = Superior = Rostral.   Refers to a structure that is nearer to, or in the direction of, the head rather than the feet. For example, the knee is superior to the foot.

Caudal = Inferior.   Refers to a structure that is nearer to, or in the direction of, the

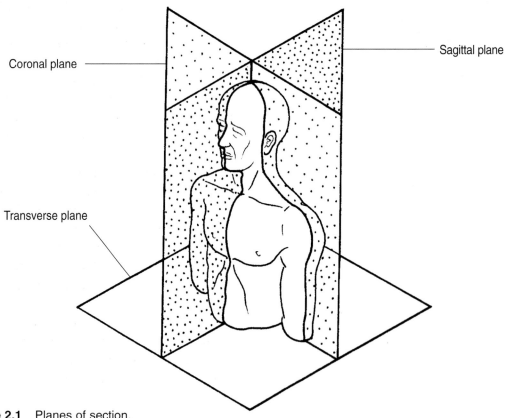

Figure 2.1   Planes of section.

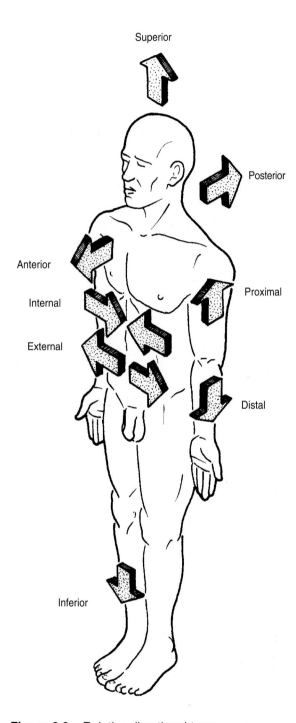

Figure 2.2   Relative directional terms.

lower part of the body. For example, the chest is inferior to the head.

Anterior = Ventral.   Refers to a structure that is closer to the front than to the back part of the body. For example, the nose is anterior to the back of the head.

Posterior = Dorsal.   Refers to a structure that is closer to the back of the body than to the front. For example, the back of the head is posterior to the nose.

Medial.   Refers to a structure that is nearer to the midsagittal plane. For example, the neck is medial to the shoulder.

Lateral.   Refers to a structure that is further away from the mid-sagittal plane. For example, the ear is lateral to the nose.

Proximal.   Refers to structures in the limbs, that are nearer to the body. For example, the arm is proximal to the hand.

Distal.   Refers to structures in the limbs that are further from the body. For example, the hand is distal to the elbow.

Superficial = External.   Refers to a structure that is further away from the interior of the body. For example, the skin is external to the muscles.

Deep = Internal.   Refers to a structure that is closer to the interior of the body. For example, the brain is internal to the skull.

Contralateral.   Refers to a structure that is on the opposite side of the body or limb, relative to the midsagittal plane. For example, on the face, the right eye is contralateral to the left eye.

Ipsilateral.   Refers to a structure that is on the same side of the body or limb, relative to the mid-sagittal plane. For example, the right eye is ipsilateral to the right ear.

3

The cardiovascular system

The cardiovascular system has three components: the heart, the blood vessels and the blood. The heart serves as a pump, causing liquid (the blood) to flow through pipes (blood vessels).

The blood vessels, and the blood that flows in them, reach every part of the body. In general terms, the cardiovascular system can be said to be the body's transport system.

FUNCTIONS OF THE CARDIOVASCULAR SYSTEM

Transport of gas

Oxygen is transported from the lungs to all tissues of the body; carbon dioxide is removed from all tissues of the body and is transported to the lungs.

If the cardiovascular system were to cease functioning, the brain cells would die within about 7 minutes due to lack of oxygen. Brain cells are the most sensitive to lack of oxygen. Cells in other tissues, however, also die if they receive no oxygen for a period of time. For example, a blockage in the blood vessels that supply the blood and oxygen to the leg causes death of the leg tissues within 4–8 hours.

Transport of nutrients and removal of waste products

Nutrients required by tissues are transported from the digestive system and from existing stores of nutrients in the body (such as fat tissue) to the various tissues. Waste products created in the tissues are removed to outside of the body via the kidneys and liver. Blood containing waste products enters the kidneys and the liver, which remove the waste products. The kidneys excrete the waste products into the ureters and the liver excretes them into the bile ducts.

Transport of hormones

A hormone is a substance produced by a gland. It is secreted into the bloodstream, reaches the target organ for which it is intended, and binds to it. The binding of the hormone to its target organ causes a change in that organ. The various hormones, which influence various target organs, circulate in the bloodstream.

Regulation of body temperature

The internal organs constantly produce heat as a byproduct of their regular activities; the external surface of the skin usually loses heat. Constriction or dilation of the blood vessels that bring blood to the skin allows this heat loss to be regulated as required. When the external temperature drops and loss of this heat to the surroundings has to be decreased, the blood vessels constrict (become narrower) and thus decrease the amount of blood flowing to the skin. When heat in the tissues becomes excessive, due either to overproduction (e.g. physical exertion) or to decreased loss (e.g. high external temperature), the blood vessels bringing blood to the skin dilate (become wider). This increases the amount of blood reaching the skin, which becomes hot and red, and heat loss to the environment is increased.

THE BLOOD CIRCULATION

The blood flows through the blood vessels via a circuit called the **blood circulation** (Fig. 3.1). The blood is pumped by the heart, which consists of two separate pumps, the **right pump** (made up of the right atrium and right ventricle) and the **left pump** (comprising the left atrium and left ventricle). The pumping sequence from left to right is as follows. The **left pump** expels blood into a large blood vessel called the **aorta**, which supplies oxygen-rich blood to all bodily tissues. The aorta divides into **arteries** which reach all the tissues of the body, in a manner similar to a tree trunk dividing into branches. They form a tree of arteries, in the shape of the body (see Fig. 3.10).

An artery is defined as a blood vessel that supplies blood to an organ. Blood in arteries always flows towards the target organs, and is usually rich in oxygen.

In the tissues, the smallest arteries branch into **capillaries**. The capillaries form a network of tiny blood vessels, which pass between the cells of the tissues. Oxygen and nutrients pass from the blood to the tissues, and waste products pass from the tissues back to the blood. The blood cells and other blood components do not leave the blood vessels, and do not come into direct contact with the tissues.

Once it has passed through the tissues, the capillary network converges to form larger vessels called **veins**. Veins are blood vessels that drain blood from the tissues. The blood in the veins (venous blood) carries relatively little

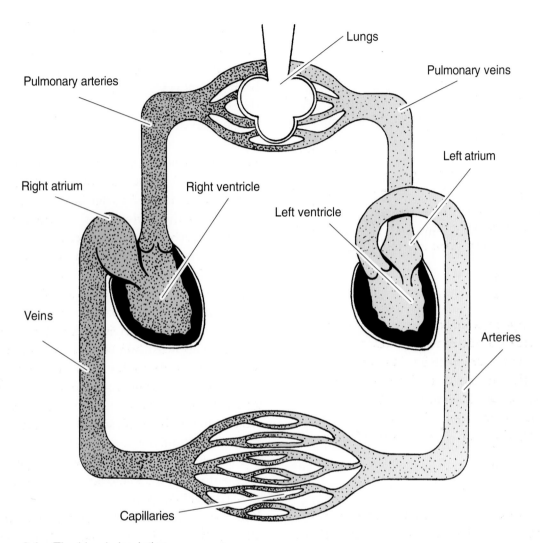

Figure 3.1   The blood circulation.

oxygen and nutrients, and is relatively rich in waste products. Blood in veins generally flows away from the organ. Veins draining blood from various regions join up to form larger veins (see Fig. 3.2).

All the venous blood from the region of the head and upper limbs drains into a large vein called the **superior vena cava**. This vein brings blood to the **right pump** of the heart. The venous blood from the remaining regions of the body drains into a large vein called the **inferior vena cava**. This vein also brings blood to the right pump of the heart. Blood flows from the right pump into a large blood vessel called the **pulmonary artery**. This vessel carries blood to the lungs, and is therefore considered as an artery despite the fact that the blood that it carries contains little oxygen. This artery branches out into two arteries, to take blood to both the lungs. Within the lungs, these arteries further branch into smaller arteries, which finally branch out into a network of capillaries, that pass between the lung's alveoli (see p. 54). In this network, an exchange of gases between the blood and the lungs occurs. Oxygen passes from the alveoli into the capillaries and carbon dioxide passes from the capillaries into the alveoli. The capillary network converges into larger vessels called **pulmonary veins**. Unlike other veins in the body, which carry little oxygen, the pulmonary veins are rich in oxygen. Blood with little oxygen enters the lungs via the pulmonary artery and oxygen-rich blood leaves the lungs via the pulmonary veins. The venous blood from each lung drains into two veins which bring it to the left pump of the heart (see Fig. 3.1).

THE HEART

Location of the heart

The heart is located in a space in the chest called the **mediastinum**. This space is located between the lungs. The mediastinum contains the heart and the large blood vessels, the esophagus, the trachea, the thymus gland and nerves. The heart is located in the center of this space, and is tilted to the left.

The location of the heart relative to other structures is as follows (Fig. 3.2): Anterior to the heart is the sternum and the costal cartilage of the ribs; posterior to the heart are the large blood vessels and the esophagus; inferior to the heart is the diaphragm. The lungs are on either side of the heart.

Layers of the heart

The heart consists of three layers. The exterior layer, enveloping the heart, is called the **peri-cardium**. The middle and major layer of the heart is the heart muscle (**myocardium**). The third layer, which coats the inner surface of the heart chambers, is called the **endocardium** (Fig. 3.3).

The pericardium consists of a number of layers. The external layer is called the **fibrous pericardium** and is constructed of thick connective tissue, strongly connected to the diaphragm and to the sternum. The second layer, called the **parietal pericardium**, is connected to the fibrous pericardium. The third layer, the **visceral pericardium**, is connected to the myocardium. Between the second and third layers there is fatty fluid under low pressure, which keeps the layers closely pressed against each other. These coatings, which envelop the heart, allow the heart to move within them with minimal friction. The coatings of the lungs constitute a similar system.

The **myocardium** takes up most of the thickness of the wall of the heart. It performs the pumping action.

The **endocardium** coats the internal surface of the heart chambers. The heart valves are part of this layer. This layer is continuous with the inner layer that coats the lumen of blood vessels.

Structure of the heart

The heart is composed of two pumps, a right pump and a left pump. Each pump is comprised of an **atrium** and a **ventricle** (Fig. 3.4). Blood enters the right atrium from the two vena cavae, which drain blood from the entire body. Blood enters the left atrium from the four pulmonary veins (two from each lung). The muscular wall of the atria is relatively thin and there is a common muscular wall between the two atria.

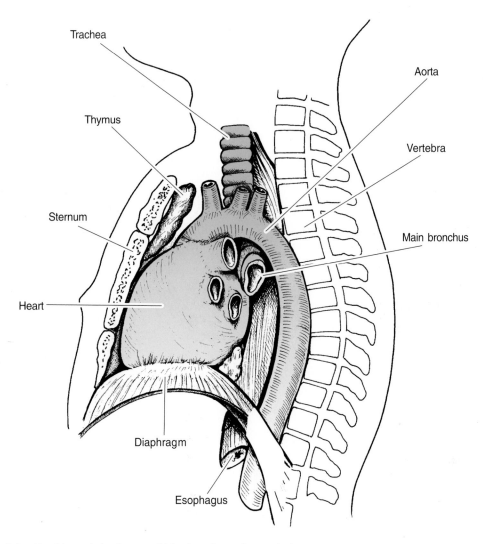

Figure 3.2   Position of the heart within the chest. Lateral view.

Between the atria and the ventricles are valves. The **tricuspid valve** is located between the right atrium and the right ventricle, and consists of three leaflets. The **mitral (bicuspid) valve** is located between the left atrium and the left ventricle, and consists of two leaflets. The function of the valves is to ensure that blood flows in one direction only when the heart contracts.

The ventricles have muscular walls. The walls of the left ventricle are three times as thick as the walls of the right ventricle. The left ventricle is thus much stronger than the right ventricle. Like the atria, the ventricles also share a common wall.

The pulmonary artery comes out of the right ventricle. The **pulmonary valve** is located between the pulmonary artery and the right

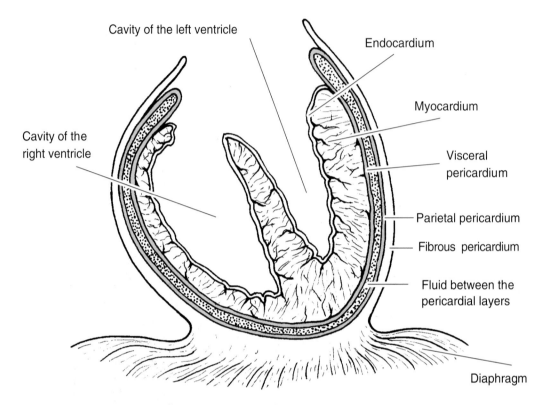

Figure 3.3   Layers of the heart. The heart is shown in coronal section.

ventricle. The **aortic valve** is located between the left ventricle and the aorta.

All four heart valves are located in a single plane, which passes between the atria and the ventricles. The blood entering the ventricles flows in a V-shaped path, because the entry to the ventricles is adjacent to the exit from the ventricles.

Function of the heart

The function of the heart valves is to prevent reverse flow of blood from the ventricle to the atrium or from the artery to the ventricle. If the pressure in the atrium is higher than the pressure in the ventricle, the valve between the atrium and the ventricle opens, in a similar fashion to swinging doors that open when pushed. If the pressure in the ventricle is higher than the pressure in the atrium, the valve closes.

When the valve between an atrium and a ventricle is closed, special mechanism prevents the opening of the valve in the direction of the atrium, similar to swinging doors equipped with a restraint to allow them to open in one direction only. This mechanism is constructed from tendons connecting the edge of the leaflets of the valve to special muscles called the **papillary muscles** (see Fig. 3.4).

When the ventricle contracts and the valve between the atrium and the ventricle closes due to increased pressure in the ventricle, the papillary muscles contract, pulling the tendons

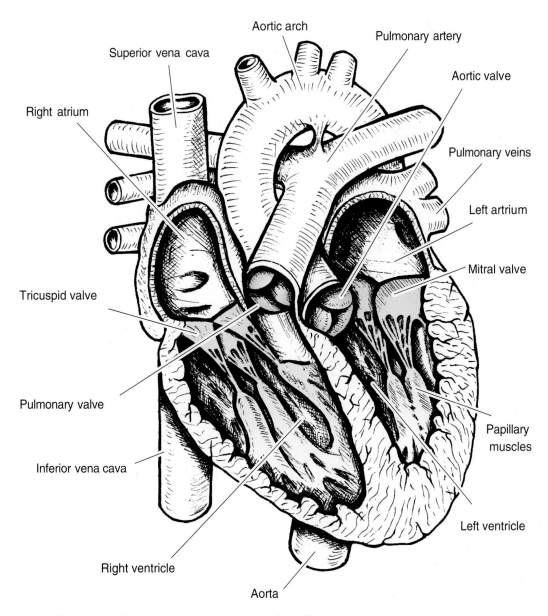

Figure 3.4   Structure of the heart as seen in coronal section.

(which are connected to the edge of the valve), and preventing the leaflets of the valve from opening in the direction of the atrium.

The valves between the ventricles and the arteries, open and close in accordance with pressure differences. Their structure differs,

however, from that of the valves between the atria and the ventricles. These valves are structures like pockets, which open in one direction only.

The principle of operation of the left pump and of the right pump is identical. The stage when the ventricle is relaxed is called **diastole**, and the stage when the ventricle is contracted is called **systole** (Fig. 3.5).

At the beginning of diastole, the muscle of the ventricle relaxes, the volume of the ventricle increases and the pressure within it decreases. This causes the valve between the atrium and the ventricle to open and blood flows in from the atrium and fills the ventricle. At the end of diastole, the atrium contracts, pushing a further amount of blood into the ventricle (the atrial 'kick').

A fraction of a second after the atrium contracts, the ventricle, now full of blood, also contracts. This contraction suddenly increases the pressure in the ventricle, and the valve between the atrium and the ventricle closes. Another fraction of a second later, the valve between the ventricle and the artery (which was closed during diastole due to the high pressure in the artery relative to the pressure in the ventricle) opens due to the high pressure created in the ventricle, and blood flows from the ventricle into the artery.

At the end of systole, the muscle of the ventricle stops contracting, the pressure in the ventricle decreases and the valve between the ventricle and the artery closes. A fraction of a second later, as a result of the drop in pressure in the ventricle following the relaxation of the

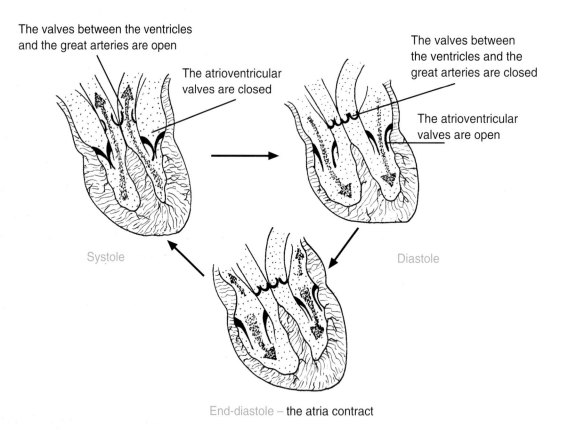

The valves between the ventricles and the great arteries are open

The atrioventricular valves are closed

The valves between the ventricles and the great arteries are closed

The atrioventricular valves are open

Systole

Diastole

End-diastole – the atria contract

Figure 3.5 Systole and diastole.

muscle of the ventricle, the valve between the atrium and the ventricle opens and the ventricle again begins to fill with blood. Contraction of the atrium contributes about 25% of the volume of blood in the ventricle. Without it, the ventricle would still fill with blood, but not as fully. In other words, the atrium is not essential, but contributes to the optimal filling of the ventricle.

The closing of the valves creates a sound similar to the slamming of a door. These sounds can be heard by pressing an ear against the chest, or with a stethoscope. The closing of the valves between the atria and the ventricles creates a sound called **the first heart sound**. Closure of the valves between the ventricles and the arteries creates a sound called **the second heart sound**.

The right pump and the left pump operate in coordination. The valves of the left pump close slightly before the valves of the right pump. The ear, however, is unable to discern that the first and the second sounds are each composed of two sounds, due to the very small interval between the sounds.

Conduction system of the heart

The heart muscle, like other muscles in the body, is activated by a change in its electrical potential. Unlike the other muscles in the body, which are activated by nerves from the nervous system (these nerves convey changes in electrical potential from the brain to the muscles), the heart is activated by an internal electrical system that is not connected to the nervous system. This is called the heart's **conduction system**.

The heart's pacemaker, called the **sinoatrial node** (abbreviated as the **SA node**), is located in the superior portion of the right atrium (Fig. 3.6). The SA node contains special cells that create changes in electrical potential at a fixed frequency; this is regulated by the nervous and endocrine systems. Every change in electrical potential spreads through the atria from the pacemaker towards the valves, causing contraction.

The valves, which are located in one plane between the atria and the ventricles, do not transmit changes in electrical potential. The change in electrical potential is thus not conveyed directly to the ventricles.

The region known as the **atrioventricular node** (abbreviated as the **AV node**), is located in the right atrium next to the tricuspid valve. A structure called the **Bundle of His,** which resembles a wire, leaves this region and conducts changes in electrical potential to the ventricles. It passes through the plane in which the valves are located, enters the muscular wall that separates the ventricles (the septum), and divides into smaller fibers, which conduct the changes in electrical potential to each ventricle.

The change in electrical potential caused by the SA node passes through the atria, causing contraction, and reaches the region of the AV node. It is delayed in this region for a fraction of a second, and is then rapidly conveyed to the muscular walls of the ventricles via the Bundle of His. As soon as the change in potential reaches the ventricles, they contract. The fact that conduction is delayed momentarily at the AV node allows the atria to contract before the ventricles. This is important for the normal functioning of the heart as a pump.

Recording of the ECG

An **ECG (electrocardiogram)** (Fig. 3.7) is the recording of the change in electrical potential

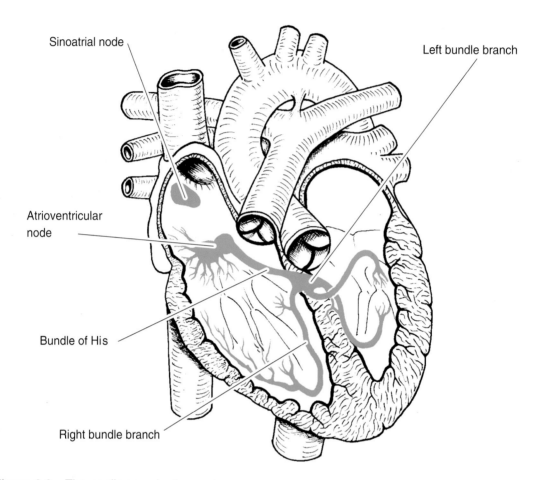

Sinoatrial node

Left bundle branch

Atrioventricular node

Bundle of His

Right bundle branch

Figure 3.6   The cardiac conduction system.

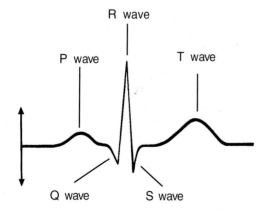

R wave

P wave

T wave

Q wave

S wave

Figure 3.7   Electrocardiogram.

that passes through the heart. The recording is taken by means of electrodes placed on the body and the different peaks and troughs in the recording correspond to the changes in the electrical potential during one beat of the heart. The **P wave** represents the change in electrical potential that progresses through the atria. The Q, R and S waves (called the **QRS complex**) represent the changes in electrical potential that progress through the ventricles. The **T wave** represents relaxation of the muscle of the ventricles.

Much can be learned from the ECG regarding the function of the heart and heart disease. Interpreting the ECG requires significant skill, and takes years to learn.

The blood supply to the heart

The coronary arteries

The **coronary arteries** are the arteries that supply blood to the heart muscle. Immediately above the valve between the left ventricle and the aorta (the aortic valve), two small arteries branch off from the aorta: the right and left coronary arteries. These arteries divide up into smaller arteries and supply blood to the heart muscle (Fig. 3.8).

The venous blood from the heart muscles drains into the **coronary veins**, which bring blood directly back to the right atrium. When the ventricles contract (at systole), the muscle fibers press on the coronary arteries, blocking them. When the heart muscle relaxes (at diastole), the blockage disappears. Blood supply to the heart muscle thus takes place while the muscle is relaxed.

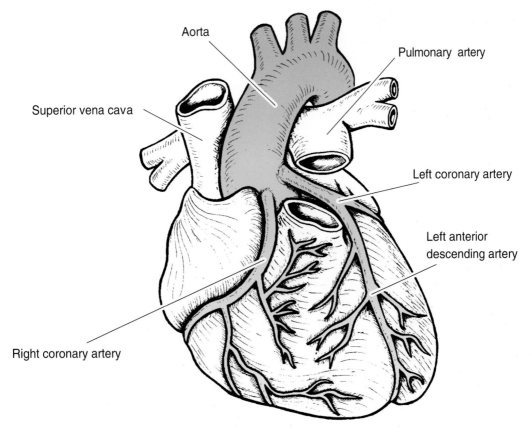

Figure 3.8   Coronary arteries and great vessels.

Cardiac output

Cardiac output is defined as the volume of blood (measured in liters) that the heart pumps per minute.

This is not the volume pumped by the right or the left pump only; both pumps pump the same volume of blood per unit of time. A normal cardiac output at rest is around 5 liters of blood per minute. This is approximately the entire volume of blood present in the blood vessels.

The **heart rate** is the number of heart-beats per minute. A normal figure would vary between 60 and 100 strokes per minute at rest.

The **stroke volume** is the volume of blood pumped per contraction. The normal volume is about 70 cm^3.

If the stroke volume is multiplied by the heart rate, the amount of blood pumped per minute is obtained – this is the cardiac output:

Cardiac output = stroke volume × heart rate

During physical exercise, the heart rate (of a young person) can reach 180 strokes per minute, and the stroke volume can reach 100 cm^3. Cardiac output thus reaches 18 liters per minute, almost four times that at rest, in order to satisfy the increased demand for oxygen by the muscles of the body during exercise. During exercise, the coronary arteries dilate and blood-flow in the coronary arteries increases, in order to satisfy the increased demand of the heart muscle for oxygen.

THE ARTERIES

An **artery** is defined as a blood vessel supplying blood to an organ or limb. With the exception of the pulmonary artery, which brings non-oxygenated blood to the lungs, all arteries carry oxygen-rich blood. The arteries are embedded within the tissues and are not seen protruding from beneath the skin.

Structure of an artery

The wall of an artery is made of a number of layers (Fig. 3.9).

The external layer is called the **adventitia**. This is an envelope of connective tissue around the artery.

The middle layer is called the **media**. This is a layer of smooth muscle. The muscle fibers wrap around the artery in a circular fashion. These muscle fibers are innervated by the autonomic nervous system (see pp. 213–215). Contraction of the smooth muscle reduces the diameter of the artery, thus reducing blood-flow through the artery.

The internal layer is called the **intima**. This layer is made of flat epithelial cells which are closely adjacent to each other, called **endothe-**

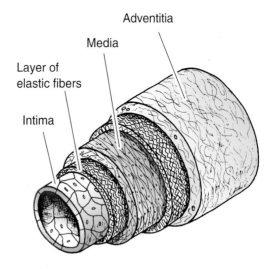

Figure 3.9   Layers of arterial wall.

lial cells. These cells are in direct contact with the blood.

Between the media and the intima is a thin layer of elastic fibers. These impart elasticity to the artery.

The arterial tree

The **aorta** emerges from the left ventricle of the heart and forms an arch known as the **aortic arch**. Arterial branches come out from this arch, supplying blood to the head, neck and upper limb regions. In the continuation of the arch, the aorta descends, running adjacent to the vertebrae, passes through the diaphragm, and enters the abdominal cavity. The aorta continues downwards, sending out large arterial branches to all of the abdominal organs. At the level of the L4 vertebra, the aorta splits up into two large arteries, called the **common iliac arteries**, which supply blood to the pelvic organs. These arteries then enter the region of the groin, and supply blood to the lower limbs (Fig. 3.10).

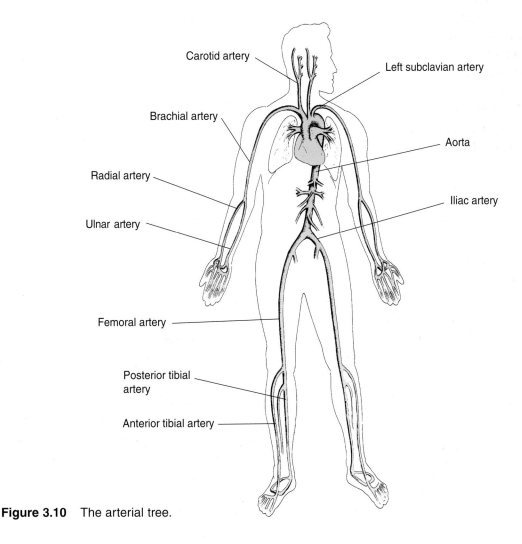

Carotid artery

Left subclavian artery

Brachial artery

Aorta

Radial artery

Iliac artery

Ulnar artery

Femoral artery

Posterior tibial artery

Anterior tibial artery

Figure 3.10   The arterial tree.

The aorta divides up into smaller and smaller arteries, like a tree trunk dividing up into progressively smaller branches. This arterial tree roughly resembles human shape. As the arteries continue to divide, they become progressively thinner. The aorta is some 2.5 cm in diameter. A medium artery is some 0.5 cm in diameter, while a small artery is some 1 mm in diameter. An artery that is not visible to the naked eye is called an **arteriole**. Arterioles are connected to the capillary network (see p. 33).

Blood pressure

Blood pressure is the pressure within the arteries. This pressure is created by the heart's left pump, and varies in a wave-like manner. During systole, the heart pumps some 70 cm³ of blood into the arterial system. As the large arteries have elastic walls, they distend, and the pressure within them increases. The maximal pressure in an artery is called the **systolic blood pressure**.

During diastole (stage of relaxation of the heart muscle), the aortic valve between the left ventricle and the aorta is closed. The pressure in the arteries begins to fall, as the blood flows into the arterioles and from there to the capillary network. The minimal pressure in the artery is called the **diastolic blood pressure**.

Normal values for blood pressure:

Systolic blood pressure:
90 – 140 millimeters of mercury (mmHg)

Diastolic blood pressure:
60 – 90 mmHg

(A millimeter of mercury is a unit of pressure.)

Blood pressure is measured with a special instrument and is usually recorded in the standard form: systolic/diastolic (for example: 120/80 mmHg).

The pulse

The **pulse** is the change in arterial pressure that can be felt. The arteries distend during systole due to entry of blood into them from the heart and this distention can be felt and measured over 1 minute. The number obtained is the heart rate. The pulse can be felt best in specific locations where arteries pass close to the skin. For example, the carotid artery in the anterior aspect of the neck and the radial artery in the volar aspect of the wrist.

Regulation of arterial blood flow

The smooth muscle in the arterial wall, which is innervated by the autonomic nervous system (the system that controls the activities of internal organs), enables the brain to control the blood supply to the various organs. The brain, via the nervous system, is able to contract the smooth muscle in the wall of a specific artery. This decreases the blood-flow in that artery, thus decreasing the blood-flow to a particular organ. For example, during exercise, the diameter of arteries bringing blood to body muscles increases (by means of relaxation of the smooth muscle in the arterial wall) and the flow of blood to the muscles thus increases. At the same time, the diameter of the arteries bringing blood to the digestive system decreases (by means of contraction of the smooth muscle in the arterial wall), thus decreasing the blood-flow to the digestive system. Due to physical laws regarding the flow of fluid in a tube, halving the diameter of an artery causes a 16-fold reduction in the flow of blood through it.

THE CAPILLARIES

The **capillaries** form a network of tiny blood vessels that pass between the cells of tissues. The exchange of substances between the blood and the tissues takes place only in the capillaries. The capillary network (Fig. 3.11) is connected to small arterioles which supply it with blood, and to venules, which drain blood from it.

Capillaries are extremely thin tubes; their diameter is 7–9 thousandths of a millimeter. The length of the capillaries varies between 0.25 and 1 millimeter. The total length of capillaries in the body reaches 96 000 km (three times the circumference of the earth). Capillaries consist of one thin layer of flat epithelial cells called **endothelial** cells.

The capillary wall is very thin to allow easy transfer of substances between the capillary and the tissues. In certain organs, such as the kidney, the spleen and the bone marrow, there are holes in the capillary walls, to facilitate transfer of particles (such as blood cells) between the capillary and the tissue. Blood flows in a continuous manner within the blood vessels from the arterioles to the capillary network, and then to the venules.

The principle of transfer of substances between capillaries and tissues

It is necessary to grasp a number of physical laws in order to understand the principle of exchange of substances between capillaries and tissues.

Hydrostatic pressure. This is the pressure exerted by water on the walls of the vessel or tube that they are in. In a system made of a pipe with tiny holes in its wall, which passes through a cell filled with water, increased pressure in the pipe will cause the transfer of water from the pipe to the surroundings.

Osmotic colloid pressure. Consider a system of two cells containing water, separated by a membrane that is permeable to water but not to large molecules such as proteins. Introduction of proteins into one of the cells raises the osmotic colloid pressure in that cell. The difference in osmotic colloid pressures between the cells initiates the movement of water from the water-filled cell into the cell containing proteins, in an attempt to equalize the pressure difference. However, increasing amounts of water in the cell containing protein causes the hydrostatic pressure in that cell to rise. This increased hydrostatic pressure resists the transfer of water into the cell. When the hydrostatic pressure in the cell containing the protein equals the osmotic colloid pressure created by the proteins, the transfer of water will stop and the system will be in equilibrium.

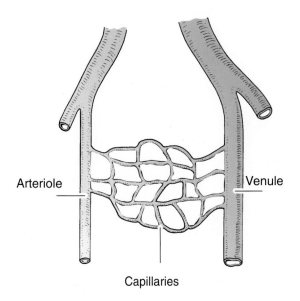

Arteriole

Venule

Capillaries

Figure 3.11   Capillary network.

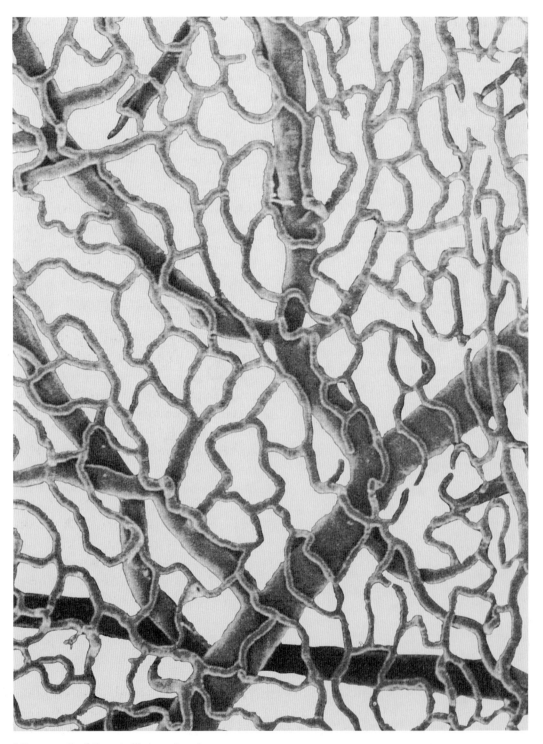

Micrograph of the capillary network.

Blood contains proteins in a higher concentration than the fluid between the cells of tissues. These proteins cannot pass through the capillary walls and the concentration difference creates osmotic colloid pressure, which draws water into the capillaries.

In the portion of the capillary network that is close to the arterioles, the hydrostatic pressure is higher than the osmotic colloid pressure. Fluid, with oxygen and nutrients, thus moves from the capillaries to the tissues. The exit of fluid from the capillaries causes a reduction in hydrostatic pressure in the capillaries and an increase in osmotic colloid pressure (due to the increased concentration of protein relative to water because of the exit of the water).

In the portion of the capillaries that is close to the venules, the osmotic colloid pressure is higher than the hydrostatic pressure. The osmotic colloid pressure thus draws fluid, which now contains little oxygen (the oxygen having entered the cells of the tissue) and which contains carbon dioxide and waste products produced by the cell, back into the capillaries.

The total amount of water leaving the capillaries is 10% higher than the amount of water returning to the capillaries. The remaining fluids return to the venous system via the lymphatic system.

THE VEINS

A **vein** is a blood vessel that normally drains blood from an organ. The capillary network connects to microscopic **venules**. These venules unite to form small veins, which in turn join up to form larger veins, and so on, to form a venous tree (Fig. 3.12). All of the venous blood from the region of the head, neck and upper limbs enters the superior vena cava, and then the right atrium. The venous blood from the remainder of the body enters the inferior vena cava, and then also the right atrium.

There are two types of vein in the body – superficial and deep. The deep veins are generally adjacent to arteries. The superficial veins pass under the skin; they can be seen as bluish streaks just under the skin. This bluish color is the color of all venous blood, which contains less oxygen than the arteries (oxygen reacts with the protein hemoglobin (see p. 37) to give arterial blood its characteristic red color).

Structure of a vein

The wall of a vein is relatively thin compared to the wall of an artery. It has three layers (Fig. 3.13).

The external layer, called the **adventitia**, is made of connective tissue and envelops the vein.

The middle layer, called the **media**, is made of round layers of smooth muscle and is thinner than the media layer of arteries.

The internal layer, called the **intima**, is composed of a single layer of **endothelial** cells and is in direct contact with the blood.

Veins contain valves (**venous valves**), which are made from folds of the intima. These valves allow the blood to flow in one direction only.

The principle of blood flow in the veins

Unlike the arteries, in which the pressure is high and variable, the pressure in veins is very low (5 mmHg) and constant. There are a number of mechanisms for blood flow in the veins.

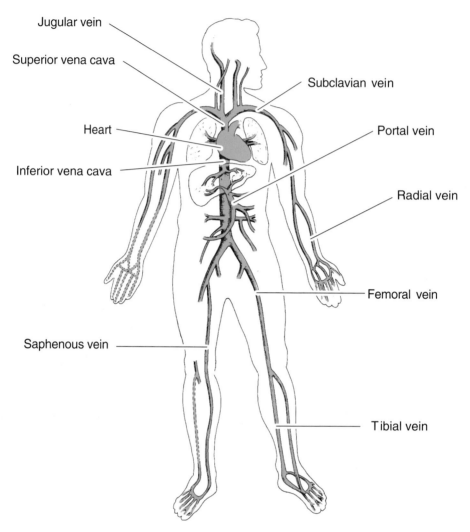

Jugular vein

Superior vena cava

Subclavian vein

Heart

Portal vein

Inferior vena cava

Radial vein

Femoral vein

Saphenous vein

Tibial vein

Figure 3.12   The venous tree.

The right pump of the heart and the vacuum created in the chest during inhalation (see p. 59), draw blood into the large veins in the region of the chest from the rest of the venous tree. The smooth muscle in the vein wall can contract and this, together with the presence of the valves (which allow blood to flow only in the direction of the heart), makes the blood flow in the desired direction.

The veins are compressed by skeletal muscles, resulting in flow of blood towards the heart. This mechanism is particularly important during physical exertion: the amount of blood that the veins must return to the heart greatly increases and the external pressure acting on the veins from the muscles assists in this.

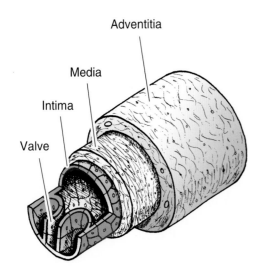

Figure 3.13   Layers of the venous wall.

THE BLOOD

An adult weighing 70 kg has 5–6 liters of blood; 45% of this blood volume is made up of blood cells, and 55% is made up of **plasma**. The ratio of the volume of blood cells to the total blood volume is called the **hematocrit**.

$$\text{Hematocrit} = \frac{\textbf{Blood cell volume}}{\textbf{Total blood volume}}$$

To measure the hematocrit in the laboratory, blood is put in a test tube, and anticoagulant (a chemical agent that prevents blood from co-agulating) is added. The blood cells eventually settle to the bottom of the test tube and the plasma collects above them. The ratio of the volume of the blood cells to the total volume of blood in the test tube yields the hematocrit. The hematocrit is low after loss of blood, such as after bleeding. If a large amount of blood is lost, the blood volume can be replenished by fluids that do not contain blood cells, and the hematocrit goes down.

Composition of the plasma

The plasma contains 90% water, 8% protein and 2% soluble substances.

Plasma proteins.   There are many proteins in the plasma. The three most plentiful proteins in the plasma are:

- **Immunoglobulins:** These proteins play an important role in the immune system (see Chapter 20, on the immune system).
- **Albumin:** This is the most abundant protein in the plasma. It plays a vital role in creating the osmotic colloid pressure and in the mechanism of exchange of substances between the capillaries and the tissues. A deficiency of albumin leads to edema (swelling) in the tissues.
- **Fibrinogen:** This protein has a critical role in blood coagulation, along with other plasma proteins that also participate in this process.

In addition to proteins, the plasma contains many other substances, such as nutrients (glucose, fatty acids, amino acids), salts (sodium, chlorine, magnesium and potassium), gases (oxygen and carbon dioxide) and hormones.

The plasma passes through all the tissues and thus constitutes a window through which one can look at what is occurring in various tissues. Hundreds of different tests are available to identify and measure the concentration of various substances in the plasma, enabling the identification of problems in various organs.

Blood cells

There are three types of blood cells: red cells, white cells and platelets; all are formed in the bone marrow.

Red blood cells (erythrocytes)

One cubic millimeter of blood contains 5–6 million red blood cells. A red blood cell resembles a disc with a depression in its center. It is about 7 thousandths of a millimeter in diameter (Fig. 3.14).

Red blood cells are continually formed in the bone marrow. They die approximately 120 days later in the 'cemetery' for old red blood cells – the spleen. Red blood cells are a special type of cell. Unlike other cells, they do not contain organelles and most of their volume is occupied by a protein called **hemoglobin**, which contains iron. The function of hemoglobin is to bind oxygen in the lungs and to release it in the tissues. Hemoglobin is the major source of oxygen reaching the tissues.

A normal hemoglobin level is 12–16 g of protein per 100 cm^3 blood in women, and 14–18 g in men.

A drop in hemoglobin level below these values constitutes **anemia**. It is important to note that anemia is not a deficiency of blood (blood is comprised of plasma and cells) but a deficiency of hemoglobin.

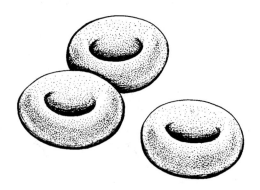

Figure 3.14   Red blood corpuscles.

White cells (leukocytes)

There are 5000–10 000 white blood cells in every cubic millimeter of blood. White blood cells are larger than red blood cells and are 12–20 thousandths of a millimeter in diameter. They are found in the bloodstream and can move between the blood and the tissues.

The white blood cells are an organized army composed of various types of cells, with the common aim of destroying foreign invaders such as bacteria. They also participate in the removal of dead body tissues. A significant deficiency of leukocytes will probably result in death from infection.

The types of white blood cell and their function will be specified in Chapter 20 (the immune system).

Platelets (thrombocytes)

There are 150 000–300 000 thrombocytes in every cubic millimeter of blood. They are disc-shaped bodies, 2–4 thousandths of a millimeter in size, and are formed in the bone marrow by huge cells called **megacaryocytes**. The thrombocytes leave the megacaryocytes and enter the bloodstream. The average life-span of a thrombocyte is 10 days.

The thrombocytes participate in the formation of clots. If a blood vessel is torn, the damaged portion secretes various substances that cause the smooth muscle in its wall to contract and to activate thrombocytes. The thrombocytes adhere to the damaged wall and to each other, thus forming a clot that stops the bleeding. The contraction of the smooth muscle in the vessel assists the thrombocytes in forming the clot by reducing blood pressure and removing blood from the vessel in the damaged region.

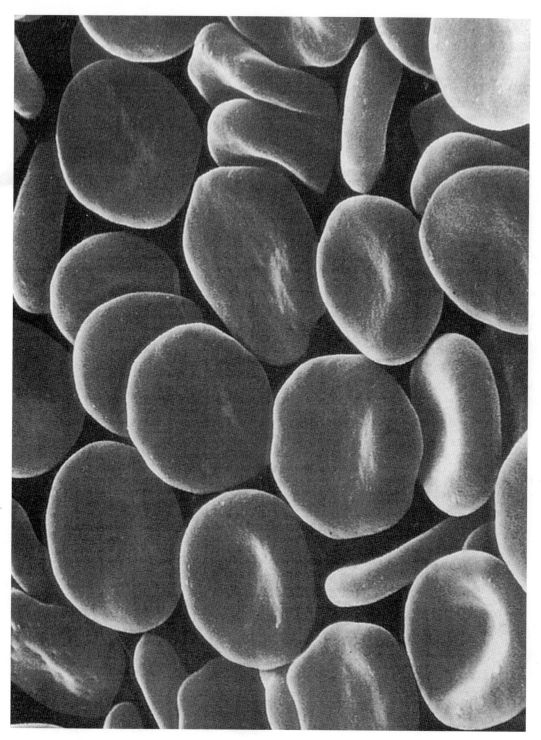

Micrograph of red blood cells.

The initial process of clot formation is called **aggregation**. During this process, the thrombocytes secrete various substances that cause other thrombocytes to join in the formation of the clot.

The thrombocyte clot is itself an unstable structure, which tends to break down after some time. There is therefore an additional coagulation mechanism, which strengthens the clot, and creates a more stable structure that blocks the hole in the blood vessel. This mechanism involves 13 proteins, known as **coagulation factors** (fibrinogen is one of them), which are activated by other substances secreted by the damaged portion of the blood vessel. Activation of this system of proteins eventually produces a network of proteinous fibers that run between the thrombocytes in the damaged portion of the blood vessel (Fig. 3.15).

The structure formed by this network of fibers and thrombocytes (and also a few red blood cells trapped between the fibers of the network) is called a **thrombus**.

A deficiency of thrombocytes or of some of the coagulation factors could lead to problems in clot formation and to uncontrolled bleeding.

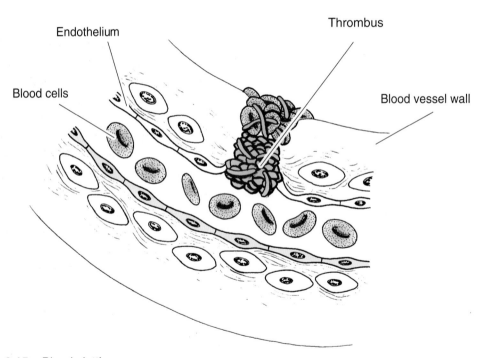

Figure 3.15   Blood clotting.

4

Diseases of the heart and blood vessels

ISCHEMIC HEART DISEASE

Ischemic heart disease is the leading cause of death in the Western world and the most important cause of chest pain in people over the age of 40.

Ischemia is defined as a lack of adequate blood supply to an organ. Ischemic heart disease is a disease that affects the coronary arteries, which supply blood to the heart muscle, and it therefore results in a lack of adequate blood supply (and oxygen) to the heart muscle. In the Western world, 40% of deaths are caused by ischemic heart disease. In China, on the other hand, only 10% of deaths are from ischemic heart disease. The precise etiology (cause) of ischemic heart disease remains unknown. However, **risk factors** for the disease can be described, many of which may be related to the Western lifestyle.

Risk factors for ischemic heart disease

High blood pressure.   This is an important risk factor, which in most cases can be treated by a change in lifestyle or by medication.

Smoking.   This is another important risk factor that is treatable. The more one smokes, the higher the risk of developing ischemic heart disease.

Cholesterol and fats (triglycerides) in the blood. Cholesterol is a fatty substance that is an essential component of all cell walls. It is also a raw material for the production of various other essential substances, such as hormones and bile acids. A high level of total cholesterol in the plasma (above 200 mg/100 ml) accelerates the process of atherosclerosis of the arteries. Cholesterol levels can be lowered to some extent by reducing the amount of saturated fat eaten in the diet (this is found mainly in animal-derived foods including cheese, cream, meat and butter).

Heredity. The risk of developing ischemic heart disease is higher in someone in whom a first-degree relative had the disease under the age of 55. This risk factor is not as amenable to treatment as those listed above.

Male gender. Ischemic heart disease is more common in males, apparently because of some protective effect of the female hormone, estrogen, which tends to 'protect' women from developing ischemic heart disease. Following the menopause, lower estrogen levels are associated with a sharp increase of ischemic heart disease in women to a level equal to men.

Age. The incidence of ischemic heart disease rises with age. Nevertheless, some people under the age of 40 have the disease.

Diabetes. There is at least a two-fold increase in incidence of myocardial infarction in people with diabetes.

Obesity. This contributes to ischemic heart disease in many individuals.

Lack of physical exercise. This also is associated with ischemic heart disease.

The more risk factors a person has, the greater the chance of developing ischemic heart disease. Generally there is not just one isolated risk factor but a combination of several factors. For example, it is common to find an overweight person who smokes, does not exercise and has a high blood level of cholesterol. The striking differences in the incidence of the disease in different countries are related to the differences in risk factors in those countries.

Pathogenesis

The process that leads to ischemic heart disease is called **atherosclerosis**. This process starts in late childhood, continues over many years and affects various arteries in the body, such as those of the legs, brain, kidneys, eye and the coronary arteries of the heart. Atherosclerosis results in the formation of blockages in the arteries. It is not known why certain arteries are more prone to this process (such as the coronary arteries), while other arteries are relatively unaffected (such as the arm arteries).

As noted above, the process of atherosclerosis starts in childhood and is caused by fatty substances and various cells forming a deposit on the internal walls of the arteries, and blocking the vessels. The various components of the sediment that cause the blockage are known as an **atheroma**. The precise reason why the sediment forms is not known but the theory is that the process starts with some damage to the inner lining of the blood vessels (the endothelium), which leads to the deposition of fatty substances and various cells in that area. Over a period of years the deposit gradually builds up and the lumen of the artery slowly becomes narrower and narrower. When more than 50% of the diameter of the artery is blocked, symptoms of ischemic heart disease may appear.

Clinical features

There are three main expressions of ischemic heart disease.

Stable angina pectoris (chest pain)

This appears when the blockage of the coronary arteries reaches a certain stage – usually over 50% of the artery's diameter. During physical exertion, the heart muscle has to work harder and therefore requires an increased blood supply. In a healthy person, the smooth muscle in the walls of the coronary arteries relaxes, the arteries widen and more blood flows to the heart. However, if there is atherosclerosis in the arteries they cannot dilate, so that during periods of physical exertion there is, temporarily, an insufficient blood-flow to the heart muscle. At rest, on the other hand, the heart requires less blood, so that even though the coronary arteries are actually partially blocked, sufficient blood gets through and the patient does not have symptoms.

The symptoms of stable angina pectoris therefore appear during physical exertion and include pressure in the chest (the patients describe it like a heavy stone or an elephant pressing on their chest), shortness of breath, fatigue and weakness. Stopping the physical exertion brings relief.

Unstable angina pectoris

This is defined as a situation where the chest pain appears at rest. This is usually caused by a blood clot that is starting to form in the area of the blockage and that quickly aggravates the degree of blockage of the artery. When the blockage is sufficiently severe, the pain is experienced because the blood supply to the heart is inadequate even when the patient is at rest. This is a dangerous situation that usually ends up with total blockage of the artery, which can precipitate a heart attack.

Myocardial infarction ('heart attack')

Infarction refers to the actual death of tissue as a result of an inadequate blood supply. Myocardial infarction occurs in most cases following complete obstruction of a coronary artery by a blood clot that forms in an area with an atheromatous deposit. The area of the heart that receives its blood supply from the diseased artery undergoes necrosis (tissue death) within 4 hours of its blood supply being cut off, and it ceases to function.

In a minority of cases, myocardial infarction is caused by an **embolus**. This is a blood clot that has formed elsewhere in the body (usually in the left atrium of the heart), has broken away from its point of formation and is swept along in the bloodstream until it gets into a coronary artery, where it lodges, blocking it completely.

A myocardial infarction can be the first sign of atherosclerosis, although usually the patient will have suffered symptoms of angina pectoris prior to it.

The symptoms and signs of myocardial infarction are severe chest pain that may radiate to the arms, neck, jaw or abdomen; shortness of breath; pallor; nausea and a feeling of apprehension.

In the short term, lack of adequate blood supply (ischemia) to part of the heart muscle can cause heart (cardiac) failure, abnormalities of the heart rhythm and death. Cardiac failure is defined as a situation in which the heart is unable to pump an adequate volume of blood to the rest of the body. In most cases of myocardial infarction the occluded artery is relatively small, so that only a small area of heart muscle is deprived of blood and undergoes necrosis, and hence, the effect on the overall functioning of the heart is not critical. If, however, a major artery is occluded, and a large area of heart muscle ceases to function, the pump function of the heart is compromised and heart failure may occur.

Disturbances of heart rhythm (dysrhythmias) are the most common cause of immediate death in a heart attack. The most serious disturbance, which is usually fatal unless treated immediately, is called **ventricular fibrillation**. In ventricular fibrillation, the heart muscle merely quivers ineffectivelly (fibrillates) and does not pump blood at all.

In the first few hours following a myocardial infarction, characteristic changes appear in the patient's electrocardiogram tracing. Moreover, proteins that are normally present within cardiac muscle cells 'leak out' of the injured cells, so that their levels in the blood rise and can be measured and monitored.

After the acute stage following the infarction, the area of muscle that underwent necrosis is gradually replaced by connective tissue called **scar tissue**. The area of the scar cannot contract and affects the heart's pumping function, depending on the size and position of the scar tissue.

A scar in the left ventricle is more serious than one in the right ventricle, because the left ventricle has to pump blood to the entire arterial system of the body. A small area of scar tissue might not affect the heart's function. A moderate-sized scar can result in a degree of heart failure when the patient undergoes physical exertion, because the heart is called upon to work harder. If the scar is large, there may be heart failure during minimal exertion or even at rest.

Diagnosis

There are various ways to diagnose ischemic heart disease.

Stress test.   The patient runs on a treadmill while, at the same time, the electrocardiogram (ECG: the electric activity of the heart) is recorded. If there is blockage in the arteries, during the exercise the supply of blood to the heart muscle will be inadequate and characteristic changes will appear on the ECG tracing.

Thallium scan.   A radioactive substance that enters heart muscle cells is injected into the bloodstream, 'marking' the cells visibly on a radio photographic image. Those areas of the heart that receive a decreased blood supply will show a fainter image than areas supplied adequately with blood. This is generally a more accurate test than the stress test.

Catheterization.   A very fine, flexible tube is inserted into the coronary artery and, under X-ray guidance, a dye is injected through the tube into the artery. The X-ray image obtained provides a clear picture of the lumen of the artery and pinpoints the precise location and extent of any blockage. This is an extremely accurate test and is used not only for diagnosis but also for treatment, because some arterial blockages can be opened, most commonly by using the catheter to insert and inflate a tiny balloon at the site of the blockage, opening up the artery. There are also miniature 'drills' which can be used to penetrate the blockage, and tiny tube-like devices ('stents') that are left inside the artery to keep it open.

Treatment

The treatment of a myocardial infarction in the acute phase (the first few hours after blockage of the artery) is aggressive and is aimed at quickly opening the blocked artery. This treatment can include the intravenous injection of substances that dissolve blood clots (e.g. streptokinase), balloon dilatation or even emergency bypass operation. If a long time has elapsed from the onset of the blockage there is no point in trying to open the blocked artery, because part of the heart muscle will have already undergone necrosis.

The treatment of angina pectoris includes medications that reduce the load on the heart, thereby reducing its requirement for blood and oxygen, and also includes dilatation and bypass surgery.

Coronary bypass surgery involves taking a portion of a vein from the leg, or of an artery in the chest region, and inserting it to bypass the blocked coronary artery.

The best treatment for ischemic heart disease is at the same time both simple and difficult. Taking care to maintain a healthy lifestyle from an early age can minimize or prevent the disease, and decrease the need for the complicated procedures discussed above. At first glance, changing one's lifestyle seems to be simple, but in practice it is very difficult for most people to change the habits of a lifetime, such as smoking and eating fatty food.

CONGESTIVE HEART FAILURE

Heart failure (or, more correctly, **congestive heart failure**) occurs when the heart is unable to pump sufficient blood for the needs of the body. Mild cardiac failure is failure evident only at times of strenous physical exertion, while severe cardiac failure appears at times of mild exertion, or even at rest.

The main clinical features of cardiac failure are fatigue and weakness, shortness of breath on exertion and swelling – particularly of the lower legs and ankles.

Many diseases can cause cardiac failure. Basically, these can be divided into three main groups:

1. diseases of the heart muscle
2. diseases of the heart valves
3. diseases of the pericardium.

Diseases of the heart muscle

The major disease that affects the heart muscle is ischemic heart disease. In addition, there are some other diseases that affect the heart muscle, which are beyond the scope of this book.

Diseases of the heart valves

The function of the valves in the heart is to direct the blood so that it flows in one direction only.

The valvular diseases can be broadly divided into:

- diseases that affect the valve's ability to open so as to allow blood to flow forward through it
- diseases that affect the valve's ability to close so as to prevent blood flowing back through it in the 'wrong' direction.

When a valve does not open adequately, this is known as **stenosis** (narrowing) **of the valve**.

Stenosis of the valve between the atrium and the ventricle (the atrioventricular valve) will obstruct blood flow from one to the other. Stenosis of the valves between the ventricles and the arteries will obstruct blood flow from the ventricles to the arterial tree.

When a valve does not close fully, this is known as **insufficiency** or **incompetence of the valve**. Insufficiency of the valves between the ventricles and the major arteries means that blood that has been expelled from the ventricles to the arteries pours back into the ventricles during diastole (when the ventricles relax and refill with blood from the atria). If the valves between the atria and the ventricles (atrioventricular valves) are incompetent then, as the ventricles contract during systole to pump blood out into the arteries, some blood will flow back into the atria instead (normally the atrioventricular valves are tightly closed during systole to prevent such backflow).

Stenosis (narrowing) or incompetence of a valve will create a distinctive sound called a **murmur** as the blood rushes through the valve. A murmur can be heard with a stethoscope and is basically the sound of blood flowing through a relatively narrow or turbulent channel. Using a stethoscope, a physician can identify the malfunctioning valve. The valves can also be observed while the heart is beating using an ultrasound examination of the heart (echocardiography).

Diseases of the pericardium

Diseases of the pericardium affect the heart's ability to contract and expand. Some consist of the accumulation of fluid between the layers of the pericardium and others involve stiffening of the pericardium, thus interfering with the heart's ability to contract and expand.

HIGH BLOOD PRESSURE

High blood pressure (**hypertension**) is defined as a state in which the pressure in the arteries is abnormally high for some length of time.

Systolic hypertension is defined as a systolic blood pressure above 140 mmHg; diastolic hypertension is defined as a diastolic pressure over 90 mmHg. Systolic hypertension is due to loss of elasticity of the large arteries, whereas diastolic hypertension is caused by narrowing of smaller arteries. (The detailed explanation for this is quite complicated and will not be discussed further.)

The cause of hypertension is usually idiopathic (i.e. unknown), but there are also some specific diseases that directly cause it.

Hypertension, particularly diastolic hypertension, over a period of years results in damage to several vital body organs:

- **Heart:** high blood pressure directly damages the heart muscle and accelerates the process of atherosclerosis of the coronary arteries.
- **Kidney:** the damaging effects of hypertension on the small arteries within the kidneys and on the main renal (kidney) arteries eventually compromises kidney function.
- **Eyes:** hypertension can damage the retinal arteries, which can lead to blurred vision.
- **Brain:** hypertension is an extremely important risk factor for the occurrence of cerebral infarction ('stroke'; see Chapters 11 and 12 on the Nervous system).

There are often no clinical signs of hypertension and most cases are, in fact, detected incidentally during the course of a routine medical examination. Hence, hypertension is known as the 'silent killer'. Severe hypertension (diastolic blood pressure above 140 mmHg) can cause severe headache and visual disturbances.

The treatment of hypertension includes changes in lifestyle (weight reduction, physical exercise, etc), and various very effective medications.

EDEMA

Edema is defined as the accumulation of fluid between the cells. An organ with edema will appear swollen. Edema occurs when the amount of fluid leaving the capillary blood vessels is greater than that entering them. The excess fluid then accumulates in the tissues in the spaces between the cells.

Edema occurs when there is a disturbance of the normal mechanisms regulating fluid and metabolite exchange between the blood vessels and the surrounding tissues.

Causes of edema

There are four main causes of edema:

1. Increase in venous pressure

As the pressure in the veins rises, the pressure in the capillaries near the venous system also rises, which interferes with the return of water from the tissues back into the capillaries. An increase in venous pressure can be caused by cardiac failure (because the heart is not pumping properly, it cannot 'suck in' the blood from the veins adequately), by obstruction of the inferior vena cava during pregnancy and by localized blockages of veins (mainly of the legs). Localized venous obstruction results in localized, rather than generalized, edema.

2. Decrease in the amount of albumin in the blood

Albumin is the major protein in plasma and it plays an important role in creating and maintaining the osmotic colloid pressure within the blood vessels, which 'pulls' fluid from the surrounding intercellular tissues into the capillaries. A lack of albumin, which can occur in liver disease (too little production), kidney disease (too much excretion) or malnutrition, leads to generalized edema of the body.

3. Abnormal permeability of the blood vessels

Various processes, such as allergy or certain diseases, can result in 'leakiness' of blood vessels. If this occurs, plasma proteins can leak out through the vessel walls into the surrounding intercellular space. As a result, the difference in concentrations of the proteins inside and outside the blood vessels is smaller and the osmotic colloid pressure within the blood vessels, which 'pulls' water into the blood vessels, is lower. Hence the water can accumulate in the intercellular space, resulting in edema.

4. Lymphatic obstruction

The lymphatic system normally drains away the small amount of intercellular fluid, and returns it to the circulatory system. Blockage of the lymphatic system can result from a cancerous growth in the lymphatic vessels or might follow inadvertent damage to the lymphatic vessels during surgery. For example, surgery to remove a large lump from the breast often also involves removing the lymph nodes (glands) from the underarm. In some cases following the surgery, edema of the arm develops, because the damaged lymphatic vessels can no longer drain the lymph fluid from the arm.

ANEMIA

Anemia is defined as a low level of **hemoglobin** in the blood. Hemoglobin is a protein present in red blood cells whose function is to transport oxygen from the lungs to the tissues.

A lack of hemoglobin affects the transport of oxygen to the tissues and results in the following clinical features: pallor, weakness, fatigue, a rapid heartbeat and rapid breathing. If the hemoglobin levels fall slowly and gradually, the body might be able to adjust to the oxygen deficiency for some time. There are cases where the hemoglobin decreases to as low as 3 g/100 ml (the normal level being approximately 12–14 g/100 ml) and yet the patient can still function. However, a rapid fall in hemoglobin, such as might occur if there is significant bleeding, causes marked problems when the hemoglobin level falls to about 8 g/100 ml.

The lifespan of a red blood cell is approximately 120 days. In order to maintain a constant hemoglobin level in the blood, the number of red blood cells being produced in the bone marrow has to equal the number of blood cells that is being destroyed in the spleen. If either the production of new blood cells is inadequate or there is excessive destruction of blood cells, anemia will result.

Causes of anemia

Inadequate production of red blood cells

This is usually the result of a deficiency of the raw materials for hemoglobin production, for example, vitamin B12 (present in animal products), folic acid (present in fruits and vegetables) or iron (found in meat and some vegetables).

The most common cause of anemia is iron deficiency, because iron is a major component of hemoglobin. In infants, iron deficiency is usually dietary in origin, so that many infant formulas and foods are fortified with iron.

In young women, a common cause of iron deficiency is loss of iron because of heavy menstrual bleeding. In adults, iron deficiency can develop from bleeding into the gastrointestinal system (often due to cancer of the bowel).

Apart from a lack of raw materials, there are other causes of inadequate production of red blood cells in the bone marrow, such as malignancies, certain drugs, infections that involve the bone marrow and some kidney diseases.

Increased destruction of red blood cells

The premature destruction of red blood cells is called **hemolysis**. Hemolysis takes place mainly in the spleen (although to some extent it also accurs within the blood vessels) and tends to occur if the red blood cells are abnormal (e.g. in a genetic disease known as thalassemia), or in diseases where the patient's immune system 'attacks' the red blood cells and destroys them.

5 The respiratory system

The respiratory system supplies oxygen (O_2) to the blood, and removes carbon dioxide (CO_2) from it. Almost every cell in the body, as it produces energy, needs oxygen and produces carbon dioxide.

The cells of the body cannot survive without oxygen. The cells that are most sensitive to lack of oxygen are the brain cells, which die if they do not receive oxygen for approximately 7 minutes.

The respiratory system starts to function immediately after birth, with the baby's first breath. In the womb, the fetus receives its oxygen supply and eliminates carbon dioxide through the placenta. It is in the placenta that the exchange of gases between the fetus' blood and the mother's blood takes place. In the womb, the fetal airways are filled with amniotic fluid, and the fetus makes breathing movements which move the amniotic fluid in and out of its lungs. This 'breathing' of the amniotic fluid is important for the normal development of the infant's lungs.

The respiratory system comprises the nasal cavities, the pharynx, the larynx, the trachea, the bronchi and the lungs.

NASAL CAVITIES

Air enters the respiratory system through the nose. The nostrils are the entrance to the nose, from which air moves to two large air-filled cavities behind the nose – the **nasal cavities.**

You can also breathe through the mouth if there is an increased demand for large volumes of air, such as during physical exertion or if the nasal air passages are blocked. In the nostrils, there are small hairs whose task it is to trap large particles and prevent them from getting into the nasal cavities. The nostrils contain cartilage, as do other parts of the nose. At the bridge of the nose, there is a bony portion made up of the two nasal bones. The floor of the nasal cavities is the roof of the oral (mouth) cavity. The front part of this floor contains bone and is called the **hard palate.** The back part does not contain bone and is known as the **soft palate.**

The **nasal septum** (from the Latin word *saeptum* = wall, fence) separates the two nasal cavities. The septum is made up partly of bone and partly of cartilage. The lateral (outer) walls of the nasal cavities are formed by portions of the skull bones. From the lateral walls, three 'shelves', known as the **conchae** (singular = **concha**), protrude into the nasal cavities. These shelves create turbulence in the air as it flows through the nasal cavities (Fig. 5.1).

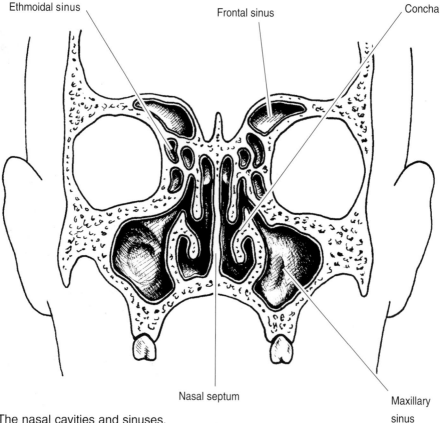

Figure 5.1 The nasal cavities and sinuses.

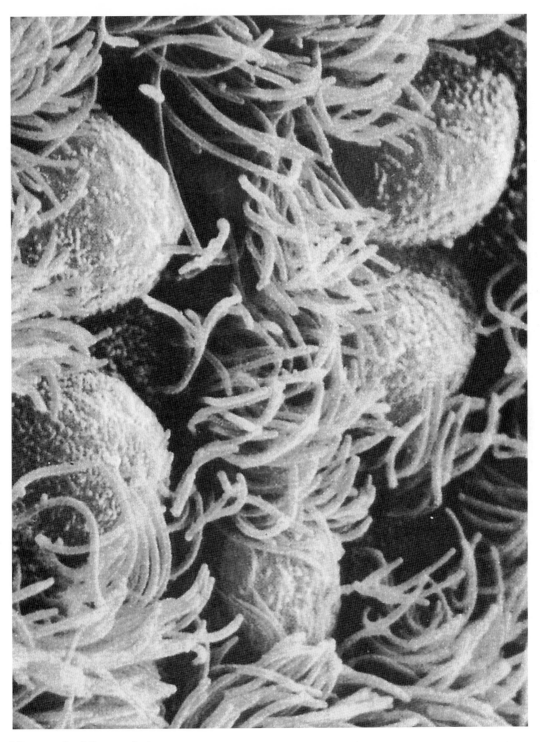

Micrograph of the respiratory mucosa.

The nasal cavities are lined with an epithelial tissue called the **respiratory mucosa,** which is continuous throughout the entire respiratory tract. There are two main types of cell in this mucosa; the most common type are cells with approximately 300 tiny hairs, called **cilia,** which project into the nasal cavity. The second type are cells that produce sticky mucus, which covers the respiratory mucosa.

The function of the nasal cavities

The structures in the nasal cavity serve several functions:

- **Filtration of the air:** as the air enters the nasal cavity it meets the conchae, which cause turbulence, causing it to swirl around in the cavity and come into contact with the walls. Any contaminating particles present in the air stick to the walls, which are coated with sticky mucus. The mucus is constantly being moved toward the nostrils by the whip-like beating action of the tiny hairs (cilia) of the mucosal cells.
- **Warming the air:** as the air comes in contact with the walls, it is warmed prior to its entry into the next part of the respiratory passages.
- **Moisturizing:** the air that leaves the back part of the nasal cavities is clean, warm, and moist.

THE SINUSES

The sinuses (see Fig. 5.1) are air spaces within the skull bones. They make the skull lighter, and play a role in resonance of the voice. The sinus cavities are lined with respiratory mucosa. Each sinus is connected to the nasal cavity via an opening in its wall.

There are three pairs of sinuses and one single sinus. These are the names and positions of the sinuses:

- **Frontal sinuses:** situated in the frontal bones (forehead), above the outer third of the eyebrows. These sinuses develop at a later age than the other sinuses, around the age of 7.
- **Maxillary sinuses:** situated in the maxillary (cheek) bones, below the eyes. They are the largest sinuses.
- **Ethmoidal sinuses:** situated in the ethmoid bones (a small bone that, together with some other bones, forms part of the lateral wall of the nasal cavities). These sinuses contain numerous air cells, in contrast to the other sinuses, which each have only one air cavity.
- **Sphenoidal sinus:** a single sinus in the sphenoid bone (one of the bones that form the base of the skull).

PHARYNX AND LARYNX

From the nasal cavities, the air passes backward into the cavity called the **pharynx** (Fig. 5.2). This cavity is divided into three parts:

- **nasopharynx:** the part immediately behind the nasal cavities
- **oropharynx:** a cavity behind the oral cavity
- **laryngopharynx:** a cavity below the oropharynx.

Only air passes through the nasopharynx, whereas both air and food pass through the other two parts of the pharynx. At the bottom of the laryngopharynx are the openings to the esophagus and trachea (windpipe).

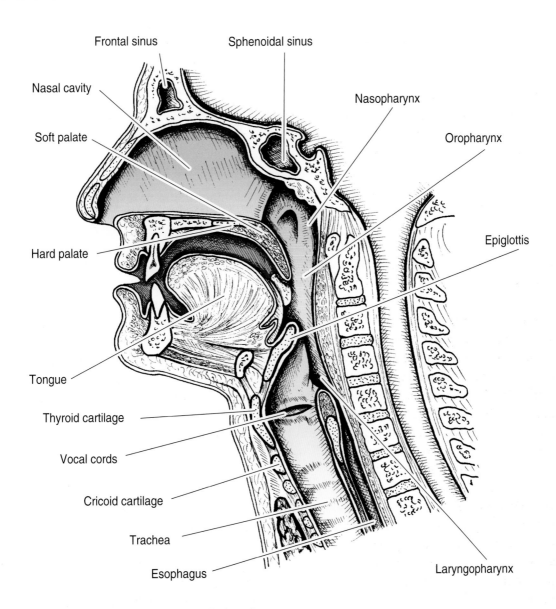

Frontal sinus

Sphenoidal sinus

Nasal cavity

Nasopharynx

Soft palate

Oropharynx

Hard palate

Epiglottis

Tongue

Thyroid cartilage

Vocal cords

Cricoid cartilage

Trachea

Esophagus

Laryngopharynx

Figure 5.2 The pharynx and larynx in sagittal section.

The **larynx** is a complex anatomic structure, made up of several cartilages; it lies in the front part of the neck. It has a mechanism to ensure that the entrance to the trachea is closed during swallowing, keeping food out of the trachea. The larynx also contains the **vocal cords**, a complex structure that enables us to produce different sounds.

The upper cartilage of the larynx is the **thyroid cartilage**, which has the shape of an open book, often referred to as the 'Adam's apple'. The lower cartilage in the larynx is known as the **cricoid cartilage**. It is ring-shaped, and the trachea starts immediately below it (Fig. 5.6). At the back of this cartilage are two other small cartilages – the **arytenoid cartilages**, which are attached to the vocal cords and to a system of muscles that move the vocal cords. The vocal cords are two folds of soft tissue at the entrance to the trachea. The muscles attached to the vocal cords can bring them close together, and thereby narrow the air opening into the trachea.

Another cartilage is called the **epiglottis**. This is attached to the back of the thyroid cartilage, and acts as a lid to seal off the trachea during swallowing. Swallowing is a complex action that requires the coordinated action of many muscles in the pharynx and larynx. The action of swallowing is described in more detail in Chapter 7, on the digestive system.

TRACHEA

The trachea is a 10-cm tube, which runs from the bottom of the cricoid cartilage (one of the cartilages of the larynx) and ends in the chest at the level of the sternal angle, where it divides.

The wall of the trachea contains 16 to 20 horseshoe-shaped cartilages, which provide rigidity so that it always remains open. The **esophagus** (gullet) is immediately behind the trachea. At the back part of the trachea, where the esophagus lies, there is no cartilage in the wall of the trachea (the open part of the horseshoe-shaped cartilages). This allows lumps of food to pass through the esophagus to the stomach by slightly compressing the rear wall of the trachea.

BRONCHI

In the chest cavity, the trachea divides into the two **main bronchi**. The left main bronchus is pushed slightly upward by the heart, which lies to the left of the midline. The walls of the bronchi are made up of three main layers (Fig. 5.4):

1. An inner lining of **respiratory mucosa**.
2. A layer containing **bands of smooth muscle**. This muscle layer can narrow or widen the diameter of the bronchi. During physical effort, when more air is needed, the muscle relaxes and the bronchi dilate. At rest the smooth muscle contracts, and the bronchi are narrower.
3. A third layer consisting of **connective tissue with pieces of cartilage** embedded in it. Within this connective tissue there are glands that secrete mucus into the lumen (cavity) of the bronchi.

The main bronchi divide into secondary bronchi, which then divide again and again, forming the **bronchial tree** (Fig. 5.3); there are approximately 22 divisions of bronchi in all. As the bronchial tree divides, the diameter of the bronchi becomes smaller and smaller, until at the lower divisions they are not visible to the naked eye.

The microscopic bronchi are called **bronchioles,** and they end in the alveoli of the lung.

ALVEOLI

The **alveoli** are microscopic air sacs in which the exchange of gases (oxygen and carbon dioxide) between the blood and the air occurs.

The number of alveoli is estimated at some 300 million; if they were all opened up and

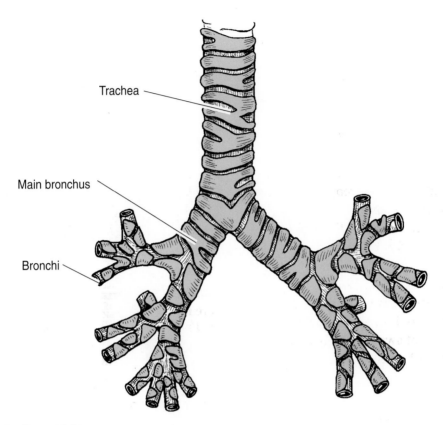

Trachea

Main bronchus

Bronchi

Figure 5.3   Bronchial tree.

laid out flat their total surface area would be about that of a tennis court. This enormous surface area greatly increases the efficiency of the gas exchange. The walls of the alveoli are extremely thin and are composed of flat cells called **pneumocytes**, which line the inner surface of the alveoli, and connective tissue containing capillaries.

As the blood flows through the capillaries in the walls of the alveoli, oxygen passes from the air in the alveolar cavity into the capillaries, and carbon dioxide passes from the blood back into the alveolar cavity. Each gas moves from an area of high concentration to an area of lower concentration.

PULMONARY BLOOD VESSELS

Alongside the main bronchus, a large blood vessel, the **pulmonary artery**, enters each lung. It carries blood with a low oxygen concentration from the right ventricle of the heart.

The blood pressure in the pulmonary artery varies in cyclic fashion, as does the blood in the general arterial system, but the actual pressures are lower in the pulmonary system, ranging from a systolic pressure of 25 mmHg to a diastolic pressure of 10 mmHg.

The pulmonary artery follows the bronchi and, as each bronchus divides, the accompanying branch of the pulmonary artery also divides. Thus, the pulmonary arterial system

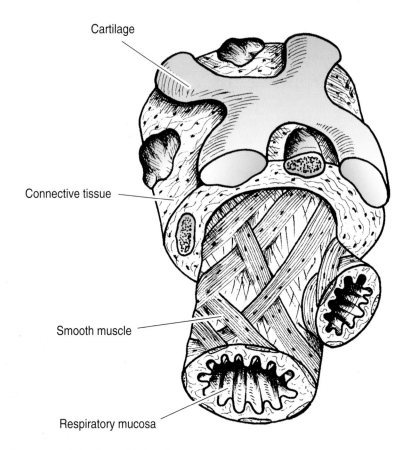

Cartilage

Connective tissue

Smooth muscle

Respiratory mucosa

Figure 5.4   Structure of the bronchial wall.

forms a branching tree similar to the bronchial tree, and each microscopic bronchiole has its accompanying microscropic arteriole. The arteriole passes through the wall of the alveolus and splits up into a network of tiny capillaries inside the alveolar wall. This capillary network then drains into a microscopic venule, which emerges from the alveolar wall and runs alongside the microscopic bronchiole and arteriole (Fig. 5.5).

The venules join other venules, forming larger and larger veins, which also run alongside the bronchi, until they eventually form large veins, the **pulmonary veins**. These carry oxygen-rich blood from the lungs to the left atrium of the heart. There are four pulmonary veins – two from each lung. Apart from the pulmonary arteries and veins, other blood vessels, which originate from the systemic arterial system (derived from branches of the aorta) enter the lung; these are the **bronchial arteries**. They supply oxygen-rich blood to all tissues in the lung that do not come into direct contact with air (the connective tissue between the alveoli, the blood vessels, the walls of the bronchi, etc.).

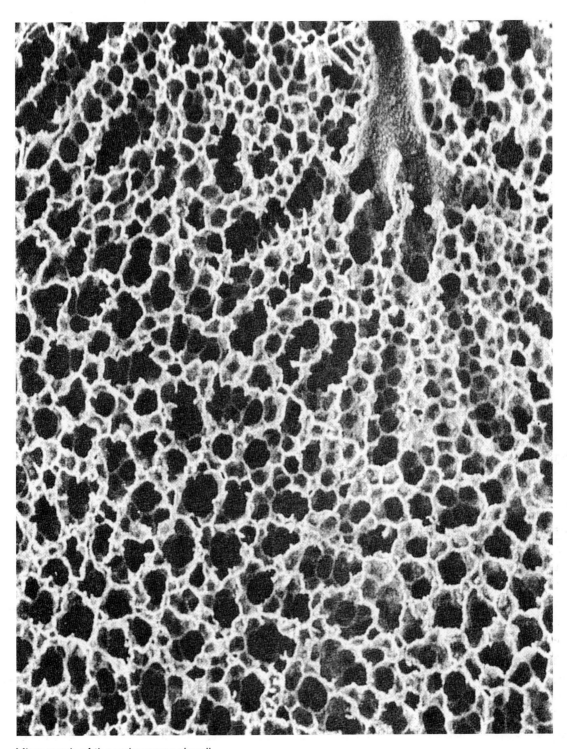

Micrograph of the pulmonary alveoli.

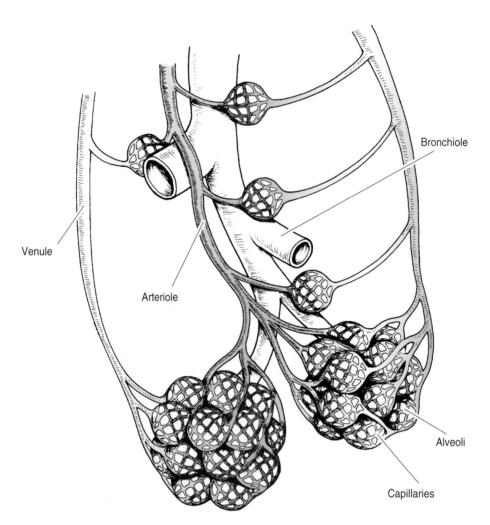

Figure 5.5 Pulmonary alveoli and blood vessels.

LUNGS

The **lungs** occupy most of the thoracic (chest) cavity. The pulmonary arteries, pulmonary veins and main bronchi all enter the lungs through the area of the lung near the heart. This region is known as the **root of the lung**.

The lungs are divided into **lobes**. Each lobe is separate, with its own bronchi and blood vessels. There are three lobes in the right lung and two in the left (Fig. 5.6). Each lobe is further subdivided into smaller portions called segments. The lobe tissue is made up of several components:

- **Blood vessels:** the pulmonary arteries bring blood from the right ventricle of the heart to the alveoli; the pulmonary veins take blood from the alveoli to the left atrium of the heart. If you look at lung tissue with the naked eye, you can see blood vessels of various sizes.

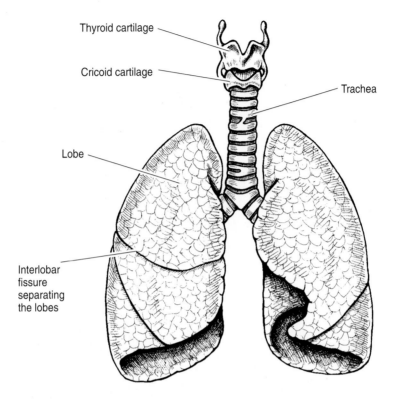

Thyroid cartilage

Cricoid cartilage

Trachea

Lobe

Interlobar
fissure
separating
the lobes

Figure 5.6   Larynx, trachea, and lungs.

- **Bronchi:** the bronchi conduct air to the alveoli. If you look at lung tissue with the naked eye, you can see bronchi of various sizes.
- **Alveoli:** the walls of the alveoli contain capillary networks. You cannot see alveoli with the naked eye because of their microscopic size.
- **Connective tissue:** between the various tissues of the lung is connective tissue.

The mechanics of breathing

Air flows in and out of the lung because of differences in the pressure in the airways and atmospheric pressure.

During **inspiration** (inhalation), the volume of the chest cavity increases (Fig. 5.7) and the pressure in the chest and the airways is thus lowered (compared to atmospheric pressure), so that air enters the lungs. During **expiration** (exhalation), the volume of the chest cavity decreases, the pressure in the chest is higher (compared to atmospheric pressure) and air leaves the lungs.

The syringe model shown in Figure 5.8 demonstrates the principle of pressure differences and airflow in the lungs. As you pull back on the syringe plunger, the volume of the space inside the syringe increases, the pressure inside the syringe is lowered, so air enters from the outside. As you push the plunger in, the volume of the space inside the syringe decreases, the pressure rises and air is expelled from the syringe.

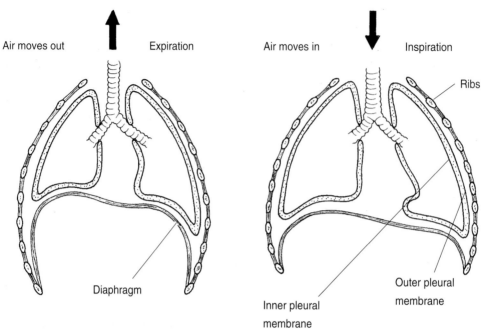

Figure 5.7   Inspiration and expiration.

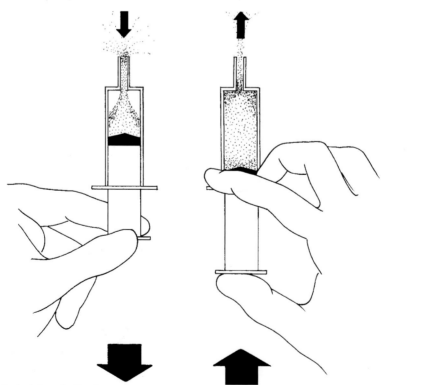

Figure 5.8   Model of airflow in the lungs.

Other organs that are also involved in breathing, apart from the lungs themselves, include the chest wall and the intercostal muscles, the diaphragm and the pleural membranes.

Chest wall and intercostal muscles

Contraction of the intercostal muscles pulls the ribs upwards and outwards, and increases the volume of the chest cavity. The respiratory muscles work constantly and are controlled via the nerves, as are all other muscles in the body.

Diaphragm

The diaphragm is a thin, dome-shaped sheet of muscle that separates the chest cavity from the abdominal cavity. The diaphragm originates from the lower borders of the ribs and the vertebral bodies, and is inserted at the central tendon at the apex of the dome (Fig. 5.9).

As the diaphragm contracts, the central tendon is pulled downwards, flattening the diaphragm. As a result of this flattening, the volume of the chest cavity expands in a downward direction. When the muscle relaxes, the diaphragm resumes its dome shape and the volume of the chest cavity decreases.

Pleural membranes

The pleural membranes cover the outside surface of the lungs and have a very important role to play in the mechanism of breathing. They consist of an outer layer, which adheres to the inside of the chest wall, the thoracic surface of the diaphragm and the pericardium,

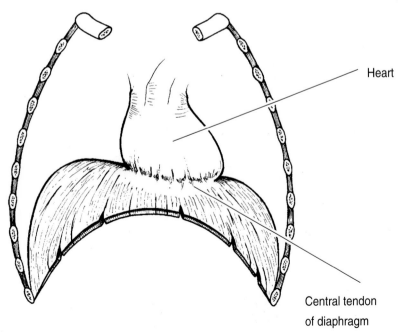

Heart

Central tendon
of diaphragm

Figure 5.9 Diaphragm.

and an inner layer adherent to the outer surface of the lung. The two layers of the pleura are close to each other, with only a small amount of **pleural fluid** between them (see Fig. 5.7). The presence of this fluid between the pleural layers creates a negative pressure, which holds them together tightly. This is similar to two sheets of glass, which can be held together tightly by a little water between them. Although the two pleural layers are tightly apposed, they can move and slide on each other. During inspiration, the chest wall rises and the diaphragm flattens. The outer pleural layer, which is tightly adherent to the chest wall and diaphragm, pulls the inner pleural layer with it because of the

negative pressure between the two layers. The inner layer, which is tightly adherent to the lungs, 'pulls out' the lungs, which increases their volume, dropping the pressure within the lungs and causing air to enter them.

Should air get in between the layers of the pleura, as for example, in the case of a penetrating injury to the chest wall, a **pneumothorax** results (Fig. 5.10). The air in the pleural cavity allows the two pleural layers to separate and eliminates the negative pressure in the pleural space. Subsequently, the lung, with its adherent inner layer of the pleura is no longer pulled out by the outer pleural layer and collapses and shrinks, separating from the chest wall and the diaphragm. During inspiration, as the chest

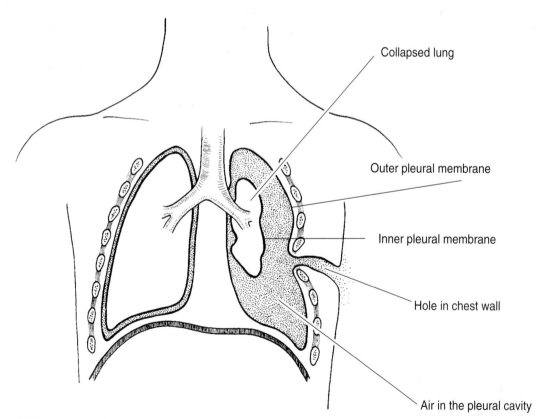

Collapsed lung

Outer pleural membrane

Inner pleural membrane

Hole in chest wall

Air in the pleural cavity

Figure 5.10   Pneumothorax as a result of a penetrating chest wound.

wall rises and the diaphragm flattens, the pressure in the chest cavity falls and air rushes into the pleural space through the opening in the chest wall. The lung itself cannot expand, remains collapsed, and does not function.

Lung volumes

During quiet relaxed breathing, the volume of air that moves in and out with each breath is approximately 500 cm^3; this is known as the **tidal volume**. The number of breaths per minute is usually between 12 and 16.

Of the total air that enters the respiratory system during inspiration, approximately 150 cm^3 fills the bronchial tree and the rest enters the alveoli.

The volume of air that fills the bronchial tree is called the **dead space** because it does not take part in the gas exchange, which occurs only in the alveoli. The largest volume that can be breathed in (or out) is called the **vital capacity;** in an adult this is 4–5 liters. The volume of air left behind in the lungs after breathing out as fully as possible is called the **residual volume**, and it is about 1 liter.

CONTROL OF BREATHING

The area of the brain known as the brainstem houses a respiratory center that controls **ventilation** (breathing). Ventilation is defined as the volume of air exchanged between the lungs and the external environment per unit time:

**Ventilation = Number of breaths per minute ×
Ventilatory volume**

The respiratory center determines the extent of ventilation in response to the level of carbon dioxide in the blood. If we deliberately stop breathing, the level of carbon dioxide in the blood rises and we feel an urge to breathe (the higher the level of carbon dioxide, the stronger the drive to breathe). We then resume breathing faster and deeper, and the lung ventilation increases. With the faster breathing rate, more carbon dioxide is 'blown off', the level of carbon dioxide in the blood falls, causing the drive to breathe to decrease, the breathing rate and volume fall, and the lung ventilation decreases.

6 Diseases of the respiratory system

Obstructive lung diseases mainly affect the bronchi. They result in narrowing of the air passages in the bronchial tree.

ASTHMA

Approximately 10% of all children and 5% of adults suffer from asthma (or bronchial asthma, as it is sometimes called). In many cases, there is a familial tendency to this illness.

Asthma is defined as a hypersensitivity of the airways to irritating stimuli. It follows from this definition that the disease affects the bronchi and that there are many causes. The affected bronchi are mainly the medium-sized ones.

When hypersensitive bronchi react to some stimulus, three processes take place:

1. The smooth muscle in the wall of the bronchus constricts. Smooth muscle is an involuntary muscle that normally relaxes when there is a need for more air to reach the lungs, such as during physical exertion. Constriction of this muscle causes narrowing of the bronchus.
2. There is excessive secretion of mucus into the lumen of the bronchus from the mucus cells. The mucus is secreted by the mucus

cells that are present in the respiratory mucosa (the inner lining of the respiratory passages), as well as by mucus glands in the wall of the bronchi.

3. Edema (swelling) of the bronchial wall occurs due to fluid accumulation in the wall of the bronchus.

Each of the above processes results in narrowing of the lumen of the bronchi, which causes some degree of obstruction to the airflow in the airways.

Causes of asthma

Allergy. This is the most common cause of asthma, accounting for some 35% of cases. Inhaled substances, called **allergens**, act on special cells, called **mast cells**, present in the wall of the bronchi. These cells are part of the immune system of the body and, when stimulated by an antigen, they secrete a substance called **histamine** (in actual fact, they secrete several substances, of which histamine is one). It is the histamine and other related substances that trigger the three processes of the hypersensitivity reaction described above.

Common antigens triggering asthma are the **house dust mite** (a tiny insect present in household dust), molds, fungi and pollens of various plants. The amount of allergen needed to trigger an attack of asthma is usually extremely small. There are people who can develop an attack of asthma when a certain plant to which they are sensitive is flowering miles away!

Physical exertion.   In some patients, the rapid breathing (particularly of cold air) that takes place during physical exertion can trigger an asthma attack.

Emotional stress.   There is a definite relationship between a patient's emotional state and the frequency of asthma attacks. The precise nature of the association between emotional state and events in the bronchi is not known.

Respiratory infection.   This mechanism is particularly important in children. Following infection of the bronchi by viruses or bacteria in sensitive people, asthma may occur.

Medications.   Various medications, such as aspirin, can trigger an attack of asthma in certain individuals.

Industrial factors.   Exposure to various dusts, such as wood dust, can trigger an attack of asthma. This is not the same as allergy, because in these cases histamine does not play a significant role in the process.

An asthmatic person's bronchi are usually sensitive to more than one trigger factor.

Clinical features

Asthma occurs in attacks, the frequency and severity of which vary from patient to patient.

The main symptom of an asthma attack is **shortness of breath** (dyspnea), which is a feeling of lack of air and difficulty in breathing. This is similar to the feeling that a normal, but unfit, person would get during strenuous physical exercise.

The asthma attack makes it especially difficult to exhale and remove air from the lungs, so that expiration tends to be prolonged. Because of the difficulty in exhaling the air from the lungs, the chest tends to be 'blown up' and overinflated by the air trapped in the lungs.

The reason that it is difficult to exhale during an asthma attack is because during inspiration, the lungs expand at the same time as the bronchi expand. However, during expiration, both the lungs and the diameter of the bronchi get smaller, increasing the obstruction to airflow during expiration.

As air passes along the narrowed bronchi during expiration, it makes a whistling sound, called **wheezing**.

Yet another symptom of an asthma attack is **cough**. Coughing occurs together with the other symptoms but, in some cases, a night-time cough by itself can be the only symptom of the disease. A severe attack of asthma can result in **cyanosis** from lack of oxygen, or even death.

Between attacks of asthma, the person is usually free of symptoms. The frequency of attacks depends on the degree of exposure to the various trigger factors, and varies from patient to patient. For example, sensitivity to plant pollens is more common in the spring. Some patients suffer from the disease virtually all the time, whereas others may have an attack only once every few years.

Diagnosis

During an attack of asthma, the diagnosis can be made by examining the patient. However, between attacks, when the patient has no symptoms, one can deliberately trigger an asthmatic attack under controlled conditions, and thereby make the diagnosis. This is done by giving inhalations of gradually increasing doses of a trigger substance. If the person is in fact asthmatic, the signs of asthma will appear after inhalation of a certain concentration of the substance. The lower the concentration at which signs appear, the more sensitive or irritable the patient's bronchi must be. Note that

high doses of these substances can produce an asthma attack even in someone who is not an asthma sufferer.

Treatment

There are various medications used for treating asthma. Some of the commonly used ones include the following.

Salbutamol. This is taken by inhalation during an attack, using a special inhaler. It dilates (widens) the bronchi by relaxing the smooth muscle in the bronchial wall.

Steroids. Steroids are commonly given by daily inhalation, to prevent asthma attacks. They are generally effective in more severe cases, and administration by inhalation rather than systemically by mouth appears to result in fewer side effects. Only severe asthmatics, who do not respond to inhaled steroids or to other medications, are given steroids by mouth.

CHRONIC OBSTRUCTIVE LUNG DISEASE

This is usually called **chronic obstructive pulmonary disease** (COPD). It is largely caused by heavy cigarette smoking over many years, or by severe air pollution.

The carbon (soot) in the cigarette smoke or polluted air damages the tiny hairs on the cells of the respiratory mucosa, which normally remove dirt and secretions from the respiratory tract. This allows mucus with carbon and other contaminants to accumulate in the airways.

For reasons that are not clear, cigarette smoke causes enlargement of the mucus glands in the respiratory mucosa, resulting in excessive mucus production in the airways in smokers. The final endpoint is obstruction of the airways.

Clinical features

The most prominent clinical feature of COPD, from its onset right through to the late stages, is cough. The cough appears initially in the morning, after the secretions have accumulated in the bronchial tree during sleep. In the morning, the patient coughs up dark phlegm, in an attempt to clear the airways and eliminate the accumulated secretions.

As the illness progresses, the walls of the bronchi are damaged and there is permanent obstruction to the flow of air. This obstruction results in shortness of breath during exertion and, as the disease progresses further, the shortness of breath appears even when at rest.

As there is obstruction to the flow of air, patients have difficulty expelling air from their lungs (expiration becomes prolonged and laborious), as occurs in asthma. The large amount of mucus that builds up in the bronchi acts as an excellent culture medium for bacteria, which get into the bronchi and cause **chronic bronchitis** with severe frequent cough and large amounts of purulent (pus) sputum. From time to time, the infection flares up, with an even greater amount of sputum being produced, more severe airways obstruction and increasing shortness of breath. The bacteria may penetrate deeper into the respiratory tract and reach the alveoli of the lungs, causing pneumonia.

In summary, patients with COPD suffer from shortness of breath on exertion, and later even at rest, from cough associated with the production of large amounts of sputum and (from time to time) from exacerbation of the respiratory problems due to infection in the airways.

In COPD, another problem may occur, called **emphysema**. Emphysema is defined as a cavity (air space) in the lungs created as the result of destruction of the walls of the alveoli. As a consequence, there are fewer functioning alveoli in the lung, which significantly affects pulmonary function.

Diagnosis

The diagnosis of COPD is based on the patient's history (chronic cough and shortness of breath in a heavy smoker), physical examination, chest X-ray and the results of laboratory tests of lung function.

Treatment

Patients with COPD are treated with medications that dilate the bronchi, medications that remove mucus from the airways and, at times of flare-ups due to infection, with antibiotics. In the more advanced stages of the disease, the patient might be confined to bed and require oxygen virtually all of the time.

CYSTIC FIBROSIS

Cystic fibrosis (CF) is a genetic (hereditary) disease and is one of the most common lethal genetic diseases in childhood in Western populations, with an incidence of about 1 per 2000 newborns. Approximately 1 in every 25 of the general population is a carrier for CF.

The disease affects mainly the respiratory tract but also involves other organs in the body, such as the pancreas, the digestive tract, the genitalia and the sweat glands. In the respiratory tract, the mucus is very thick and sticky. The tiny hairs lining the respiratory mucosa are unable to clear away this mucus effectively and it accumulates in the airways.

People with CF suffer from chronic (continuous) shortness of breath, cough and often from severe respiratory infections.

The average lifespan of these patients is of the order of 20 years, and at present, the most effective treatment is lung transplantation.

INTERSTITIAL LUNG DISEASES

Interstitial lung diseases involve the alveoli, the pulmonary blood vessels and the interstitial tissue between the alveoli. This is in contrast to the diseases we have discussed thus far (asthma, chronic obstructive pulmonary disease and cystic fibrosis), which affect mainly the bronchi.

There are many different interstitial pulmonary diseases (some 180 of them), most being quite rare. Some are the result of exposure to certain industrial dusts and pollutants (e.g. asbestos, silicone), some are caused by exposure to certain organic substances in the air (e.g. flour, pigeon droppings) and some appear for no obvious reason. All interstitial lung diseases present with a chronic dry cough and progressively worsening shortness of breath.

PNEUMONIA

Pneumonia is an infection of the alveoli of the lung. It is usually caused by viruses or bacteria and, occasionally, by other microorganisms.

The bacteria get into the lung tissue through the air passages. The alveoli in the infected area of the lung fill up with an inflammatory fluid that contains bacteria as well as cells from the immune system (basically, a form of pus).

The part of the lung involved (which may be part of a lobe, an entire lobe or a larger area of the lung) cannot function normally because of the infection. The clinical features of pneumonia depend to some extent on the type of organism causing the infection. As an example, the effects of a common bacterium called *Pneumococcus* are described below.

Clinical features

The illness starts fairly abruptly with high fever and shaking chills. Next, a troublesome cough with green–yellow purulent sputum appears, often with pain in the chest (caused by irritation of the pleura of the lung) and shortness of breath.

Diagnosis

The diagnosis can be made by examining the patient and by chest X-ray. Superficially, the symptoms of pneumonia (infection of the alveoli) are similar to those of acute bronchitis (infection of the bronchi not involving the alveoli), and the two illnesses usually cannot be distinguished from each other without detailed physical examination and an X-ray.

Treatment

In the past, many patients who had pneumonia (particularly infants and the elderly) died from the disease. Today, death from pneumonia is rare because of antibiotic treatment. Although the vast majority of patients will recover from pneumonia even without antibiotics, one cannot predict who will and who will not recover spontaneously and it is therefore essential to treat every patient with antibiotics.

PULMONARY EMBOLISM

Pulmonary embolism is a blood clot that forms initially on the inner wall of one of the large veins (usually in the thigh or pelvis), breaks away from the vein wall and is swept with the blood towards the heart. It reaches the right atrium, then passes through the right ventricle and into the pulmonary artery. It then lodges in the pulmonary artery or one of its branches in the lungs, blocking it. Such blood clots usually form in people who are immobile for prolonged periods (e.g. following an operation, especially orthopedic operations such as replacement of the head of the femur, following a severe traffic accident or sometimes even after sitting for a long time on a lengthy air flight).

Clinical features

The typical picture of a pulmonary embolism is sudden onset of shortness of breath, an increase in the breathing rate and pulse, cough (sometimes with blood-stained sputum) and pain in the chest related to breathing. The severity of the illness depends on the size of the artery that has become blocked. If the main pulmonary artery becomes blocked, the patient may die very quickly.

Diagnosis

The diagnosis is based on the use of special tests that are beyond the scope of this book.

Treatment

If the patient is in a serious condition, medications that dissolve blood clots can be given in an attempt to open the blocked pulmonary artery. Most patients who are not in a life-threatening situation are treated by giving oxygen and medications that prevent the formation of blood clots.

PULMONARY EDEMA

Pulmonary edema is the filling of the alveoli with fluid. The most common cause is acute failure of the pump of the left side of the heart, such as may occur as the result of an inadequate supply of blood to the heart muscle due to atherosclerosis. The impaired left ventricle cannot expel the volume of blood that enters it, causing the pressure in the pulmonary veins to rise ('back pressure') and, as a result, the pressure in the capillaries in the alveolar walls to rise. This increase in pressure within the alveolar capillaries causes fluid to leak out into the alveolar cavity, which then fills up with fluid.

Clinical features

The clinical features include severe shortness of breath, cyanosis (blue color of the skin) and a cough with frothy pink sputum. Pulmonary edema is a life-threatening condition.

Diagnosis

The diagnosis can be made by examining the patient and by characteristic chest X-ray features.

Treatment

The treatment includes oxygen and intravenous medications that reduce the amount of fluid in the alveoli.

7 | The digestive system

CHAPTER CONTENTS

The **digestive system** basically consists of the digestive tract, which starts at the mouth and ends at the anus, together with a series of glands that secrete digestive juices into the tract. In the developing embryo, the digestive system starts off as a simple tube that changes its shape until, by the end of the process, all of the digestive organs have formed. The digestive tract is made up from the mouth and pharynx, esophagus, stomach, small intestine (bowel), large intestine, rectum, and anus (Fig. 7.1).

The glands involved in the digestive system are the salivary glands, the pancreas and the liver. Both the liver and the pancreas have other important functions unrelated to the digestive system.

The task of the digestive system is to break down the food we eat and to absorb the components into the bloodstream. The breakdown is both **mechanical** – by means of crushing – and **chemical** – by means of the **digestive enzymes**. Only after the food has been broken down chemically is it **absorbed** into the bloodstream.

THE MOUTH

The mouth (Fig. 7.2) fulfills an important task in speech as well as its role in digestion.

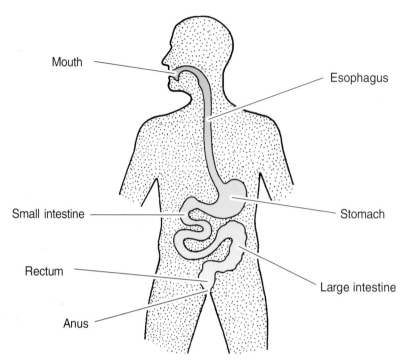

Figure 7.1   Digestive tract.

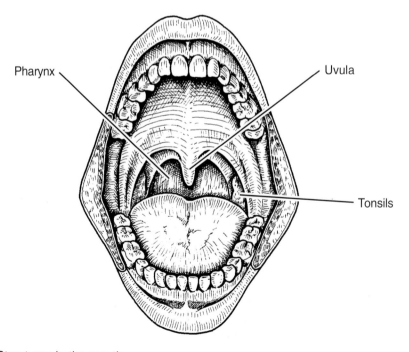

Figure 7.2   Structures in the mouth.

Mechanical breakdown of the food takes place in the mouth. The chewing muscles, the teeth and the tongue all play a part in the process of **mastication** (chewing), in which the food is broken down into small pieces and mixed with saliva to form a pasty, chewed lump called a **bolus**.

Salivary glands

Many microscopic salivary glands are scattered throughout the mucosal lining of the mouth.

There are also three pairs of large salivary glands, which together can secrete a total of about 1 liter of saliva per day (Fig. 7.3).

The largest pair of glands – the **parotid** glands – are situated at the angle of the jaw, just in front of the lower part of the ear. The saliva secreted by these glands passes through a narrow duct that ends at the outer side of the upper gum, just near the second molar tooth (this is where your dentist places a cotton wool tampon to soak up the saliva that emerges from this duct). Another pair of glands is situated under the jaw, called the **submandibular** glands. These secrete saliva onto the floor of the mouth through a small duct (one duct from each gland). Under the tongue is another pair of glands, called the **sublingual** glands, whose secretions are discharged through a number of small ducts onto the floor of the mouth. Sometimes you can actually see the saliva coming out of the tiny openings on the floor of the mouth (dentists put a tube into the mouth

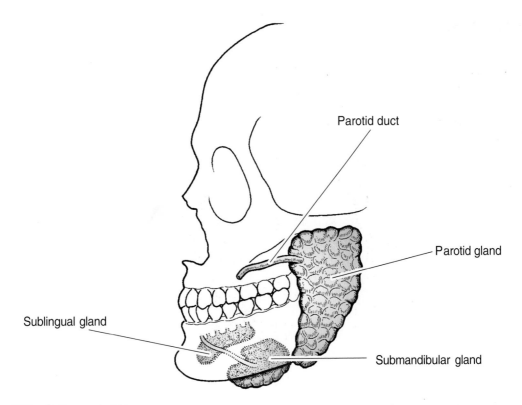

Figure 7.3   Salivary glands.

to suction the saliva from the floor of the mouth).

Saliva has several functions:

- Liquefaction of the food.
- Protection of the teeth and cleaning the mouth. The teeth are constantly bathed in saliva, which contains substances that protect the covering of the teeth.
- Combating bacteria by means of immunologically active substances present in saliva.
- Breaking down starch into glucose by means of an enzyme called **amylase**, which is secreted in saliva. Only 5% of the starch in food is digested in the mouth. If you chew bread for a long time, you will feel a sweet taste in the mouth as the starch is broken down to glucose.

The tongue

The tongue is made of six muscles and is covered by a special mucous membrane.

The tongue helps in chewing, swallowing, and cleaning the teeth. It contains the organs for sense of taste (the taste buds) and is involved in producing voice sounds.

The posterior third of the upper surface of the tongue contains lymphoid tissue (lymphoid tissue is part of the immunologic system). The tongue is covered with epithelial tissue and, over its anterior two-thirds, there are small bump-like projections. These bumps give the tongue its rough feeling and contain the **taste buds**. The taste buds are part of the nervous system and nerve fibers lead from them to the taste center in the brain. Most of the taste buds are in the tongue (about 2000 in number); the rest are found in the palate and the throat. Different areas of the tongue

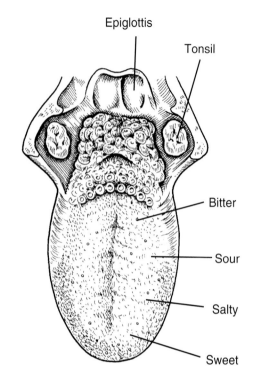

Figure 7.4   The tongue.

contain different sorts of taste buds (Fig. 7.4). In order from the front of the tongue to the back, the taste areas are: sweet, salty, sour and bitter. Pungent (hot, peppery) is not a taste but a slight irritation of the mucosa of the mouth. The sensation of taste is actually a combination of the effect of the taste buds, together with the smell and texture of the food.

The **frenulum** is the strip of tissue joining the undersurface of the tongue to the floor of the mouth.

The teeth

Each side of the jaw normally contains eight teeth and the entire mouth contains 32 teeth. Each side contains two **incisors**, one **canine**, and five **premolar** and **molar** teeth. The last molar tooth is known as the wisdom tooth. The 20 deciduous (or 'milk') teeth of childhood precede the permanent teeth.

A tooth comprises a section called the **crown**, which is outside the gum, and the **root**, which is within the gum. The crown is covered by a hard substance called enamel (Fig. 7.5). **Enamel** is an extremely resistant connective tissue that protects the other layers of the tooth from various agents, such as bacteria, in the mouth. It can withstand temperatures of 2000°C, and is the only tissue that remains after a body has been burnt at high temperatures. Under the enamel is a layer called the **dentin**, from which the crown and root of the tooth are formed. Dentin is a softer connective tissue than enamel, and also contains nerves. If the enamel is damaged, the nerves in the underlying dentin can be stimulated, causing pain (as occurs, for example, when drinking something cold). Deeper inside the root of the tooth is the **red pulp**. This contains the blood vessels that nourish the tooth and its nerves. Damage to the red pulp interferes with the blood supply to the tooth, and the tooth may die.

PHARYNX

The pharynx is the passageway through which:

- food passes on its way from the mouth to the esophagus

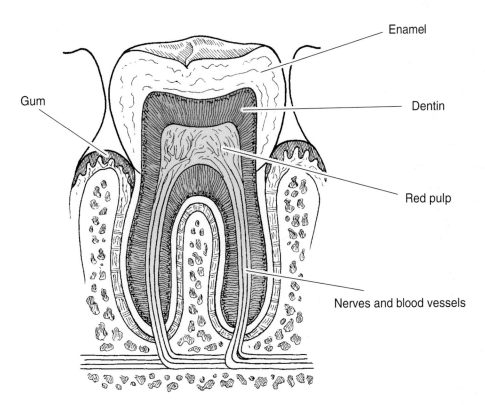

Figure 7.5 Structure of the tooth.

- air passes on its way from the nasal passages and mouth to the trachea.

Food moves into the esophagus by means of the **swallowing reflex**. To initiate this reflex, the tongue pushes the chewed food towards the pharynx (Fig. 7.6A). The moment that the food touches the back wall of the pharynx, the pharyngeal muscles contract, closing off the opening to the upper part of the pharynx (the nasopharynx) and pushing the food into the esophagus. At the same time as the pharyngeal muscles contract, the muscles of the larynx also contract, the cover of the larynx (the epiglottis) snaps shut and food is thereby prevented from entering the trachea (Fig. 7.6B). The swallowing reflex, which involves a complex series of coordin-ated muscular contractions of the pharynx and the larynx, is controlled by a center in the brain stem.

ESOPHAGUS

The esophagus is a muscle-walled tube about 25 cm long. It starts at the lower part of the pharynx, passes through the chest along-side the back of the trachea and the back of the heart, then through the diaphragm into the abdominal cavity, where it connects to the stomach.

Food moves down the esophagus by means of waves of muscular contractions of its wall, known as **peristaltic waves** (Fig. 7.7). It is peri-staltic waves that move food along the entire length of the digestive tract. Solid food and

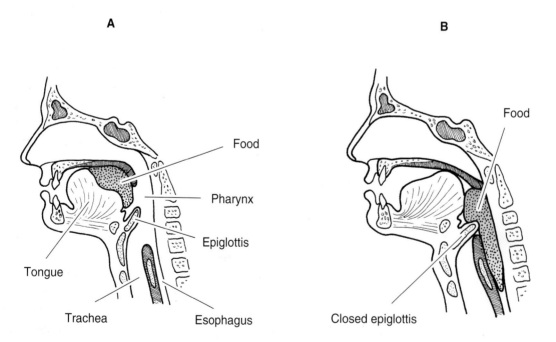

A

B

Food

Pharynx

Epiglottis

Tongue

Trachea

Esophagus

Food

Closed epiglottis

Figure 7.6   Swallowing. **A** shows the initiation of swallowing. In **B** (the continuation of the swallowing process) the cover of the larynx (the epiglottis) is closed, and the food slides down the esophagus.

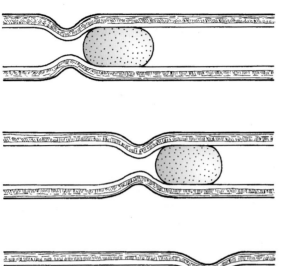

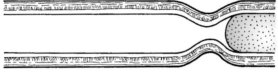

Figure 7.7   A peristaltic wave.

liquids are moved along the esophagus by an active process and not just by gravity; hence one can drink water standing on one's head.

STOMACH

The stomach is a muscular bag with a capacity of about 2 liters (it is, in effect, a widening of the digestive tract). It is situated in the upper left area of the abdominal cavity, anteriorly. Most of the anterior surface of the stomach is covered by the lower ribs.

Structure of the stomach

Food passes from the esophagus into the stomach through an upper opening, called the **cardia**. At the lower end of the stomach is another opening, called the **pylorus** (the Greek word **Pylorus** = gatekeeper), through which food leaves the stomach and enters the small intestine. Around the pylorus is a circumferential muscle, which acts as a sentinel at this stomach opening. At the cardia there is no circumferential muscle, but the anatomic structure of this area prevents food from being regurgitated from the stomach back up into the esophagus. The stomach itself is divided into three areas known as the **fundus**, which normally contains only air; the **body**, which is most of the stomach; and the **antrum**, which lies between the body and the pylorus (Fig. 7.8).

The wall of the stomach is composed of three layers. The outermost layer, called the **serosa**, is a thin membrane that covers the stomach and is part of the peritoneum. The middle layer, called the **muscularis**, comprises three layers of smooth muscle – a longitudinal layer, a transverse layer and an oblique layer. Contraction of these muscles 'kneads' the food within the stomach and mixes it with the stomach juices. The innermost layer of the stomach, the **mucosa**, has many folds and ridges (which can be seen with the naked eye) and contains several different types of cells. Between this layer and the muscular layer is connective tissue.

The gastric (stomach) mucosa

If you were to look at the gastric mucosa under a microscope you would see a layer of cells with depressions between them. These depressions are called **gastric pits** and are formed as a result of mucosal cells that penetrate into the underlying connective tissue. At the bottom of the gastric pits are glands containing various types of cells (Fig. 7.9).

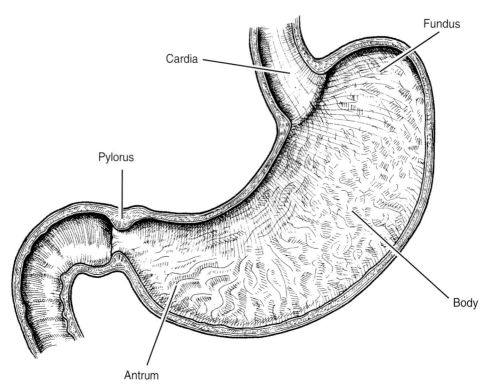

Figure 7.8   The Stomach.

Cells of the gastric mucosa

The superficial (top) layer of the gastric mucosa and the gastric pits is made of a layer of **mucous cells**. These cells produce mucus, which contains an alkaline substance that coats the gastric mucosa and protects it from the acid in the stomach.

The glands within the stomach contain three types of cell:

1. **Parietal cells:** produce a strong acid (hydrochloric acid; HCl).
2. **Chief cells:** produce an enzyme called **pepsin**, which breaks down proteins.
3. **G cells:** found in the glands in the region of the antrum. They produce a hormone called

gastrin, which is secreted in response to food entering the stomach. Gastrin stimulates the parietal cells to produce hydrochloric acid.

There is a constant turnover of the cells in the gastric mucosa, with new cells being formed all the time. The average lifespan of a mucosal cell is a few days.

Function of the stomach

Regulation of the release of food to the rest of the digestive tract. Food that contains fat stays in the stomach for a relatively long time – approximately 6 hours, food that contains protein remains for about 4 hours and

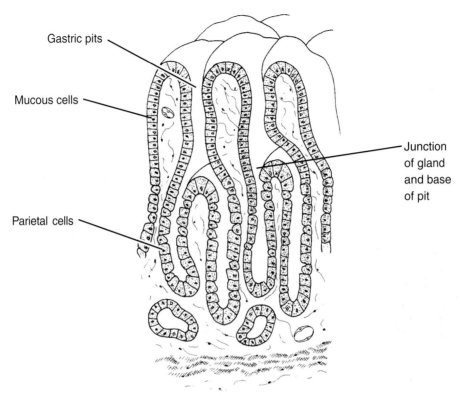

Gastric pits

Mucous cells

Parietal cells

Junction
of gland
and base
of pit

Figure 7.9   Gastric mucosa.

food that contains carbohydrate for about 2 hours; water stays in the stomach for 15 minutes. The time that a complete meal remains in the stomach therefore depends on the composition of that meal. The stomach retains foods such as fat for a longer period because their digestion takes a relatively long time. It will 'release' quickly those foods whose digestion in the bowel is faster. If, for example, the stomach has been removed surgically, the main problem is the incomplete digestion of foods (mainly fats) that pass in large amounts from the esophagus directly to the small bowel. This is because the small bowel is only able to digest fats in small quantities.

Mechanical breakdown of the food.   The stomach is a muscular sac that kneads the food and mixes it with the gastric juices. The acid in the stomach breaks down the food and turns it into a watery mixture.

Chemical breakdown of the food.   The pepsin in the stomach juice breaks down some of the proteins in the food into amino acids. This process helps in the digestion of meat. In addition to the breakdown of protein by pepsin, there is also some breakdown of fats and carbohydrates in the stomach. It should be pointed out that even in the absence of a stomach, the chemical digestion of food is unaffected, provided that the meals are small.

The absorption of water, salts and alcohol.   As alcohol is absorbed directly into the blood stream from the stomach, its effects can be felt within minutes of drinking it.

Protection against the entry of bacteria. The high acidity of the stomach, as a result of the secretion of hydrochloric acid by the gastric glands, kills bacteria that get into it. There are, however, some bacteria that are resistant to the stomach acid.

SMALL BOWEL

The small intestine is a tube, approximately 5 m long, in which most of the chemical break-down and absorption of food into the blood-stream takes place. The small intestine is the most important part of the digestive system – a person cannot survive without a small bowel (unless feeding is done intravenously).

The small intestine is divided into three segments. The first part is called the **duodenum**, and is approximately 25 cm long. The second and third parts are the **jejunum** and **ileum**, respectively, and comprise two-fifths and three-fifths of the length of the small bowel (Fig. 7.10).

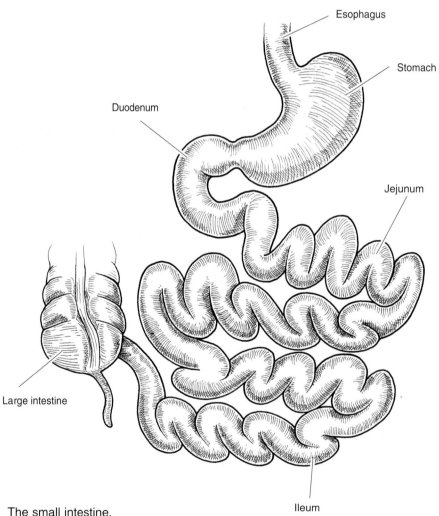

Figure 7.10   The small intestine.

The duodenum, which is horseshoe-shaped, is situated towards the back of the abdominal cavity and encircles the head of the pancreas. The pancreatic duct and the bile duct, through which digestive juices pass into the small bowel, enter the middle part of the duodenum (see Fig. 7.18).

Apart from the duodenum, most of the small intestine is covered by a membrane called the **mesentery**, which is attached to the back of the abdominal cavity. The blood vessels and nerves leading to the small intestine pass along this membrane. (Fig. 7.11).

Structure of the wall of the small intestine

The wall of the small intestine is composed of three major layers (Fig. 7.12):

1. The outermost layer is called the **serosa**, and is part of the peritoneal membrane that surrounds the intestine.
2. The middle layer is the **muscularis**, made up of two layers of smooth muscle – a longitudinal layer and a circular (circumferential) layer.

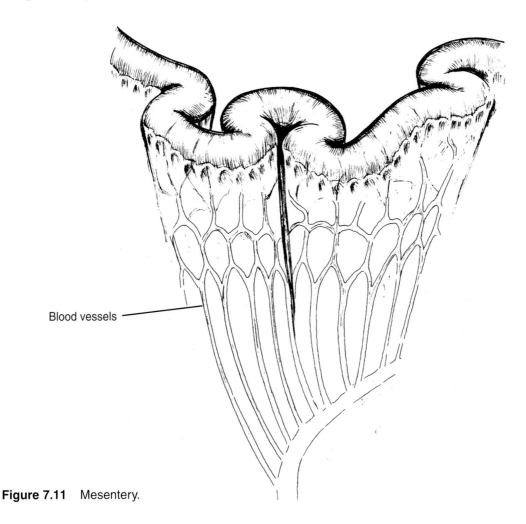

Blood vessels

Figure 7.11 Mesentery.

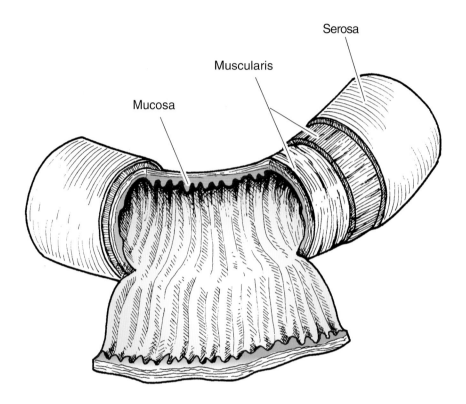

Figure 7.12   Structure of the wall of the small intestine.

3. The innermost layer is called the **mucosa.** There is also connective tissue between the mucosa and muscularis.

Mucosa of the small intestine

The processes of chemical breakdown of the food and its absorption take place at the small intestinal mucosa. This layer has a special structure that greatly increases its total surface area and maximizes the efficiency of digestion and absorption.

With the naked eye, the mucosa can be seen to have many transverse ridges and folds. Under the microscope, one can see millions of finger-like projections from the mucosa, called **villi** (singular = villus) (Fig. 7.13). These pro-jections are made up of the mucosal cells. **Goblet cells,** a specialized type of mucosal cell, secrete a mucus that lubricates the internal surface of the digestive tract. The majority of the cells of the mucosa are the **absorptive cells**. Each of these cells contains some 3000 tiny projections, called **microvilli**, which protrude into the cavity of the intestine. It is on the surface of these projections that the processes of digestion and absorption of food occur (Fig. 7.14).

Function of the small intestine

Nearly all of the proteins, fats and carbohy-drates that enter the small intestine undergo chemical breakdown and are absorbed into the

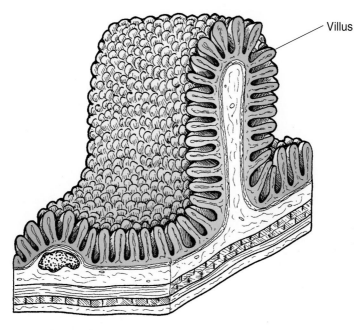

Villus

Figure 7.13   Mucosa of small intestine.

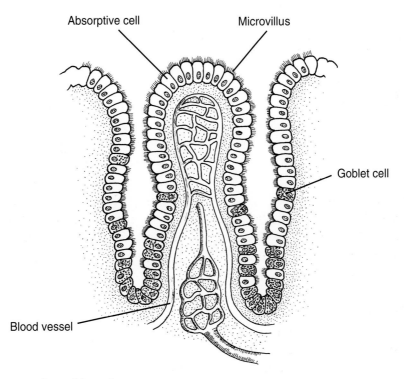

Absorptive cell

Microvillus

Goblet cell

Blood vessel

Figure 7.14   Mucosa of small intestine.

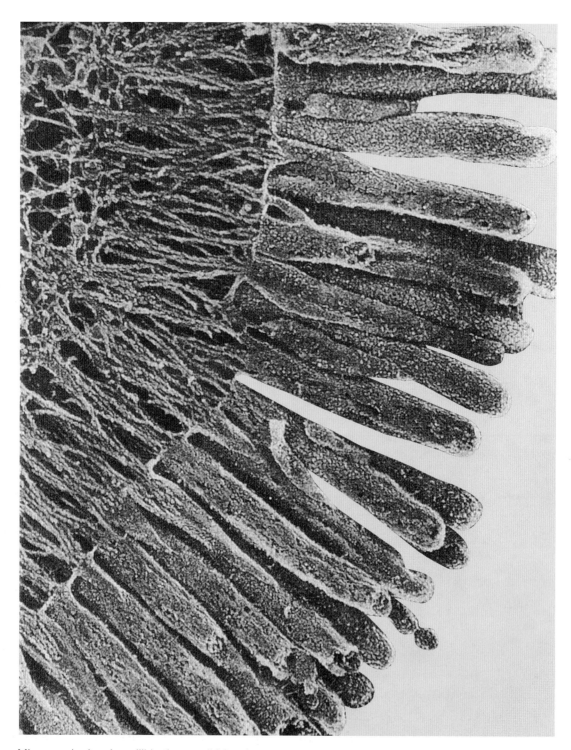

Micrograph showing villi in the small intestine.

bloodstream. Cellulose found in the food is neither digested nor absorbed in the small intestine, and passes on to the large intestine intact.

The various food components are broken down by digestive enzymes. Some of the digestive enzymes are secreted by the pancreas into the duodenum, and some are produced by the small bowel mucosa. These enzymes break down the major food constituents into their components:

Proteins → Amino acids

Fats → Fatty acids + Glycerol

Carbohydrates → Monosaccharides

Only after the food has been broken down into its components can it pass into the absorptive cells, and from there into the network of capillaries within the villi of the mucosa.

The food passes along the intestine by means of waves of contraction that proceed along the muscles of the wall of the intestine, the **peristaltic movement**. Apart from the orderly and regular peristaltic waves, the intestinal wall also contracts randomly to mix the food in the intestinal cavity.

LARGE INTESTINE

The large intestine, also called the **colon**, is the final part of the digestive tract. Its major task is the absorption of water and salts, leaving feces. The large intestine is divided into several segments (Fig. 7.15).

The **cecum** is a sac-like enlargement at the junction of the small and large intestines, in the lower right-hand side of the abdomen. There is a small, blindly ending tube, approx-imately 0.5 cm in diameter and about 5 cm long, attached to the cecum. This is the **appendix**, whose function in man is unclear.

At the area of the junction between the small and large intestines is an anatomic valve called the **ileo-cecal valve**, which prevents the contents of the large bowel from passing back into the small bowel. On the right side of the abdomen is the **ascending colon**, which heads upwards, then becomes the **transverse colon**, situated across the breadth of the upper abdomen, anteriorly. The colon then heads downwards, to become the **descending colon**, which is situated on the left side of the abdomen. The next segment is the **sigmoid colon**, which descends into the pelvis. Within the pelvis, immediately in front of the sacrum, is the **rectum**, which functions as a reservoir for feces, terminating at the **anus**.

Structure of the wall of the large intestine

The wall of the large intestine is composed of three main layers, as is the rest of the digestive tract. However, unlike the layer of smooth muscle in the small intestine (which consists of longitudinal and circular muscles that go all the way around the wall of the bowel) in the large intestine, the longitudinal muscle layer is only found along part of the wall, and forms three strips of muscle called the **tenia coli**.

Large intestinal mucosa

The mucosa of the large intestine is a flat surface containing many glands, which give it a pitted appearance. It consists of two main types of cells – cells that secrete mucus and absorptive cells.

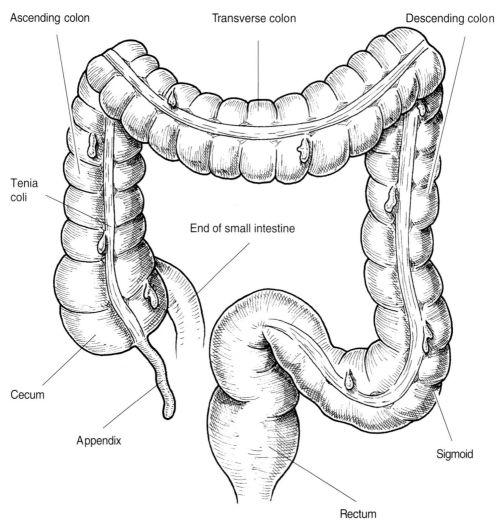

Figure 7.15   Large intestine.

Function of the large intestine

The contents of the first part of the large intestine are essentially those of the small intestine – mainly water, salts, cellulose and small amounts of food that was not absorbed in the small intestine. As this material moves along the large intestine, water and salts are absorbed, and the bowel contents become progressively more solid.

Towards the end of the large intestine, feces are formed. These accumulate in the rectum. They are composed of 75% water and 25% solid material, which consists of cells, bacteria and food remnants. When the rectum becomes full of feces, it produces a sensation of pressure, and then, if the circumstances are appropriate, the feces are expelled by a peristaltic wave coordinated with relaxation of the ring muscles ('sphincter muscles') around the anus. This is the process of **defecation**. Within the large intestine are enormous numbers of bacteria, which are 'permanent residents' of the bowel.

LIVER AND BILIARY TRACT

The liver is a large vascular (filled with blood) organ in the upper abdominal cavity on the right side, immediately below the diaphragm. Most of the liver is covered by the lower ribs.

Several tubes and vessels are connected to the liver (Fig. 7.16):

- The **hepatic artery** supplies arterial blood to the liver.
- The **hepatic vein** drains venous blood from the liver.
- The **portal vein** brings venous blood to the liver. Although a vein is defined as a blood vessel that drains blood from an organ, the portal vein is unique in that it brings

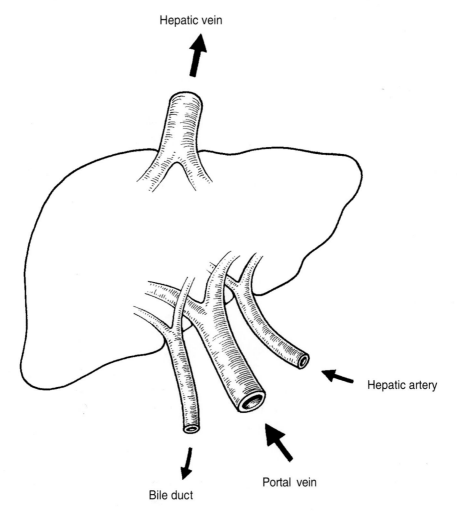

Hepatic vein

Hepatic artery

Portal vein

Bile duct

Figure 7.16 Tubes and vessels connected to the liver. The arrows show direction of drainage.

blood to the liver. Veins converge from the stomach, small intestine, large intestine, pancreas and spleen to form the portal vein which enters the liver. The venous blood from the digestive system, which contains the various substances that were absorbed into the bloodstream, does not return directly to the right atrium of the heart, but first passes through the liver.

- The **common bile duct** is a tube transporting bile, produced in the liver, to the gallbladder and then to the duodenum.

Liver tissue

If you look at liver tissue under the microscope, you can see many hexagonal structures, called **lobules** (Fig. 7.17). At the angles of these lobules is an arteriole (derived from the hepatic artery), a venule (derived from the portal vein) and a biliary duct. The arteriole and the venule both discharge their blood into small canals that pass between the liver cells. In these

canals, there is mixing of arterial blood and venous blood from the portal vein.

In the center of each lobule is a venule, into which blood from the canals drains. These venules join together to form larger and larger vessels, to eventually become the hepatic vein, via which the blood leaves the liver to pass into the inferior vena cava.

Liver cells, or **hepatocytes**, are in direct contact with the blood flowing between them in the canals, and perform various chemical processes on the substances in the blood. The biliary ducts at the angles of the lobules of the liver drain the bile that is formed by the hepatocytes into the bile duct, which ultimately drains the bile into the duodenum.

Function of the liver

The liver is a vital organ that carries out many important functions in the body. One cannot live for long without a liver and, to date, no machine has been invented that can replace

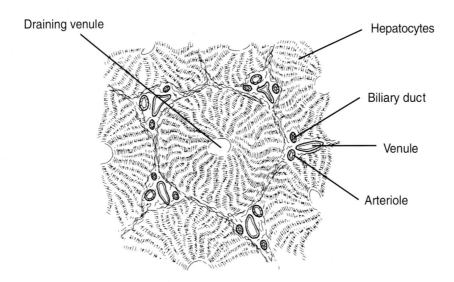

Figure 7.17   Liver tissue. This illustration shows a hexagonal liver lobule with a draining venule in its center.

the liver. Below are some details of the various functions of the liver.

Production of many proteins found in the blood. The liver cells produce plasma proteins, such as coagulation (clotting) factors and a protein called albumin. Liver malfunction will therefore affect blood clotting, leading to bleeding because of lack of some of the coagulation factors. It also will result in edema (accumulation of fluid) in the body because of lack of albumin.

Neutralization of poisons and their excretion into the bile. The liver is involved in neutralizing or detoxifying toxins produced in the body, as well as those found in food and many medications. It acts as a filter for the blood passing through it, including both arterial blood entering via the hepatic artery and all of the venous blood from the digestive tract via the portal vein. The blood in the portal vein contains various toxins that were absorbed from food. These pass through the liver, which filters them out and neutralizes them, thereby preventing them from entering the bloodstream.

Bilirubin is produced from the breakdown of old red blood cells (a normal process that is going on all the time). It is a yellow-colored substance, which, in high concentrations, is poisonous to body tissues. It is neutralized and excreted into the bile by the liver. In the digestive tract, bilirubin undergoes chemical change as a result of the action of intestinal bacteria, and acquires a brown tint – giving feces their brown color. If bilirubin is not excreted normally and accumulates in the body, it causes **jaundice** (a yellow discoloration of the skin and mucous membranes).

Regulation of levels of nutrients in the blood. The liver acts as an important center of metabolism. For example, during a fast, the liver produces glucose in order to maintain a normal sugar level in the blood, even if no glucose is available from food.

Manufacturing red blood cells. The liver is not normally involved in making blood cells but, under emergency circumstances of a severe deficiency of red blood cells, the liver is able to produce them.

Production and excretion of bile. Liver cells secrete **bile**, and excrete it through the bile ducts into the duodenum. Bile contains several components:

- **An alkaline substance**: needed to counteract the acidity of the food that emerges from the stomach.
- **Bile salts**: substances chemically and functionally similar to soap, and important in the digestion of fats. Bile salts turn fat into tiny droplets known as an emulsion, which greatly enlarges the surface area available for contact between the fat and the enzymes that break it down into its chemical components. Bile salts are made from cholesterol. They are excreted into the small intestine and approximately 90% of the bile salts is subsequently reabsorbed in the lower part of the small bowel, to be returned to the liver for re-use.

THE BILIARY TRACT

The **gall bladder** is a hollow organ, of about 50 cm³ capacity, with a muscular wall that serves as a reservoir for bile.

The gall bladder lies immediately under the liver, with its edge sticking out beyond the liver margin. A tube called the **cystic duct** leads from the gall bladder to the bile duct. Between meals, the gall bladder fills up with

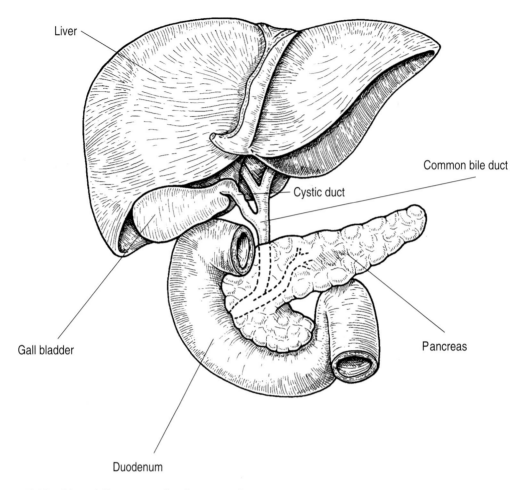

Figure 7.18   Liver, biliary tract, duodenum and pancreas.

bile (formed in the liver) and, when food reaches the duodenum, the gall bladder contracts and pours bile via the cystic duct and the bile duct into the duodenum (Fig. 7.18).

THE PANCREAS

The pancreas is an oblong-shaped organ in the posterior part of the abdominal cavity, behind the stomach. It has a wide end, the **head** of the pancreas, which is encircled by the duodenum,

a central section called the **body** of the pancreas, and a thin end called the **tail** of the pancreas (Fig. 7.19).

Structure of the pancreatic tissue

The tissue within the pancreas consists of two types of gland. One type is related to the endocrine system, which secretes hormones into the blood (see Chapter 15, on the endocrine system); The second type excretes

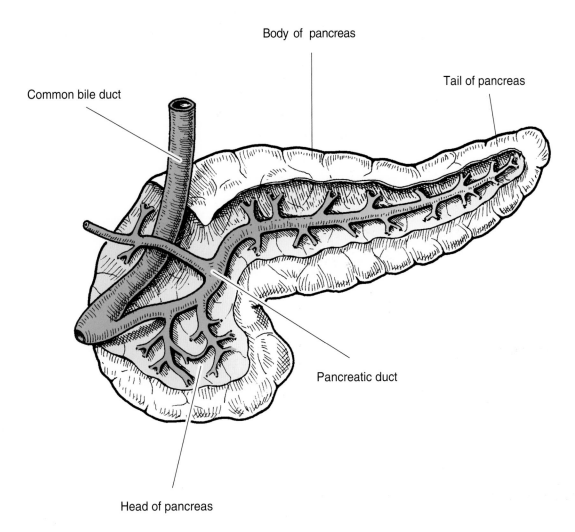

Body of pancreas

Tail of pancreas

Common bile duct

Pancreatic duct

Head of pancreas

Figure 7.19 Pancreas.

digestive juices into a tube, called the **pancreatic duct**, which passes along the length of the pancreas and eventually enters the duodenum. Occasionally, this pancreatic duct joins the common bile duct before it enters the duodenum, and the two ducts then share a single point of entry into the duodenum (see Fig. 7.19).

Role of the pancreas in digestion

The pancreas secretes approximately 2 liters of digestive juices into the duodenum per day. This juice contains two main constituents:

- An **alkaline substance**: this substance neutralizes the acidity of the food as it leaves the stomach, similar to bile.

● **Digestive enzymes**: amylase breaks down starch to glucose; lipase breaks down fats to fatty acids and glycerol; carboxypeptidase and related enzymes break down proteins into amino acids.

When food reaches the duodenum, the pancreas and the gall bladder excrete digestive juices into the duodenum. This occurs in response to signals from the nervous system and from the endocrine system.

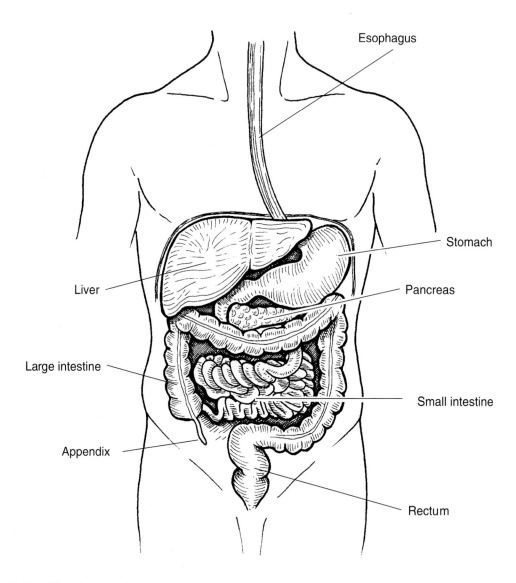

Figure 7.20   The abdominal organs.

Diseases of the digestive system

DISEASES OF THE ESOPHAGUS

Reflux esophagitis

'Reflux' refers to stomach content that flows back into the esophagus, and 'esophagitis' means inflammation of the esophagus. Normally, the anatomic structure of the lower end of the esophagus, where it enters the stomach, prevents stomach contents flowing 'backwards' into the esophagus. In reflux esophagitis, which is a common disease that usually appears after the age of 40, this mechanism is faulty and acidic stomach content is able to flow back into the esophagus, where it causes inflammation of the mucosa.

The clinical features include a feeling of **heartburn**, pain when swallowing (**odynophagia**) and difficulty in swallowing (**dysphagia**). Sometimes, stomach content refluxes into the esophagus while the patient is asleep, reaches the pharynx, and from there overflows into the air passages and the lungs. This causes coughing and a choking feeling at night, and sometimes even pneumonia.

The esophageal mucosa is attacked by the acid from the stomach and can bleed or develop fibrosis and scarring leading to a permanent narrowing of the esophagus known as a **stricture**.

Reflux esophagitis is diagnosed mainly on the basis of the typical symptoms and the nature of the pain. A special fiberoptic instrument called an **endoscope** can be inserted into the esophagus and the inflamed area examined and photographed.

Treatment of the disease involves alteration of the lifestyle to some extent: not eating for several hours before going to bed and not lying down totally supine (on the back) while asleep. Various medications are available to decrease the amount of acid secreted in the stomach and thus lessen the damage to the esophageal mucosa. In some cases, an operation can be performed to prevent reflux of food from the stomach back to the esophagus.

Carcinoma of the esophagus

This cancer occurs usually in males over the age of 50 and is particularly common in certain countries, such as China, Iran and South Africa. It appears to be related to the diet of the people in these countries, and is also related to excessive alcohol use and smoking.

The cancerous growth starts in the mucosa and gradually grows until it becomes a large mass that eventually blocks the cavity of the esophagus. Subsequently, the cancerous cells also spread to adjacent organs, such as the trachea, the larynx and the heart.

The main symptom of carcinoma of the esophagus is increasing difficulty in swallowing (**dysphagia**). At first, there is difficulty in swallowing large lumps of food. It then becomes difficult to swallow even small lumps, and eventually the patient is unable to swallow liquids. Marked weight loss is a striking feature of this disease. As the cancer spreads to nearby organs, other symptoms can appear, such as hoarseness and shortness of breath.

Definitive diagnosis is by means of endoscopy – a tube (endoscope) inserted into the esophagus. Through the endoscope, the interior of the esophagus can be viewed or photographed, and if a suspicious area is seen, a sample of tissue (a **biopsy**) can be taken from it. A pathologist then examines the biopsy specimen under the microscope to establish the precise diagnosis.

Treatment of esophageal carcinoma involves removal of the esophagus. Usually, by the time it is diagnosed, the disease has spread to adjoining organs, making it incurable. The prognosis (outlook) for patients with carcinoma of the esophagus is extremely poor.

DISEASES OF THE STOMACH AND DUODENUM

Peptic ulcer disease

Peptic ulcer disease is commonly called 'ulcer'. This disease is more common in males than females and usually appears in adult life, although it can occur in childhood. It is estimated that approximately 10% of the population have peptic ulcer disease.

An ulcer is a 'sore' in the mucosa. Although the common lay term is a 'stomach ulcer', most ulcers are in the duodenum, with only a minority actually in the stomach. The mucosa of the stomach and duodenum is protected against the extreme acidity of the stomach by a layer of mucus, which coats it. If there is excessive acidity, or if the protective mucus layer is deficient, the strong acid and other components of the stomach juice (such as pepsin, an enzyme that breaks down proteins), attack and 'digest' the mucosa, creating an ulcer.

Alcohol, smoking and certain medications such as aspirin or steroids increase the risk of developing an ulcer. Recently, a bacterium by the name of *Helicobacter pylori* has been found to be present in the stomach and is now recognized to be responsible for most cases of peptic ulcer disease not attributable to medications.

The clinical features of peptic ulcer disease include a characteristic pain at the top of the abdomen (epigastrium), which appears between meals or which wakes the patient in the middle of the night. The pain appears between meals or at night because the stomach is empty at those times and the stomach juices come into direct contact with the ulcer in the mucosa. Eating or drinking something basic (i.e. alkaline – the opposite of acidic) relieves the pain because the food or liquid 'dilutes' the stomach juices and the base neutralizes the acid. Sometimes the pain is associated with nausea and vomiting, or with a feeling of fullness in the stomach and hiccoughs.

Peptic ulcer disease can produce complications that can on occasion require urgent surgery. For example, perforation of the stomach or duodenum, with stomach contents leaking into the abdominal cavity; bleeding as a result of exposed blood vessels in the floor of the ulcer; obstruction of the outlet of the stomach because of swelling (edema) or fibrosis of the stomach wall in the area around the ulcer.

Peptic ulcer disease can be diagnosed on the basis of the symptoms and with the use of X-rays, gastroscopy and other imaging techniques.

In summary, the treatment of the disease is by medication, although in some cases surgery has to be used. The medications used are antacids (to counteract the acid) or medica-tions that decrease the secretion of acid, as well as antibiotics to eliminate the *Helicobacter pylori* bacteria. Surgery involves cutting the nerves to the stomach that control acid secretion, or closing the ulcer directly.

Carcinoma of the stomach

This form of cancer usually appears in males over the age of 50. It is particularly common in Japan, China, Colombia and Finland. Eating certain types of food, such as smoked and salted meat, pickled and preserved foods, are thought to increase the risk of developing carcinoma of the stomach. The cancer begins in the stomach mucosa and usually causes an ulcer or a lump that grows into the stomach cavity. Subsequently, the tumor cells invade other organs around the stomach, and may also invade distant organs, such as the liver.

The clinical features of cancer of the stomach are very similar to those of peptic ulcer of the stomach.

The diagnosis of stomach cancer can be established by means of X-rays of the stomach and by taking biopsies (samples of tissue) from the area of the lesion for microscopic examination. Treatment involves complete or partial removal of the stomach.

In most cases, surgery does not provide a total cure and the prognosis is very poor.

DISEASES OF THE SMALL INTESTINE

Acute gastroenteritis

This is an infection of the small (and sometimes the large) intestine, caused by various infectious agents, such as viruses and bacteria.

Gastroenteritis is the second most common disease in mankind (the 'cold' being the most common), and it is estimated that some 40% of the population suffers from it at least once a year. It is caused by eating food that is contaminated with viruses, bacteria, bacterial toxins or other organisms such as amebae and parasites.

The clinical features are usually stomach pain, nausea, vomiting and diarrhea.

The diagnosis of gastroenteritis is based essentially on the patient's history. Samples of the stool can be taken to identify the cause precisely. The treatment is based on replacing the lost fluids and electrolytes, and antibiotics are given as necessary.

In the Western world, gastroenteritis is usually not considered a serious illness, because most patients – mainly children with diarrhea – get appropriate fluid and electrolyte replacement. However, in developing countries, many children die every day from acute gastroenteritis. The main cause of death is severe loss of fluid and electrolytes from the body.

Small bowel obstruction

Because of its narrow lumen and its considerable length, the small bowel is the most common site of obstruction of the digestive tract.

Small bowel obstruction can be caused by a lump of food that gets stuck, or by something pressing on the bowel from the outside. Following any abdominal surgery, it is not uncommon for bands of fibrous tissue (called **adhesions**) to form between different areas of the peritoneum (the membrane that covers all the abdominal organs). These fibrous bands encircle parts of the bowel and effectively cause a blockage by external pressure. Other causes of small bowel obstruction include twisting of the bowel or cancerous growths in the abdomen.

The clinical features of small bowel obstruction are:

- Colicky abdominal pain: as each peristaltic wave tries to get past the obstruction, the pressure in the bowel increases sharply, causing waves of severe pain.
- Nausea and vomiting.
- Abdominal swelling and tenderness: the abdomen swells due to the accumulation of fluid and gases in the bowel above the obstruction.
- Lack of passage of stools or gas.

The treatment of bowel obstruction depends to some extent on the cause. However, in every case the patient should be hospitalized and the treatment will include intravenous fluids and close observation, and possibly surgery to relieve the obstruction.

Complete bowel obstruction, if untreated, is fatal, because of the severe loss of fluids into the bowel cavity (from the blood vessels in the bowel wall) and because of bacteria from the bowel, which enter the bloodstream and cause overwhelming infection.

Inflammatory bowel disease

This term includes two diseases that bear certain similarities to each other. The first is **Crohn's disease**, which can affect any region of the digestive tract from the mouth to the anus; it usually involves the small bowel. The second is **ulcerative colitis**, which affects mainly the large bowel.

These diseases are caused by the body's own immunologic system, which, for some reason, attacks the bowel and causes severe inflammation.

Crohn's disease tends to occur in 'attacks', and presents with diarrhea, weakness, abdominal pain, fever and weight loss. Other organs or systems can also be affected, such as the joints, (arthritis), the eyes and the skin.

Ulcerative colitis also occurs in 'attacks', and presents mainly with bloody diarrhea, abdominal pain and weight loss. Patients with ulcerative colitis that has been present for more than 10 years are at increased risk of developing cancer of the large bowel.

Both of these diseases can cause severe damage to the bowel, with serious complications, such as perforation or obstruction.

The diagnosis of inflammatory bowel disease is based on X-rays of the bowel, and direct inspection of the lining of the bowel by a procedure known as **colonoscopy**. This involves inserting a flexible tube containing optic fibers through the anus, along the large bowel, up to the end of the small bowel.

The treatment of inflammatory bowel disease involves changes in diet (to a diet low in fiber and in milk products) and various medications.

Celiac disease

This disease is caused by sensitivity to a wheat protein called gluten. If foods containing wheat flour are eaten by a person with celiac disease, inflammation and severe damage to the mucosa of the small bowel occurs. Celiac disease usually appears at the age when the child starts eating solids containing wheat products. Affected children develop diarrhea, possibly a swollen abdomen, and their rate of growth decreases.

In adults, the disease presents with diarrhea, swelling of the abdomen and weight loss. Treatment involves a special gluten-free diet.

Lactose intolerance

This disease is common in black populations. It is caused by the lack of an enzyme called **lactase,** which is produced by the cells in the small bowel mucosa. This enzyme breaks down lactose (milk sugar). If a person with lactase deficiency drinks milk, the sugar in the milk is not broken down and absorbed into the blood and the person develops abdominal pain and distension, gas and diarrhea.

The treatment is the addition of the enzyme lactase to any milk product or avoidance of milk products.

Malabsorption

Normally, 95% of the fat, protein and sugars that enter the digestive system is broken down chemically and absorbed into the bloodstream. These processes normally take place in the small bowel and, if they fail, diarrhea results, due mainly to the large amount of fat that reaches the large intestine. This diarrhea is called **steatorrhea**. The stool is typically bulky, has a very offensive odor, is pale yellow, and tends to float on water, sticking to the sides of the toilet bowl.

Malabsorption leads to weight loss and eventually to symptoms and signs of deficiencies of various dietary components, such as certain vitamins. Diseases of the pancreas, liver and the bile system, all of which are involved in fat absorption, as well as diseases of the small bowel, where absorption takes place, can all cause malabsorption.

DISEASES OF THE LARGE BOWEL

Irritable bowel syndrome

This disease occurs more frequently in women and might be related to psychologic stress. It is the most common cause of chronic diarrhea.

The diarrhea typically occurs upon awakening or immediately after meals. The stool is mucousy and, after having a bowel motion, there is a feeling of not having emptied the bowels fully. Sometimes the diarrhea is associated with abdominal pain (usually in the left lower part of the abdomen) and sometimes with abdominal swelling, gas, nausea, headache, depression or anxiety. From time to time there might be constipation. It is important to note that patients with the irritable bowel syndrome do not lose weight, do not have diarrhea at night, and do not have blood in the stool.

The cause of this syndrome is not known but there is an association between the various features of the illness and situations of psychologic stress. The direct cause of the diarrhea is apparently excessively active peristalsis of the bowel (the waves of muscle contraction in the bowel wall).

In essence, the diagnosis is based on excluding other causes of chronic diarrhea.

Treatment is based on psychologic support and medications that slow down peristalsis.

Acute appendicitis

This common disease occurs mainly between the ages of 15 and 25. The usual cause is obstruction of the appendix by a piece of firm bowel contents; the appendix then becomes inflamed, bacteria multiply inside it and infection ensues.

Perforation of the appendix, with spillage of pus into the abdominal cavity can occur 24 hours after the onset of clinical signs and can result in a dangerous situation called **peritonitis**.

The features of appendicitis develop gradually. At first, there is pain in the central part of the abdomen and loss of appetite. Later, the pain 'moves' to the lower right abdomen, becomes more localized and more severe, and is aggravated by coughing or deep breathing. There is also usually fever, nausea, vomiting and occasional constipation.

The diagnosis is based on the history and the physical findings on examination of the patient. The treatment is surgical removal of the appendix.

Carcinoma of the colon (large intestine)

This form of cancer is common in the United States, Canada, Europe and Israel, and quite uncommon in the developing countries and in Japan. It usually occurs in older individuals.

It appears that the differences in the frequency of the disease in different countries are related to diet. A diet rich in animal fats and deficient in fiber increases the risk of developing carcinoma of the colon. There is also a familial tendency to develop the disease.

The cancer starts in the mucosa of the colon, in most cases in the last part of the large bowel near the anus. The cancer grows into a large mass that gradually obstructs the bowel. At a later stage the cancerous cells invade adjacent tissues and metastases (cancerous cells that break off from the main tumor and spread to distant sites in the body) travel to the liver and other organs.

The clinical features of carcinoma of the colon include:

- Changes in bowel habit: these changes could include diarrhea, constipation (or alternating diarrhea and constipation every few weeks), blood in the stools and changes in the thickness of the stools.
- Anemia: this occurs because of gradual bleeding from the cancerous tissue into the bowel.
- Weight loss.

The diagnosis of cancer of the large intestine is based on X-rays of the bowel and by direct inspection of the bowel mucosa through a colonoscope.

Early detection of the disease enables a cure of about 80% by means of surgery. The operation involves removing that portion of bowel where the growth is situated and rejoining the cut ends of the intestine.

Hemorrhoids

Hemorrhoids are dilated (widened) veins that bulge out under the skin of the rectum and anus. They usually occur over the age of 30, or in pregnant women.

Constipation is one factor that contributes to the appearance of hemorrhoids as a result of the increased pressure in the veins of the rectum when straining during defecation. Hemorrhoids cause bleeding (bright, fresh blood) during defecation and pain in the anal area.

The treatment consists of applying ointment to the area to soothe the irritation and laxatives to soften the stool. In severe cases, the hemorrhoids can be removed surgically.

DISEASES OF THE LIVER AND BILIARY TRACT

Viral hepatitis

This is an inflammation of the liver caused by a virus, it is the most common liver disease, in the world today.

Various viruses can affect the liver, the most common are **Hepatitis A** and **Hepatitis B** viruses. Infection with Hepatitis A virus occurs following the ingestion of food contaminated by the feces of a Hepatitis A patient (for example, if a cook has Hepatitis A and does not wash the hands properly after going to the toilet).

Infection with Hepatitis B virus usually occurs as the result of sexual intercourse with an affected partner, receiving a transfusion of infected blood, or using an infected injection needle.

The usual clinical features of viral hepatitis are fever, weakness, loss of appetite, a revulsion to cigarettes (even in smokers), nausea, vomiting and jaundice (yellowing of the skin).

In most cases, Hepatitis A resolves without any treatment. However, some patients suffer from fatigue that continues for months and in a small percentage of patients, the disease progresses to destruction of the liver and death.

Unlike Hepatitis A, the Hepatitis B virus can remain in the patient's liver for years. In some cases, there is gradual destruction and scarring of liver tissue, known as **cirrhosis**. This can lead to liver failure and is characterized by gradual shrinking of the liver, progressive deterioration of liver function and the appearance of fibrous tissue within the liver. Patients with cirrhosis develop a characteristic appearance, with muscle atrophy (shriveling-up of the muscles), generalized edema (swelling due to fluid accumulation), a swollen abdomen due to fluid accumulation in the peritoneum (**ascites**) and jaundice.

Viral hepatitis can be diagnosed on the basis of blood tests or liver biopsy. There are few effective treatments and these are very expensive and not widely available, thus the management of hepatitis is often only supportive treatment. If the disease is very severe, with significant liver damage, the only treatment is a liver transplant.

There are now vaccines available that immunize against Hepatitis A and B. In many countries, these are given routinely to all children.

Gallstones (cholelithiasis)

This condition is particularly common in white, overweight, fertile women in their 40s (medical students have a saying 'Fair, fat, fertile females of forty').

Gallstones usually consist of cholesterol. They develop if there is an imbalance in the chemical composition of the bile; the reason for such an imbalance is unclear. The presence of stones in the gall bladder does not necessarily cause pain or other symptoms or signs and a person could have gallstones for many years without any clinical manifestations.

The pain associated with gallstones usually appears when a stone starts to pass from the gall bladder into the bile ducts. As it travels down the bile ducts, it causes severe colicky pain in the right upper part of the abdomen, occasionally associated with nausea and vomiting. Fatty foods stimulate the gall bladder to contract and secrete bile, and so may trigger the onset of the pain. If the stone lodges in the **cystic duct** which drains the bile from the gall bladder to the bile duct, the gall bladder becomes distended and inflamed, a condition known as **acute cholecystitis**. The pain in the upper right abdomen now becomes constant rather than occurring in waves and fever develops, often with nausea and vomiting. After several hours, the gall bladder might perforate.

The presence of gallstones is diagnosed by means of an ultrasound examination of the gall bladder.

The treatment of cholelithiasis is the surgical removal of the gall bladder (an operation called **cholecystectomy**).

It is important to note that cholecystectomy is usually carried out only if the gallstones cause symptoms.

9

The locomotor system

The locomotor (movement) system is made up of bones, joints, ligaments, muscles and tendons. All these components combine to produce movement of the body.

The locomotor system is under the control of the nervous system. Nerves in the muscles, joints and tendons are continuously passing information to the brain regarding the position, degree of tension, and so on, of those components. Signals pass in the opposite direction – from the brain to other nerves in the muscles – to activate them and bring about movement.

For movement to occur, all of the components of the locomotor system must act in coordination. This coordination is extremely complex, because any given movement usually requires the coordinated activation of many muscles in the correct sequence. When you carry out a movement (such as passing a comb through your hair), you are aware only of the movement itself, not of the coordinated activation of the muscles in the arm, for example.

Malfunction of the locomotor system can arise from injury or disease affecting any part of the locomotor system or the nervous system.

FUNCTIONS OF THE SKELETON

The skeleton (Fig. 9.1) has several functions:

Support of the body tissues and organs. The shape of the skeleton determines the shape of the body. The body organs are positioned either within spaces created by skeletal structures (e.g. the organs of the chest and the abdomen) or around skeletal structures (e.g. the limbs).

Levers for movement. The long bones of the body, connected to each other by joints, form a system of levers that allows movement.

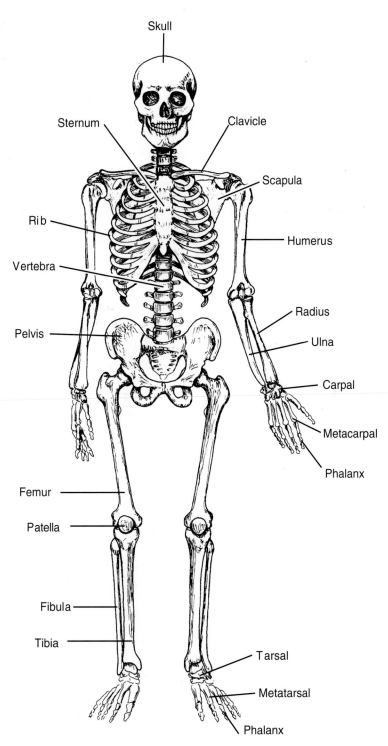

Figure 9.1   The skeleton.

Protection of internal organs. The hard bones protect the internal organs from external trauma. For example, the brain tissue is soft and, without the skull to protect it, a slight blow to the head could cause severe brain damage. Also, the organs within the chest (e.g. the heart and lungs) and the organs within the abdomen (e.g. the liver and spleen) are protected from injury by the bony skeleton.

Production of blood cells. Within the bones (particularly the pelvis, the spinal vertebrae and the sternum) there is bone marrow. Blood cells are manufactured in the bone marrow. Severe damage or illness affecting the bone marrow (e.g. following irradiation) can be fatal.

Storage of minerals. The bones contain an enormous amount of calcium and phosphorus.

TYPES OF BONE

There are several different types of bones in the skeleton:

Long bones. These are found in the limbs and are generally cylindrical in shape. Examples of long bones are the thigh bone (femur), the bone of the upper arm (humerus) and the bones of the fingers.

Short bones. These generally have a rectangular or square shape. Examples of short bones are the bones of the wrist and the hindfoot.

Flat bones. These are shaped like curved plates. Examples of flat bones are the bones of the pelvis, the skull bones and the ribs.

Special bones. These are bones that cannot be classified in any of the above categories and have complex shapes, such as the spinal vertebrae.

MACROSCOPIC STRUCTURE OF BONE

The macroscopic structure is the appearance of the bone to the naked eye.

Bones are covered on their outer surface by a layer of dense connective tissue, called the **periosteum** (from the Greek words: *Peri* = around and *osteon* = bone). This layer contains nerves that are involved in the transmission of pain sensation. When pain is felt from a bone, it arises in the periosteum. Stretching the periosteum causes intense pain, hence a complete fracture of a bone can be less painful than a partial fracture, in which the periosteum is constantly under tension.

The periosteum, which is highly developed in children, contains young bone cells, called **osteoblasts**. These cells are responsible for producing new bone tissue as part of growth, and for the repair of bone following a fracture.

Under the periosteum is a layer of very dense, hard bone called **compact bone** (the outer shell of the bone). Underneath this layer there is **spongy bone**. This tissue looks like a sponge, and is made up of bony partitions surrounding many hollow spaces that are filled with bone marrow. This arrangement of a thick, dense outer layer and a spongy inner section creates a strong, yet light, structure.

A flat bone is made up of two layers or plates of compact bone, with spongy bone between them.

The end of a long bone is called the **epiphysis** and the main portion (the shaft) is the **diaphysis** (Fig. 9.2). The portion between them is the **metaphysis**. The diaphysis is a hollow cylinder consisting of a thick compact bone around the periphery, surrounding a space filled with fatty tissue, called the **medullary**

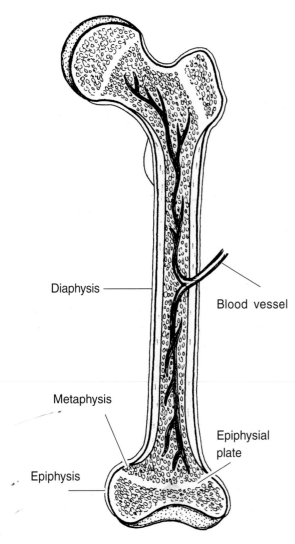

Diaphysis

Blood vessel

Metaphysis

Epiphysial plate

Epiphysis

Figure 9.2 Macroscopic structure of bone.

cavity. The epiphysis and metaphysis consist of a thin compact bone, surrounding spongy bone.

While the long bones are still growing there is a layer of bone-producing cells between the epiphysis and the diaphysis, the **epiphysial plate**. The epiphysial plate continues to produce new bone as long as the bone is growing. At the end of the growth period, the epiphysial plate disappears and growth of the bone ceases. The epiphyseal plates can be seen on an X-ray, and can be used to determine whether a bone still has the potential for growth.

STRUCTURE AND COMPOSITION OF BONE

Bones retain their external shape for years after death but, in fact, the composition of living bone is different from that of dry, dead bone. A living bone is much heavier than a dry bone because it contains many components not present in a dry bone. Living bone contains bone cells, an intercellular substance between the bone cells, and minerals contained within the intercellular substance but which are considered to be a separate component.

Bone cells

Bone cells are called **osteocytes** (from the Greek words *osteon* = bone and *kytos* = cell); they have an elongated body with thin processes coming out of it.

In the compact bone, the cell bodies of the osteocytes are arranged in an orderly fashion, at specific distances from each other. Near the periphery of the bone they are arranged in layers; nearer the center of the bone they are arranged in concentric circles. Between the cell bodies of the osteocytes are the intercellular substance and the cell processes that form connections with each other (Fig. 9.3).

The reason for this orderly arrangement of the cells is related to the relatively poor blood supply in bone. Compared to other tissues, which receive a rich blood supply from a network of capillaries between the cells, the

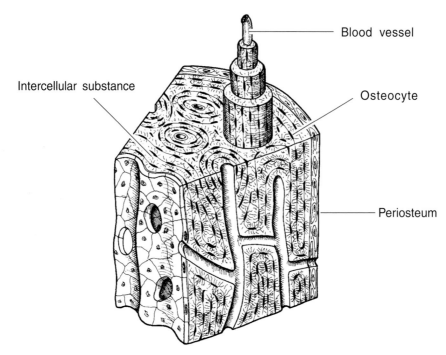

Blood vessel

Intercellular substance

Osteocyte

Periosteum

Figure 9.3   Microscopic structure of compact bone.

blood supply to compact bone tissue is extremely sparse. Within the bone tissue, there are tiny canals that contain blood vessels, and the osteocytes are arranged in concentric circles around those canals. The innermost circle of cells, nearest to the canal that contains the blood vessels, receives its blood supply directly from those blood vessels. However, the cells further away from the central canal receive their oxygen and nutrients via the inner circle by means of the fine processes joining the cells.

The intercellular substance

The intercellular substance is a jelly-like substance that contains protein fibers called **collagen fibers**, which contribute to the bone's strength.

During the development of bone tissue, the young osteocytes, which are close together, produce the intercellular substance. As this substance accumulates, the cells are pushed further and further apart, creating spaces between them. At a certain point, the young cells stop producing intercellular substance and become mature osteocytes surrounded by intercellular substance.

Mature bone is an active, living tissue that is constantly undergoing a process of destruction and rebuilding. The destruction of bone is carried out by special cells called **osteoclasts** (from the Greek words *osteon* = bone and *klastos* = broken). These are phagocytic (devouring) cells that are constantly creating microscopic channels within the bone, like boring a tunnel through rock.

Other special cells, called **osteoblasts** (Greek *osteon* = bone and *blastos* = germ, sprout) enter these channels. Osteoblasts are young osteocytes that can produce intercellular substance. They enter the microscopic channels carved out of the bone by the osteoclasts, produce the intercellular substance that surrounds them and then become mature osteocytes.

The mineral

The mineral of bone is made up of crystals of a molecule containing calcium and phosphorus. Within the human body, there is approximately 1 kg of calcium and 1 kg of phosphorus, most of which is present in the bones. The mineral is present in the intercellular substance, and it is what makes bones rigid. The admixture of the mineral and the intercellular substance creates an extremely strong structure; a bone without mineral becomes soft and weak.

After death, the bone cells and the intercellular substance disappear, and only the mineral is left. A dry (dead) bone is therefore much lighter and weaker than a living bone.

JOINTS

A joint is defined as an area where two different bones are connected to (the medical term is 'articulate with') each other. There are three types of joint:

1. **Fibrous joint**: this is a joint that cannot move. For example, the junctions between the various bones of the skull are fibrous joints. In a fibrous joint, there is connective tissue between the bones, which acts as a sort of glue.

2. **Cartilaginous joint**: this is a joint with a limited degree of movement. For example, the joints between the ribs and the sternum, or the anterior joint between the hip bones, are cartilaginous joints. The bones are connected in this case by **cartilage**, which is actually attached to each of the bones. The slight flexibility of cartilage allows a limited degree of movement at these joints. Cartilage is made up of cartilage cells surrounded by connective tissue, similar to the structure of bone. The major difference between bone and cartilage is that bone contains mineral, which makes it rigid.

3. **Synovial joint**: this type of joint has a wide range of movement, the shoulder or the knee, for example. A synovial joint has a special structure that allows movement between bones with a minimum of friction. The ends of the bones that make up the joint are covered by a layer of cartilage, called **articular cartilage** (articular = related to a joint) (Fig. 9.4). This cartilage is very smooth and the two opposing surfaces of the joint are perfectly matched. Between the two cartilages there is a fluid called **synovial fluid**, which greatly reduces the friction between the two parts of the joint. The articular capsule is composed of two layers. Its delicate inner layer is the **synovial membrane**, which produces the synovial fluid. The fibrous connective tissue of its outer layer, called the **fibrous capsule**, is attached to the bones just beyond the limits of the joint cavity. The synovial membrane acts as a barrier to keep the synovial fluid free of foreign matter or infection, and also keeps it enclosed within the joint.

Ligaments are tough, fibrous bands that are attached to the end of one bone, pass over the

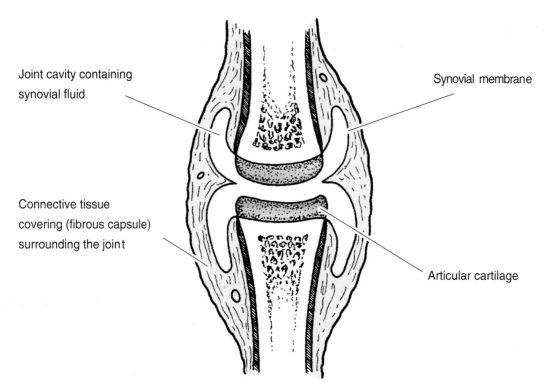

Figure 9.4   Structure of a synovial joint.

joint, and attach to the end of the second bone, to hold the two articular cartilages firmly together. They can be part of their fibrous capsules or separated from them. Ligaments have a certain degree of elasticity, which enables them to stretch and thus allows the joint to move. Like bone and cartilage, ligaments are composed of cells and intercellular substance, although in this case the intercellular substance contains protein fibers, called **elastin** fibers, that are slightly elastic. If the ligaments should tear, the articular cartilage surfaces that make up the joint will separate one from the other. In other words, the joint will dislocate.

There are several types of joint that have a wide range of movement. The actual nature of the movement depends on the shape of the joint and on the stabilization of the ligaments. The elbow joint allows movement in one plane only, like a hinge, whereas the shoulder joint can move in all directions.

SKULL

The skull is made up of a number of bones connected at junctions called **sutures**. These are joints that do not allow any movement between the bones. Between the bones, in the sutures, is connective tissue that acts like a glue. In a dry (dead) skull the jagged, tooth-like shape of the sutures keeps the bones together, but as there is no longer any glue between them, the bones of a dry skull can be pulled apart and separated without much effort.

The one joint in the skull that is the exception to this is the jaw joint, which has a considerable range of movement.

There are a number of holes in the skull (called foramina; singular = foramen), through which nerves and blood vessels pass in and out of the skull. At the base of the skull is the largest foramen, called the **foramen magnum**, through which the spinal cord passes.

The bones of the skull are divided into two groups: the bones of the **face** and the bones of the **cranium**.

The cranium is egg-shaped, which is not just coincidence. An egg is an extremely strong structure, despite having thin walls. The bones of the skull vary in thickness from 2 to 4 mm, yet despite that, the skull is able to withstand strong blows.

Cranial bones

Frontal bone. This bone is the front of the skull. The forehead, the roof of the eye sockets and the front part of the base of the skull are all part of the frontal bone. The portion of the frontal bone above the eyebrows is hollow, forming two air-filled spaces. These are the **frontal sinuses**, which develop at a relatively late age (7–10 years of age).

Parietal bones. These two bones meet in the midline at the top of the skull at a suture called the **sagittal suture** (Fig. 9.5). The parietal bones are connected to the frontal bone in front at a suture called the **coronal suture**.

Occipital bone. This bone forms the back of the skull and also comprises the major portion of the base of the skull. It contains the foramen magnum. In front, it is joined to the parietal bone at the **lambdoid suture**.

Temporal bones. These bones are at the sides of the skull (the temples) (Fig. 9.6). They make up part of the base of the skull and contain the external ear canals as well as the middle and inner ears. The temporal bone has a small projection behind the ear called the **mastoid process**.

Facial bones

Mandible. This is the lower jawbone (Figs 9.6, 9.7 and 9.8). It articulates with the temporal bone at a joint that allows a wide range of movement. This joint (the temporomandibular joint) is a complex synovial joint that allows the lower jaw to open, to close and to move sideways, backwards and forwards.

Maxilla. This is the bone of the upper jaw. It forms part of the orbit (socket) of the eye and part of the hard palate. Within the maxillary bone, underneath the orbits, is a large air space known as the **maxillary sinus**.

Zygomatic bones. These are the cheekbones. They form the lateral wall of the orbit of the eye. From the back of the zygoma, a piece of the bone projects to join up with a projection from the temporal bone, forming the **zygomatic arch**.

Sphenoid bone. This bone has a butterfly shape and forms part of the base of the skull, part of the orbit of the eye and part of the side wall of the cranium in front of the temporal bone (Figs 9.6, 9.7). Within the sphenoid bone is an air space called the **sphenoidal sinus**.

Nasal bones. These are the bones of the nose. Most of the nose is composed of cartilage, and only the base is bone.

Ethmoid bones. These are two small bones in the center of the orbits of the eyes, with air spaces within them – the **ethmoidal sinuses**.

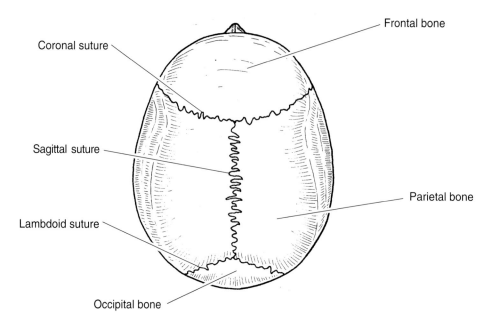

Figure 9.5   View of skull from top.

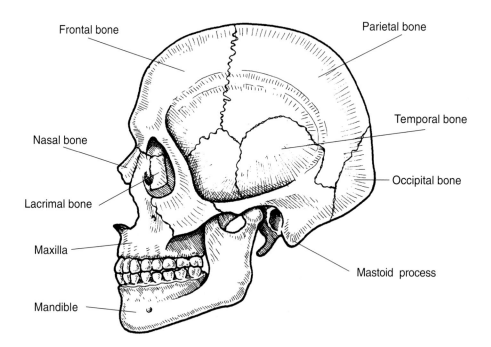

Figure 9.6   Lateral view of skull.

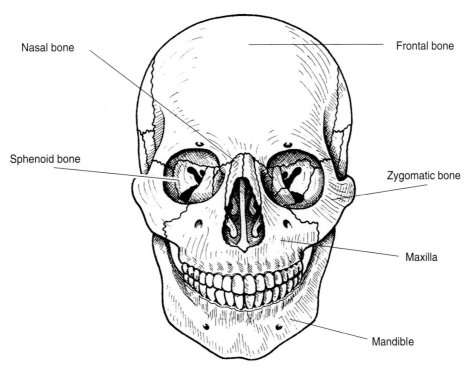

Figure 9.7   Anterior view of skull.

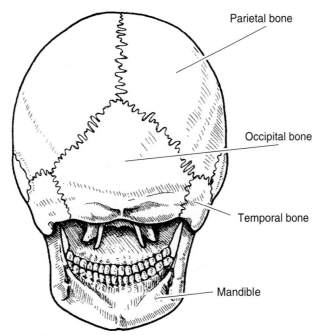

Figure 9.8   Posterior view of skull.

Vomer bone. This small bone forms the bony part of the nasal septum (the 'wall' that divides the nose into left and right halves).

Orbit. This is the eye socket. It is cone-shaped and made up of the following bones: the frontal bone in its roof, the zygomatic bone at its (outer) side wall, the maxillary bone in its floor and inner wall, the ethmoid and lacrimal bones in its inner wall, and the sphenoid bone at the rear (the apex of the cone).

SPINAL COLUMN (SPINE)

The spinal column is a flexible structure made up of 33 vertebrae (Figs 9.9 and 9.10). It is the central axis of the body and protects the spinal cord that passes through its center.

The spine has to support considerable weight for long periods of time and, in the Western world, 80% of the population suffer from backache (mainly the lower back) at some point in their lives.

The spine has natural curves in the coronal plane (i.e. it curves in a fore-and-aft direction, but not sideways) which enable it to function as a shock absorber, like a spring. The forward curvature in the region of the abdomen and a backward curvature at the chest level give the spine an S shape. An excessive backward curve at the chest level is called **kyphosis** and is seen mainly in the elderly as a result of degenerative changes in the spinal column. An exaggerated forward curvature at the abdominal level is called **lordosis**. Mild lordosis is normal in pregnant women and in children between 2 and 3 years of age. A sideways curvature of the spine is called **scoliosis**. As the spine normally has no lateral curves, any such curvature is pathological. It occurs primarily in adolescents, particularly females.

The vertebrae

The vertebrae are numbered from top to bottom. There are 7 vertebrae in the neck, called the **cervical** vertebrae, numbered C1–C7 (Fig. 9.10) 12 vertebrae in the chest region, called the **thoracic** vertebrae, numbered T1–12;

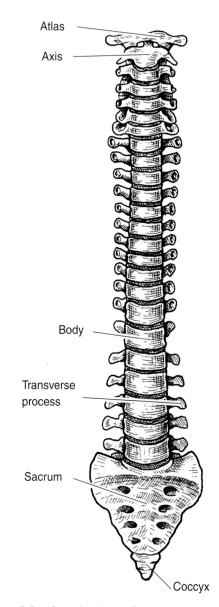

Figure 9.9   Anterior view of spine.

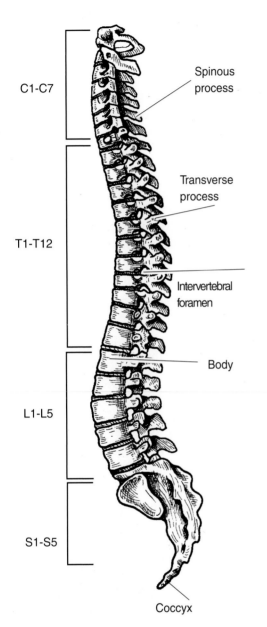

C1-C7

Spinous process

T1-T12

Transverse process

Intervertebral foramen

Body

L1-L5

S1-S5

Coccyx

Figure 9.10   Lateral view of spine.

and 5 vertebrae in the lower back, called the **lumbar** vertebrae, L1–L5. The **sacrum** is made up of 5 vertebrae (S1–S5) that have fused into one bone. The tail bone is called the **coccyx**, which is made up of 4 tiny vertebrae (Fig. 9.10).

The vertebrae all have the same basic structure, except for the first two cervical vertebrae, which have a unique shape.

Each vertebra consists of a **body** and an **arch** arising from it (Fig. 9.11). The arch and body form a round opening called the **vertebral foramen**, through which the spinal cord runs. There are projections arising from the arch: the **spinous process**, or spine, arises from the back, and there are **transverse processes** at the sides. Two projections pointing upwards are called the **superior articular processes**, and two other downward-pointing projections are called the **inferior articular processes** (see Fig. 9.14).

The first cervical vertebra is called the **atlas** (Fig. 9.12). It is ring-shaped (it lacks a body) and is connected to the occipital bone of the skull at the atlanto-occipital joint.

The second cervical vertebra is called the **axis** and is made up of a small vertebral body, an arch and one process arising from the body, pointing upwards, called the **dens**. This process passes upwards through the arch of the atlas, with which it articulates, and functions as an axle around which the atlas can rotate.

The cervical vertebrae have small bodies because they do not have to support much weight. On the other hand, the vertebral foramen is quite large, to accomodate the relatively thick spinal cord at that level. The thoracic vertebrae have larger bodies because they support more weight, and their spines point downward. The lumbar vertebrae have even thicker bodies because they have to support even more weight, and they have short, straight spines.

The only parts of the vertebrae that can be felt through the skin are the spines that point backwards. If the neck is bent forward, the first

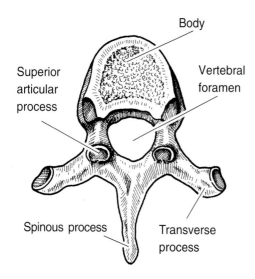

Body

Superior articular process

Vertebral foramen

Spinous process

Transverse process

Figure 9.11   Structure of a vertebra.

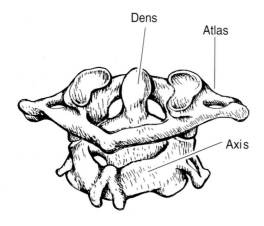

Dens

Atlas

Axis

Figure 9.12   The atlas and axis.

and most obvious protrusion that can be seen (and felt) at the back of the neck is usually the spine of C7. The transverse processes cannot be felt because they are covered by a thick layer of muscle. In very thin people, it is sometimes possible to feel the bodies of the lumbar vertebrae through the abdomen.

Intervertebral joints

The joints between vertebrae are unique, and are of two types. The combination of the two types of joint provides the spine with its flexibility and enables it to function as a shock absorber.

Between every two vertebral bodies is an **intervertebral disc** (Figs 9.13 and 9.14). This is a cartilaginous joint with limited movement. The disc is made up of a fibrous ring, called the **annulus fibrosus** around the perimeter and the center is filled with a gelatinous substance called the **nucleus pulposus**.

The intervertebral disc is a very sophisticated shock absorber. The body weight presses on the vertebral bodies and they, in turn, press on the discs. The gel in the center of the disc is compressed and absorbs the pressure. The fibrous ring ensures that the gel stays in place. If it is torn or damaged the gel can escape – a not uncommon occurrence referred to as a 'slipped disc'.

There are also synovial joints between the vertebrae. These allow some range of movement. As is the case with all synovial joints, these joints also contain articular cartilage, synovial fluid and ligaments. They lie between the

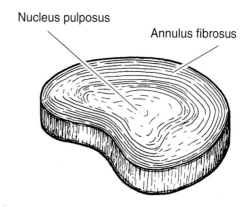

Nucleus pulposus

Annulus fibrosus

Figure 9.13   Intervertebral disc.

superior articular process of one vertebra and the inferior articular processes of the vertebra directly above it (Fig. 9.14). When the vertebrae are connected in this way, between every two vertebrae is an opening at the sides called the **intervertebral foramen** (see Fig. 9.14). These foramina allow the passage of the nerves that emerge from the spinal cord to all parts of the body.

Each intervertebral synovial joint is reinforced by ligaments. There are also large, thick, tough ligaments that run along the entire length of the spinal column and reinforce it. Along the anterior surface of the vertebral column is the **anterior longitudinal ligament**. The supraspinous ligament runs along the entire spinal column between the spines of the vertebrae.

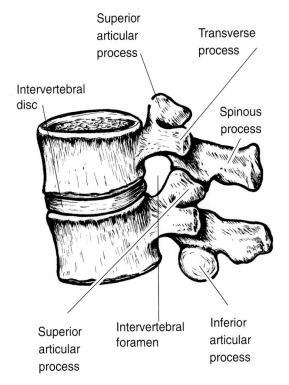

Figure 9.14   The intervertebral joints.

CHEST

The **thoracic cage** (Fig. 9.15) is made up of the **sternum** (breastbone) and **costal** (rib) **cartilages** anteriorly, the **ribs** laterally and posteriorly, and the **spinal column** at the back.

The thoracic cage protects the organs within the chest and two abdominal organs (the liver and spleen) and is essential for the act of breathing.

The **sternum** is made up of three parts: the upper part called the **manubrium**, a central part called the **body** and a sharp projection at the lower end, called the **xiphoid**, which is made of cartilage rather than bone. Between the manubrium and the body is a protrusion that can usually be felt in the front of the chest; this is the **sternal angle**. The second costal cartilage joins the sternum exactly at this point. (The sternal angle has no special significance but it is an easily felt and useful landmark in the chest for the position of the second rib.)

The **ribs** are flat bones. There are 12 pairs of ribs, all of which are connected by synovial joints to the spine at the back. The first 10 ribs are also connected to the sternum via the costal cartilages in front. Those joints do have limited movement, which allows the thoracic cavity to change its volume during breathing. The lower edge of the **costal cartilages** (the bottom of the rib cage) can be felt quite easily and is known as the **costal margin**.

Ribs 11 and 12 are not connected to the sternum in front and are therefore the **floating ribs**. The ends of these ribs can sometimes be felt.

UPPER LIMB GIRDLE

The **clavicle** (collarbone) is connected to the sternum medially and to the scapula (shoulder

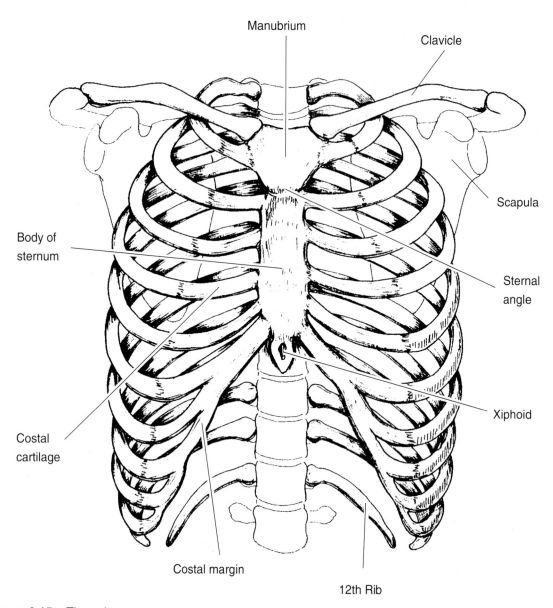

Figure 9.15   Thoracic cage.

blade) laterally. At the top end of the sternum, between the ends of the two clavicles, is a depression called the **suprasternal notch**. The trachea can be felt through the suprasternal notch, and pressing on the notch usually causes the person to cough.

The **scapula** (shoulder blade) is a flat, triangular bone that lies over the ribs at the upper part of the back of the chest (Figs 9.16 and 9.17). It is connected to the clavicle and to the humerus (upper arm bone), but not to the ribs.

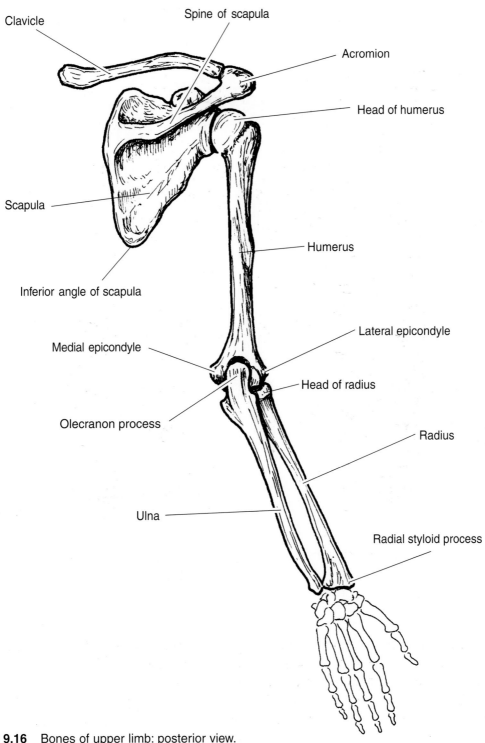

Figure 9.16   Bones of upper limb: posterior view.

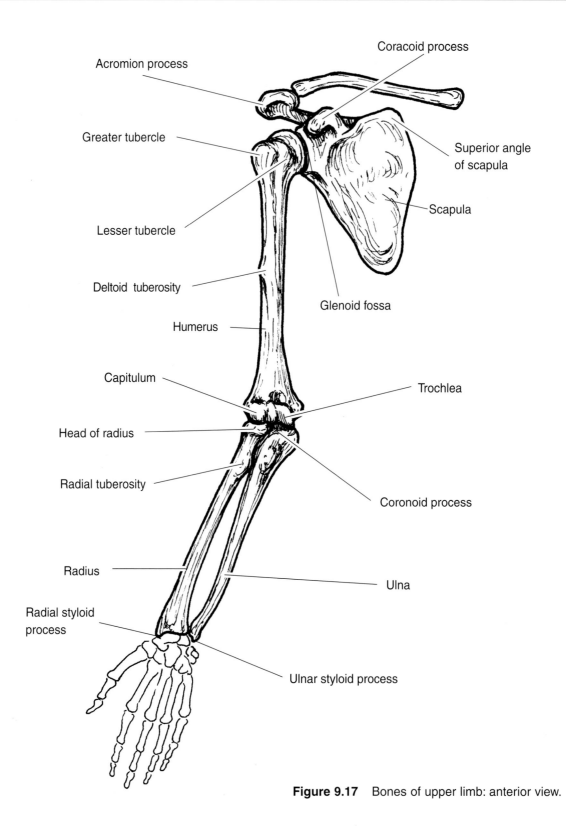

Figure 9.17   Bones of upper limb: anterior view.

The scapula is held in position by strong muscles that can move it in all directions. As the humerus is connected to the scapula, any movement of the shoulder also moves the upper limb, which contributes to the extraordinary variety of movement of the upper arm.

The lower angle of the scapula (the **inferior angle of the scapula**) is at the level of the T7 vertebra; its upper angle (the **superior angle of the scapula**) is at its medial side.

At the lateral side of the scapula is a cartilage-covered socket called the **glenoid fossa**, which articulates with the humerus.

There is a shelf-like ridge projecting out from the back of the scapula, and which can be felt through the skin, called the **spine of the scapula**. At its lateral end this spine ends in a protrusion called the **acromion process**, which articulates with the clavicle. There is another protrusion from the superolateral side of the scapula, which points anteriorly. This is the **coracoid process**, and is a point of attachment for muscles.

Humerus

The bone of the upper arm is the **humerus**. At its proximal end is a rounded portion covered by a layer of cartilage, called the **head of the humerus**, which articulates with the glenoid cavity of the scapula to form the shoulder joint. Just below the head are two prominences – the **greater tubercle** on the lateral side and the **lesser tubercle** on the anterior side. These prominences form attachment points for muscles. In the middle of the bone, anteriorly, there is another prominence, called the **deltoid tuberosity**, to which the deltoid muscle is attached.

There are two prominences at the distal end of the humerus: the **medial epicondyle** medi-ally, and the **lateral epicondyle** laterally. These can both be felt quite easily.

Also at the distal end of the humerus are anatomic structures covered with a layer of cartilage, which articulate with the bones of the forearm – the **capitulum**, which articulates with the radius, and the **trochlea,** which articulates with the ulna.

Forearm bones

The lateral forearm bone is called the **radius**. This articulates with the humerus, with the medial forearm bone and with the wrist bones. At its proximal end is a rounded portion covered by articular cartilage, called the **head of the radius**, which articulates with the humerus to form the elbow joint.

Just below the head of the radius is a projection called the **radial tuberosity**, which is a point of attachment for the biceps muscle. At the distal end is a projection laterally called the **radial styloid process**, which can be felt.

The medial forearm bone is called the **ulna** and articulates with the humerus and with the radius. The ulna has no articulation at the wrist joint.

At its proximal end is a projection anteriorly, called the **coronoid process**, and a posterior projection felt at the back of the elbow, called the **olecranon process**.

The proximal end of the ulna articulates with the humerus to form a joint that functions like a door hinge. This type of joint allows movement in one plane only – flexion and extension of the elbow. At the distal end of the ulna is also a projection called the **ulnar styloid process**.

The proximal end of the ulna articulates with the head of the radius at the elbow and the distal end of the ulna articulates with the distal end of the radius at the level of the wrist.

Between the shafts of the radius and ulna there is a ligament (the interosseous membrane) that joins them together firmly.

The radius can perform unique rotational movements called **supination** (turning the palm of the hand up) and **pronation** (turning the palm of the hand down). To carry out those movements, the head of the radius rotates on its axis, while its distal end 'climbs' around the distal end of the ulna (see Fig. 9.35).

Bones of the wrist and hand

There are eight bones in the wrist, called the **carpal bones**. These are all short bones and are connected to each other, to the radius and to the bones of the hand by many small joints.

The pea-shaped **pisiform bone** (from the Latin *pisum* = pea and *forma* = appearance) is one of the wrist bones on the medial side of the wrist (Fig. 9.18); it can be felt through the skin.

There are five bones in the hand itself (the palm), known as the **metacarpal bones**. They articulate at their proximal ends with the carpal bones and at their distal ends with the bones of the fingers.

The finger bones are called **phalanges** (singular = phalanx). In every finger, apart from the thumb there are three phalanges – a proximal phalanx, a middle phalanx and a

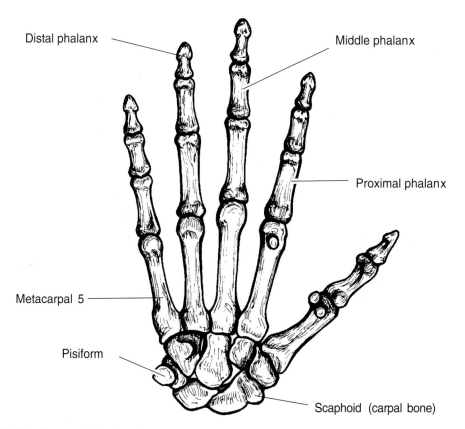

Distal phalanx

Middle phalanx

Proximal phalanx

Metacarpal 5

Pisiform

Scaphoid (carpal bone)

Figure 9.18   Bones of the hand.

distal phalanx. The thumb has only two phalanges.

LOWER LIMB GIRDLE

Pelvis

This is a funnel-shaped structure, and is made up of three bones – the **sacrum** posteriorly, and two other bones called the **hip bones**. The joint between the sacrum and the hip bones is a synovial joint that allows little movement. In a pregnant woman, towards the end of the pregnancy, certain substances are secreted that increase the range of motion of that joint, allowing the pelvis to stretch a little to help the infant pass through. The two hip bones are joined by a cartilaginous joint called the **symphysis pubis**, which allows a limited amount of movement (Fig. 9.19).

Each hip bone is composed of three bones that have fused together into one: the **ischium** at the lower (inferior) part of the hip, the **pubis** anteriorly and the **ilium** superiorly (Fig. 9.20 and 9.21). Although the bones were originally formed separately, they are now fused together at an imaginary joint in the area of a socket at the lateral side of the pelvis, the **acetabulum**. The inner surface of the acetabulum is covered by a layer of articular cartilage, which forms part of the hip joint.

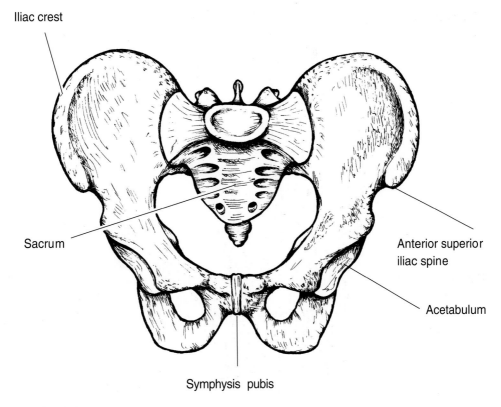

Iliac crest

Sacrum

Anterior superior iliac spine

Acetabulum

Symphysis pubis

Figure 9.19 Pelvic bones.

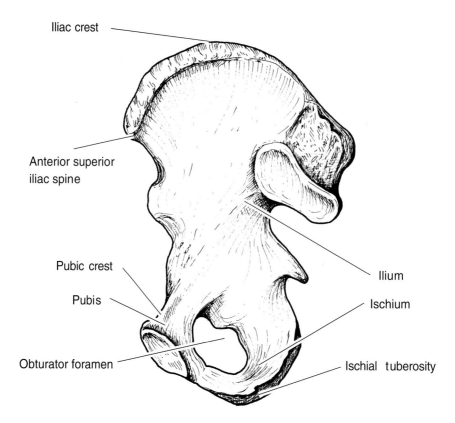

Iliac crest

Anterior superior
iliac spine

Pubic crest

Pubis

Obturator foramen

Ilium

Ischium

Ischial tuberosity

Figure 9.20 Hip bone: medial view.

The iliac bone has a ridge along its upper edge, the **iliac crest**, which is the bony hip that can be easily felt along its entire length. At the anterior end of this ridge is a small protrusion that can be felt through the skin, the **anterior superior iliac spine**.

The pubic bones form a bony ridge anteriorly, which can be felt, called the **pubic crest**. The ischium also has a fairly large protrusion (the **ischial tuberosity**), which can be felt through the skin and which serves as a point of attachment for muscles. (These are the parts of the pelvis that are sore after riding a bicycle!) At the inferior part of the pelvis is a large opening called the **obturator foramen**,

through which pass nerves and blood vessels. The presence of the foramen lessens the overall weight of the pelvis.

Thigh

The thigh bone is called the **femur**, and it is the largest bone in the body. There is a very close correlation between the length of the femur and a person's height. In forensic medicine, this fact is often helpful in identifying the skeleton of a missing person. The length of the femur of a fetus can be measured by ultrasound to determine its gestational age and growth.

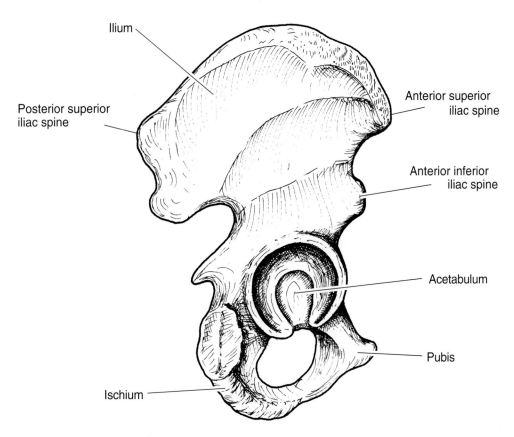

Ilium

Posterior superior
iliac spine

Anterior superior
iliac spine

Anterior inferior
iliac spine

Acetabulum

Pubis

Ischium

Figure 9.21   Hip bone: lateral view.

The femur has a **head,** which is covered by articular cartilage and is part of the hip joint (Figs 9.22 and 9.23). The covering cartilage corresponds precisely to the cartilage lining of the acetabulum of the pelvis (a ball and socket joint). This enables movement in all planes.

Below the head of the femur is the **neck of the femur,** at the base of which there are two protuberances. The larger is called the **greater trochanter,** which points laterally, and the smaller is called the **lesser trochanter,** directed medially. These two bony projections are points for muscle attachments.

The angle between the neck of the femur and the shaft (135 degrees) is an anatomically

weak point. As the body weight presses down on the head of the femur, considerable leverage is exerted on the base of the neck of the femur. For example, when someone lands on their feet from a jump, a force of hundreds of kilograms may be exerted at that point.

A roughened ridge called the **linea aspera** runs along the posterior surface of the shaft of the femur and serves as an area for muscle attachment. At the lower end of the femur are two large projections: the **medial condyle** and the **lateral condyle.** The ends of these condyles are covered by a layer of articular cartilage and form the upper part of the knee joint. The anterior surfaces of the condyles are also

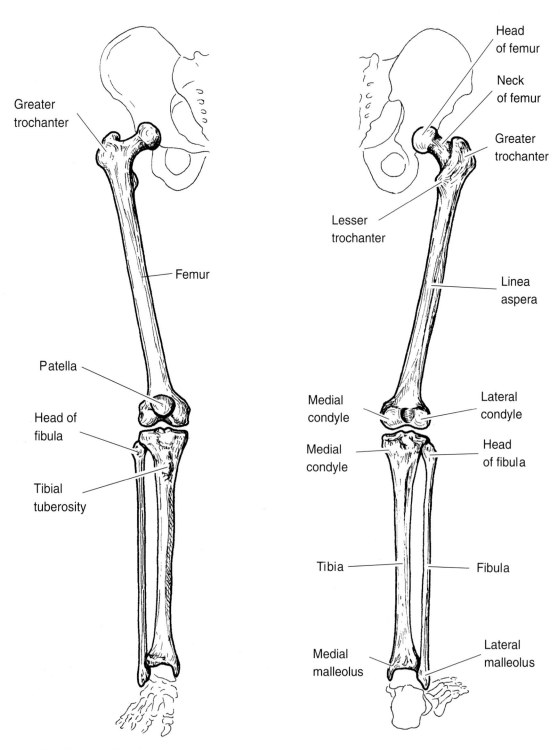

Figure 9.22   Bones of lower limb: anterior view.

Figure 9.23   Bones of lower limb: posterior view.

covered by cartilage, and articulate with the bone known as the **patella** (the kneecap). The patella plays an important part in the function of the thigh muscles.

Bones of the leg

There are two long bones in the leg. The larger is called the **tibia** which articulates with the femur above, with the other bone of the leg (the fibula), and with the talus bone at the ankle.

There are two protuberances at the upper end of the tibia: the **medial condyle** and the **lateral condyle**.

At the upper end of the tibia, on its anterior surface, is a prominence called the **tibial tuberosity**, to which the major thigh muscle is attached. The medial surface of the shaft of the tibia lies directly under the skin and can be felt along its entire length. This is the 'shinbone' and, because it is not covered by muscle but only by skin, when it is injured it is quite painful. At the lower end, on the medial side of the tibia, is a prominence called the **medial malleolus** (see Fig. 9.23).

The smaller of the two leg bones is the **fibula**. At its proximal end is the **head**, which articulates with the tibia and which can be felt at the lateral side of the knee, toward the back. At the distal end is a prominence called the **lateral malleolus** (see Fig. 9.23). The distal surface of the tibia, the inner surface of the medical malleolus and the inner surface of the lateral molleolus are covered by a layer of cartilage and articulate with the talus to form the ankle joint (Fig. 9.25). The tibia and fibula are joined together tightly by a tough ligament along their length.

Foot bones

The basic structure of the foot is similar to that of the hand; the differences arise from their different functions. In animals that walk on four limbs, the task of both the forelimbs and the

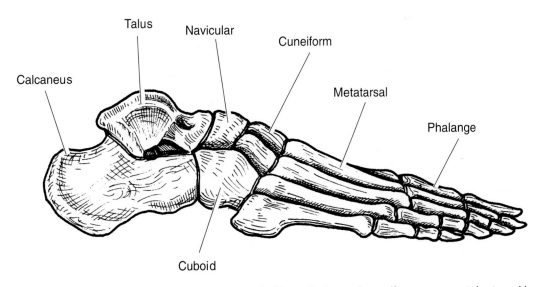

Figure 9.24   Bones of the foot. Calcaneus, talus, cuboid, navicular and cuneiform represent the tarsal bones.

hindlimbs is to bear the weight of the body. In the process of evolution, animals progressed gradually to walking on two limbs – on what used to be the hindlimbs, which bear the weight of the body – and the forelimbs became available for carrying out more complex tasks.

There are seven **tarsal bones** in the hindfoot and midfoot (Figs 9.24 and 9.25). The **talus** is the bone that articulates with the tibia and fibula to create the ankle joint (Fig. 9.25). This joint is capable of movement in one plane only, like a door hinge.

The heelbone is called the **calcaneus** and the protrusion at the back of the heel, the **calcaneal tuberosity**, can be easily felt. This prominence is the point of attachment of the Achilles tendon. The other tarsal bones are called the **cuboid**, the **navicular**, and the three **cuneiform bones**. The bones of the sole of the foot are called the **metatarsal bones**, and the bones of the toes are called **phalanges**, just as are the bones of the fingers.

The foot has to bear enormous weight, up to hundreds of kilograms when jumping, for example, and it also has to be able to carry lesser weights but for prolonged periods of time. This requires the structure of the foot to be extremely strong. Furthermore, the foot has to adapt its shape, to some extent, to its undersurface and thus must have considerable flexibility in addition to strength. This requirement for flexibility combined with strength seems quite daunting, but the foot meets it superbly. Foot pain is much less common than back pain.

The 'secret' of the foot's success lies in the principle of the **arch**. The arch is a structure that provides strength and flexibility, as well as excellent shock absorption. The foot has two arches – a medial arch, which is high, and a shallower lateral arch (Fig. 9.26).

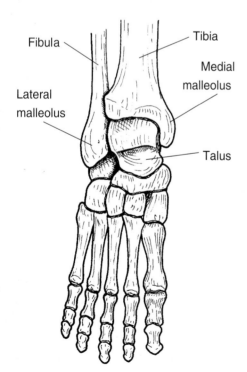

Figure 9.25　Ankle.

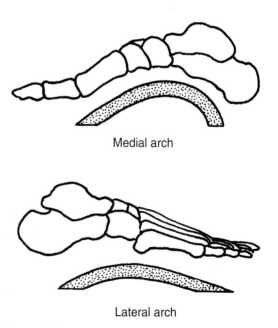

Medial arch

Lateral arch

Figure 9.26　Arches of the foot.

Most of the weight of the body is applied to three points:

1. the bottom of the calcaneus bone
2. the distal end of the first metatarsal bone
3. the distal end of the fifth metatarsal bone.

Points 1 and 2 form the high medial arch, while points 1 and 3 form the shallower lateral arch.

The shapes of the arches of the foot are maintained by a series of ligaments and tendons (bridge building makes use of similar supportive techniques). For example, the ligament known as the plantar fascia under the metatarsals is attached to the calcaneus and to the phalanges, and prevents the arch from collapsing.

MUSCLES

Muscle tissue is made up of fibers that have the ability to contract (contractile fibers).

Skeletal muscles. These are voluntary muscles that are activated by a conscious 'command' from the brain.

Cardiac muscle. This is a unique type of muscle found only in the heart. Its basic structure is similar to that of skeletal muscle but it is not activated voluntarily and it works non-stop from the fourth gestational week in the embryo until death.

Smooth muscles. These muscles are found mainly in the walls of 'tubes' in the body, such as in blood vessels, the digestive tract, the urinary system and the respiratory tree. Their contraction is involuntary and is part of the overall function of internal organs.

Structure of skeletal muscle

The entire muscle is enclosed in a tough layer of connective tissue. When this covering is removed, the muscle can be seen to be made up of bundles called **muscle fasciculi** (Fig. 9.27). Each fasciculus is a bundle of microscopic **muscle fibers**. Each microscopic fiber is a single cell, which can be up to 30 centimeters long and between 10 and 100 microns wide (a micron is a thousandth of a millimeter). Under the microscope, each muscle cell (or fiber) can be seen to contain a series of transverse stripes across its width. Because of these stripes, skeletal muscles are also known as **striated** (striped) **muscles**.

Within each muscle fiber are many tiny fibers called **myofibrils**. These contain protein filaments that contract and shorten, and it is the orderly, regular arrangement of these protein filaments that produces the striations visible under the microscope. There are two types of protein filament, **actin** and **myosin**.

The number of muscle cells does not change during a person's lifetime. Muscle building and exercise make the existing muscle fibers thicker and wider by increasing the amount of contractile protein in each cell. In people who stop exercising or reduce their food intake, the muscles become wasted and thin because of a decrease in the number of protein filaments but there is no decrease in the overall number of muscle cells.

A muscle is attached to a bone at a point called its **origin**. It then passes over one or more joints and finally attaches to another bone at a point called its **insertion** (Fig. 9.28). The body of the muscle itself is called the **belly**. In general, the origin of a muscle is nearer the center of the body, where the muscle

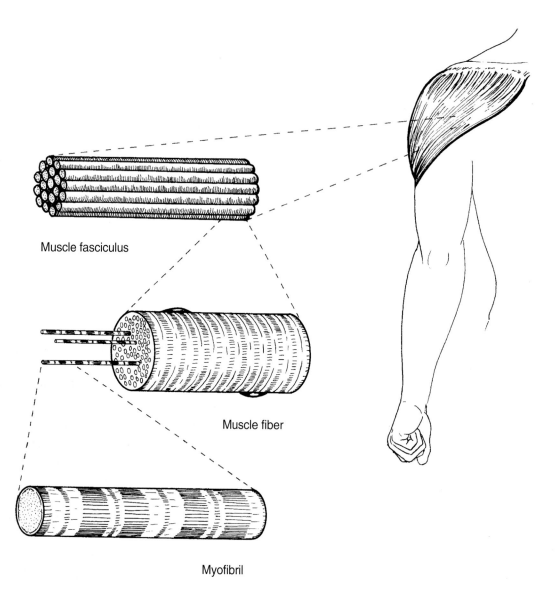

Muscle fasciculus

Muscle fiber

Myofibril

Figure 9.27 Structure of muscle.

is attached directly to the bony surface. Its insertion is generally further away from the center of the body and the muscle is often attached to a bone via a structure called a **tendon**.

A tendon is a piece of connective tissue that joins a muscle to a bone. Unlike a muscle, it cannot contract or shorten. When the muscle contracts, it pulls on its tendon (which is attached to a bone) and, because the muscle passes across a joint, the joint moves when the muscle shortens.

Every joint has several muscles that move it in different directions. The more movements

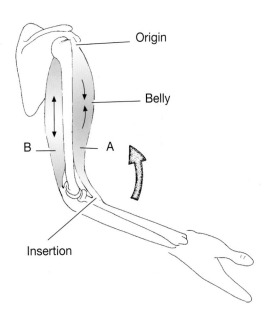

Figure 9.28 Principle of muscular action in joint movements. During flexion of the elbow muscle, **A** is the agonist and muscle **B** the antagonist.

that a joint can make, the more complex is the muscle system involved.

When considering a specific movement, such as flexing the elbow, the muscles that cause the flexion are defined as the **agonist muscles** (prime movers) for flexion of the elbow. These muscles contract and shorten in order to flex the elbow. At the same time as these muscle contract, however, the muscles that normally extend (straighten) the elbow must relax and lengthen to allow the movement. These latter are called the **antagonist muscles** for elbow flexion (see Fig. 9.28).

Some movements, such as flexing the wrist, require several muscles to contract (the agonist muscles for that movement) and, simultaneously, other muscles must relax (the antagonist muscles for wrist flexion).

Fixator muscles steady the proximal parts of the limb (e.g. the arm) while movements are occurring in distal parts (e.g. the hand). If an agonist muscle passes more than one joint and the movement involves only the distal joint, other muscles, called **synergist muscles**, come into play and prevent the proximal joints from moving. For example, in closing the fist, the tendons of the agonist muscles that flex the fingers pass in front of the wrist joint. To stabilize the wrist and prevent its flexion while the fingers are flexed, the extensors of the wrist (i.e. the synergist muscles) must contract simultaneously.

Activation of a muscle

Muscles are activated by the nervous system. Every muscle is innervated by nerves called motor nerves. Each motor nerve has many **axons** which enter the muscle and form **synapses** (junctions) with the individual muscle cells. An action potential (see p. 203) moves down the axon and reaches the muscle fibers, causing them to contract. As a muscle fiber contracts, it uses up energy. Those muscle cells that are innervated by a single axon are called a **motor unit** (Fig. 9.29).

All of the muscle fibers in a motor unit contract simultaneously. The smaller a motor unit (i.e. the fewer muscle cells that are innervated by a single axon), the more precise and delicate will be its action. The smallest motor units are in the muscles that move the eyeball (each axon innervates only a few muscle cells). In contrast, the muscles of the back have very large motor units, with each axon innervating hundreds of muscle cells.

The brain can control the strength of a muscle contraction by controlling the number of motor units that it activates. When a muscle contracts weakly, only a fraction of its motor

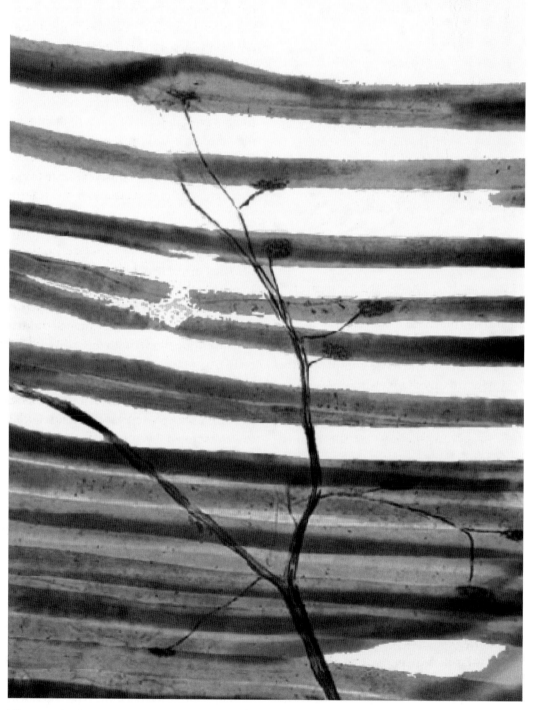

Micrograph showing branching of a small nerve innervating muscle fibers.

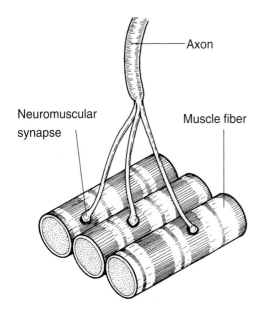

Axon

Neuromuscular synapse

Muscle fiber

Figure 9.29 A motor unit. This illustration shows the end of an axon (part of a neuron) innervating three muscle fibers.

units is activated. When it contracts maximally, all of its motor units are activated.

When a joint is moved passively, the length of the muscles alters but the contractile proteins are not activated and no energy is expended.

If a muscle is cut off from its motor nerves, it very rapidly (within weeks) becomes thin and weak (a process called **atrophy**), for reasons that are not clear.

In addition to the motor nerves that activate the muscle, there are tiny organs within muscle, called **muscle spindles**, that are connected to the endings of sensory nerves, which continuously transmit information to the brain regarding the current status of the muscle fibers (their degree of tension, length, etc.). There are similar nerves in tendons and joints, which transmit information to the brain continuously regarding the position, tension, etc. of those structures.

Even when muscles are at rest, a certain amount of tension usually remains. This tension is required for maintenance of posture (e.g. sitting on a chair) and is called **muscle tone**. Skeletal muscle tone is produced by a low rate of nerve impulses from the spinal cord.

MOVEMENTS

Movement is basically a change in the position of a joint. Every joint is able to carry out certain movements, depending on its anatomical shape and structure.

For example, the shoulder joint, which comprises the rounded head of the humerus and the surface of the scapula (the glenoid fossa), is capable of many movements in multiple planes. The very fact of its having such a wide range of movements makes the shoulder joint somewhat unstable, and it can be dislocated relatively easily.

On the other hand, the elbow joint allows movement in only one plane, like a door hinge, and is therefore quite a stable joint, with dislocation being less common (Fig. 9.30).

The movements of **flexion** and **extension** occur in the sagittal plane. It can be said that, in general, when flexion occurs at a joint, the body tends to take a fetal position (Fig. 9.31). The opposite movement, extension, results in the body looking like a long-jumper in mid-air, with all the limbs straightened. (Fig. 9.32).

The movements of **abduction** and **adduction** take place in the coronal plane. When a limb is abducted, it moves away from the central axis of the body, and adduction occurs when a limb is brought toward the central axis of the body (Fig. 9.33)

The movements of **external rotation** and **internal rotation** take place around an axis.

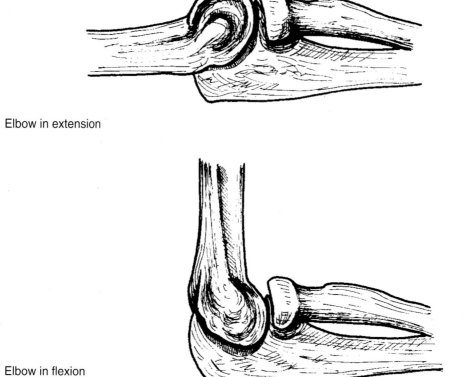

Elbow in extension

Elbow in flexion

Figure 9.30   Movement of the elbow. The structure of this joint allows movement in only one plane.

External rotation is rotation outwards from the midline of the body, and internal rotation is rotation inward toward the midline of the body (Fig. 9.34).

Only the radius can carry out the movements of **supination** and **pronation**. Supination is the movement of turning the palm of the hand upwards, while pronation is the movement of turning the palm of the hand downward (Fig. 9.35).

Inversion and **eversion** refer to movements of the foot (not the ankle). Inversion occurs when the sole of the foot is turned inward, towards the midline of the body, while ever-

sion is the reverse – the sole of the foot is turned outward (Fig 9.36).

The movements of **plantarflexion** and **dorsiflexion** occur at the ankle. Dorsiflexion occurs when the angle between the top (dorsum) of the foot and the leg is decreased (bending the foot up toward the shin), while plantarflexion is the reverse movement – increasing the angle between the dorsum of the foot and the leg (bending the foot down, away from the shin) (Fig 9.37).

Circumduction is a combination of successive movements of flexion, abduction, extension and adduction in such a way that the distal

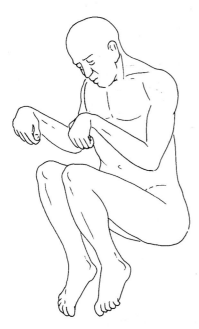

Figure 9.31   Flexion results in the body adopting the position shown.

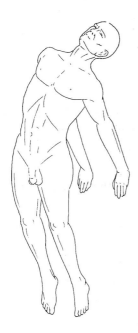

Figure 9.32   Extension results in the body adopting the position shown.

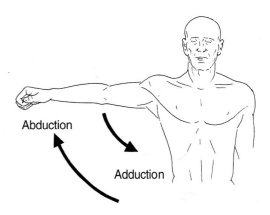

Abduction

Adduction

Figure 9.33   The movements of abduction and adduction.

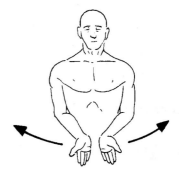

External rotation

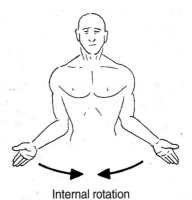

Internal rotation

Figure 9.34   The movements of external rotation and internal rotation.

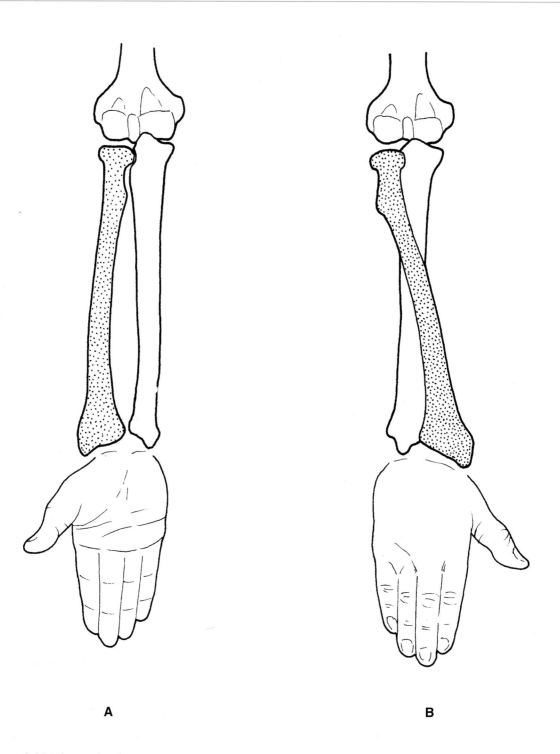

A

B

Figure 9.35 In moving from position **A** to position **B** the forearm is carrying out pronation. In moving from position **B** to position **A** it is carrying out supination.

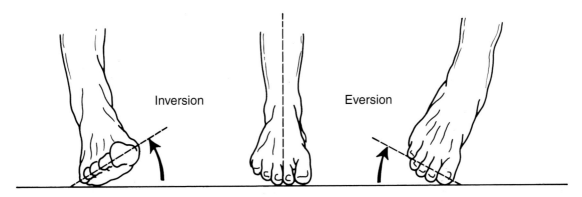

Figure 9.36   Inversion and eversion.

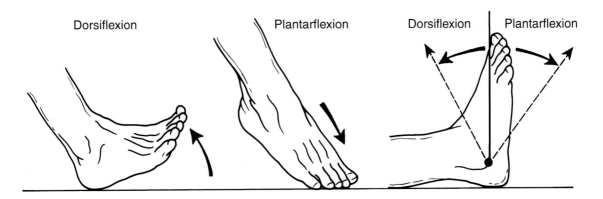

Figure 9.37   Dorsiflexion and plantarflexion.

end forms a circle. It can occur in the shoulder, hip and the wrist (Fig. 9.38).

MUSCLES OF THE BACK

Trapezius (Fig. 9.39)

Origin.   From the posterior portion of the skull and the spines of vertebrae C1–T12.

Insertion.   Into the lateral third of the clavicle, the acromion process and the spine of the scapula.

Innervation.   Accessory nerve.

Action.   The upper fibers raise the scapula, the middle fibers bring the scapula nearer to the spinal column, and the lower fibers lower the scapula.

Latissimus dorsi (Fig. 9.39)

Origin.   From the posterior portion of the iliac crest, the spines of vertebrae L5–T7 and from the lower 3 or 4 ribs.

Insertion.   To the anterosuperior part of the humerus.

Innervation.   Thoracodorsal nerve.

Action.   This very large muscle arises from the back and inserts into the arm, hence moving the shoulder joint. The muscle takes part in extension, adduction and medial rotation of the

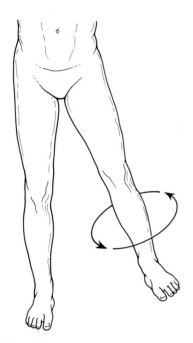

Figure 9.38   Circumduction.

shoulder. Monkeys use the latissimus dorsi muscle when climbing trees but it is not used extensively in humans, so it cannot usually be seen. Development of this muscle produces the triangle of chest muscle seen in body builders.

Rhomboids (Fig 9.39)

Origin.   From the spines of vertebrae C6–T5.
Insertion.   The medial border of the scapula.
Innervation.   Dorsal scapular nerve.
Action.   Brings the scapula closer to the spine.

Levator scapula (Fig.9.39)

Origin.   From the transverse processes of C1–C4.

Insertion.   To the superomedial border of the scapula.
Innervation.   Dorsal scapular nerve
Action.   Raises the scapula and pulls it medially.

Deep back muscles

This large, interwoven group of muscles creates a thick band that fills the spaces between the spines and the transverse processes of the vertebrae (Fig. 9.40). Each muscle in this group has its own origin and insertion. In some of the muscles, the fibers are arranged parallel to the spinal column, while in others they run at an angle to the spine. The muscles are attached to various anatomic structures, such as the spines and transverse processes of the vertebrae and the ribs.

The deep back muscles are very important in maintaining the normal curvatures of the spine. When they contract, they produce extension of the spinal column (straightening of the back).

Quadratus lumborum (see Fig. 9.58)

Origin.   From the posterior portion of the iliac crest, and the transverse processes of L1–L5.
Insertion.   Into the lower border of the 12th rib.
Innervation.   Lumbar plexus.
Action.   Bending the spinal column sideways (a movement called lateral flexion).

Layers of the back muscles

The most superficial muscles are under the skin of the back – the trapezius and latissimus

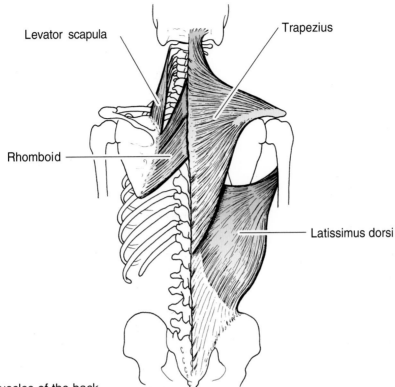

Figure 9.39   Muscles of the back..

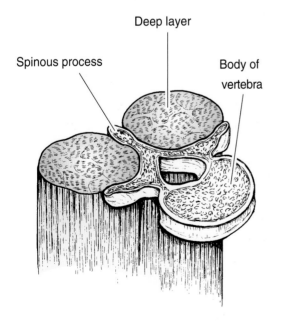

Figure 9.40   Deep muscles of the back.

dorsi (the upper part of which is covered by the trapezius). Next are the rhomboids and the deep layer of back muscles. The rhomboids are superficial to the deep muscle layer. The quadratus lumborum lies underneath the deep muscles and, in effect, forms part of the posterior wall of the abdomen.

MUSCLES OF THE CHEST AND ABDOMEN

Pectoralis major (Fig. 9.41)

Origin.   From the medial two-thirds of the clavicle and the sternum.

Insertion.   To the anterosuperior part of the humerus.

Innervation.   Pectoral nerve.

Action.   Adduction, extension and internal rotation of the shoulder. This muscle is well developed in monkeys, who use it in climbing trees.

Pectoralis minor

This muscle lies underneath pectoralis major.

Origin.   From the anterior surface of ribs 3, 4 and 5.

Insertion.   Into the coracoid process of the scapula.

Innervation.   Pectoral nerve.

Action.   Pulls the scapula downwards and forwards.

Serratus anterior (Fig. 9.41)

Origin.   From the upper eight ribs.

Insertion.   Passes between the scapula and the ribs and inserts into the medial border of the scapula.

Innervation.   Long thoracic nerve.

Action.   Pulls the scapula forwards, thereby bringing the shoulder forward.

Rectus abdominis (Fig. 9.42)

Origin.   From the pubic crest.

Insertion.   To the xiphoid and the costal cartilages of ribs 5, 6 and 7. The two rectus abdominis muscles (right and left) are joined along their length exactly in the midline of the body, at a band called the **linea alba** (Latin = white line) made up of connective tissue.

Innervation.   Thoracic nerves.

Action.   Flexion of the spinal cord. These muscles are the antagonists of the deep spinal muscles of the back and play an important role in stabilizing the spinal column.

The abdominal wall contains three layers of broad, thin muscles: the external oblique is the superficial layer, the internal oblique is in the middle, and the transversus abdominus is the deep layer.

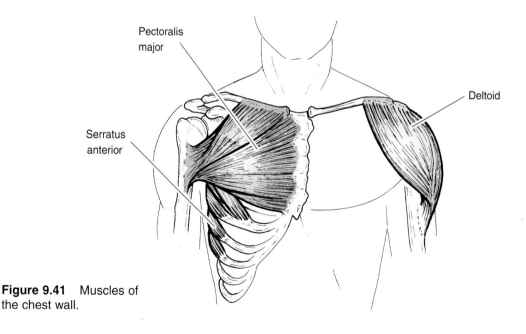

Figure 9.41   Muscles of the chest wall.

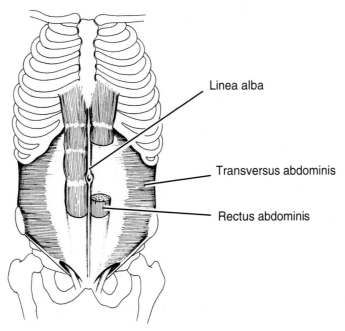

Figure 9.42   Transversus abdominis and rectus abdominis.

External oblique (Fig. 9.43)

Origin.   From the inferior portion of the lower eight ribs.

Insertion.   Into the anterior portion of the iliac crest, the pubic crest and the linea alba.

Internal oblique (Fig. 9.44)

Origin.   From the anterior two-thirds of the iliac crest and the lower three ribs.

Insertion.   Into the pubic crest and the linea alba.

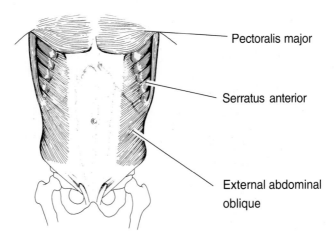

Figure 9.43   External oblique.

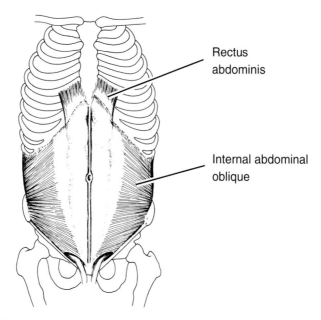

Rectus abdominis

Internal abdominal oblique

Figure 9.44   Internal oblique.

Transversus abdominis (see Fig. 9.42)

Origin.   From the anterior two-thirds of the iliac crest and the costal cartilages of ribs 5–10.

Insertion.   Into the linea alba and the symphysis pubis.

Innervation.   Intercostal nerves.

Action.   This muscle and the two described before it make up the muscular wall of the abdomen. When these muscles contract, they increase the intra-abdominal pressure, which occurs during urination, defecation, coughing or laughing.

When these muscles become flaccid, they result in a 'potbelly' (even in thin people), because the abdominal organs push out the weak abdominal wall.

When the abdomen must be opened surgically, the incision should be made through the linea alba, if possible, so as to minimize damage to the abdominal wall muscles.

MUSCLES ACTING ON THE SHOULDER

Deltoid (see Fig. 9.41)

Origin.   From the lateral third of the clavicle, the acromion process and the spine of the scapula.

Insertion.   Into the deltoid tuberosity of the humerus.

Innervation.   Axillary nerve.

Action.   The middle part of the muscle abducts the shoulder, while the anterior and posterior parts stabilize the arm to stop it from moving forwards or backwards.

Supraspinatus (Fig. 9.45)

Origin.   From the spine of the scapula.

Insertion.   Into the upper part of the greater tubercle of the humerus.

Innervation.   Suprascapular nerve.

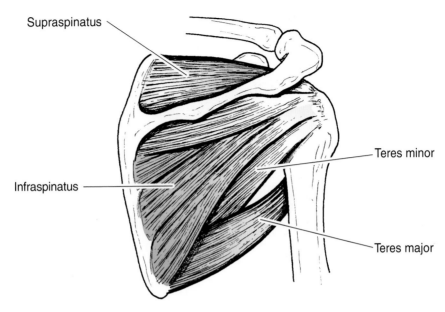

Figure 9.45 Muscles of the shoulder.

Action. Abduction of the shoulder. This muscle prevents superior migration of the humeral head when the deltoid abducts the shoulder.

Infraspinatus (Fig. 9.45)

Origin. From the posterior surface of the scapula, below the spine.
Insertion. Into the greater tubercle.
Innervation. Suprascapular nerve.
Action. External rotation of the shoulder.

Teres major (Fig. 9.45)

Origin. From the inferolateral border of the scapula.
Insertion. Into the anterosuperior part of the humerus.
Innervation. Subscapular nerve.
Action. Adduction and internal rotation of the shoulder.

Teres minor (Fig. 9.45)

Origin. From the medial border of the scapula.
Insertion. Into the greater tubercle.
Innervation. Axillary nerve.
Action. External rotation of the shoulder.

Subscapularis

Origin. From the anterior surface of the scapula.
Insertion. Into the lesser tubercle.
Innervation. Subscapular nerve.
Action. Internal rotation of the shoulder.

The subscapularis, teres minor, supraspinatus and infraspinatus muscles together comprise the **rotator cuff** which stabilizes the shoulder during its movements.

MUSCLES OF THE UPPER ARM

Biceps (or biceps brachii) (Fig. 9.46)

Origin.   This muscle has two origins from two different bony points and thus 'two heads' – hence its name (Latin *bi* = two and *caput* = head). One head is called the **long head**, and it arises above the glenoid fossa of the scapula. The second head is called the **short head**, and it arises from the coracoid process of the scapula. The two heads combine into one muscle belly.

Insertion.   Into the radial tuberosity.

Innervation.   Musculocutaneous nerve.

Action.   Flexion and supination of the elbow. This muscle is the major muscle for supination of the forearm.

Brachialis (Fig. 9.46)

Origin.   From the anterior surface of the humerus.

Insertion.   Into the projection called the coronoid process on the anterior surface of the upper end of the ulna.

Innervation.   Musculocutaneous nerve.

Action.   Flexion of the elbow (bending the arm).

Triceps (Fig. 9.47)

Origin.   This muscle originates from three different skeletal points, hence its name (Latin *tri* = three and *caput* = head). The long head originates underneath the glenoid fossa of the scapula, the lateral head originates from the lateral border of the upper humerus and the medial head originates from a large portion of the posterior surface of lower humerus.

Insertion.   The three heads combine into one muscle that is inserted into the olecranon process of the ulna (the back of the elbow).

Innervation.   Radial nerve.

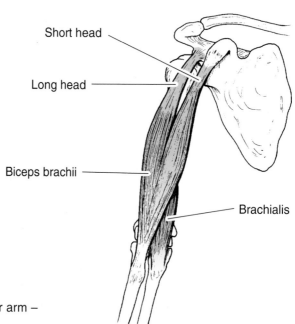

Short head

Long head

Biceps brachii

Brachialis

Figure 9.46   Muscles of the upper arm – anterior compartment.

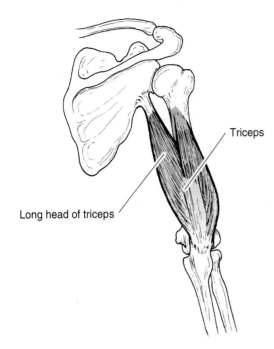

Figure 9.47   Muscles of the upper arm – posterior compartment.

Action.   Extension of the elbow (straightening out the arm).

FOREARM MUSCLES

Anterior compartment

Brachioradialis (Fig. 9.48)

Origin.   From the lateral side of the lower humerus.

Insertion.   Into the styloid process of the radius.

Innervation.   Radial nerve.

Action.   Flexion of the elbow.

Pronator teres (Fig. 9.48)

Origin.   From the medial epicondyle of the humerus.

Insertion.   Into the superolateral surface of the radius.

Innervation.   Median nerve.

Action.   Pronation of the forearm.

Flexor carpi radialis (Fig. 9.48)

Origin.   From the medial epicondyle of the humerus.

Insertion.   Into the bases of the second and third metacarpals.

Innervation.   Median nerve.

Action.   Flexion and abduction of the wrist.

Palmaris longus (Fig. 9.48)

Origin.   From the medial epicondyle of the humerus.

Insertion.   Into the connective tissue that covers the palm of the hand. This insertion is unique in that it does not attach to a bone but instead to a sheet of connective tissue.

Innervation.   Median nerve.

Action.   Flexion of the wrist.

Flexor carpi ulnaris (Fig. 9.48)

Origin.   From the medial epicondyle of the humerus and from the olecranon.

Insertion.   Into the base of the fifth metacarpal.

Innervation.   Ulnar nerve.

Action.   Flexion and adduction of the wrist.

The last four muscles described form the superficial layer of the anterior forearm muscles, which can be seen upon removing the skin of the forearm. Deep to those muscles is another layer of muscles, which flex the fingers.

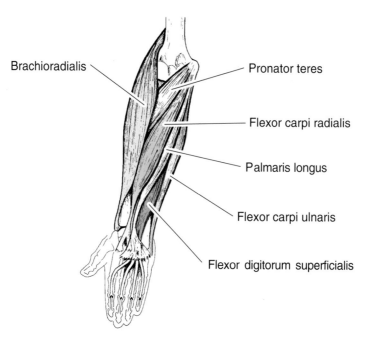

Figure 9.48   Muscles of the forearm – anterior compartment.

Flexor digitorum superficialis (Fig. 9.48)

Origin.   From the medial epicondyle of the humerus and the anterior surface of the upper radius. It has two heads.

Insertion.   The main body of the muscle divides into four tendons that attach to the bases of the middle phalanges of fingers 2–5 (but not the thumb).

Innervation.   Median nerve.

Action.   Flexion of the fingers.

Flexor digitorum profundus

Origin.   From the anterior surface of the ulna.

Insertion.   The body of the muscle divides into four tendons that pass through an opening in the tendons of flexor digitorum superficialis and then insert into the distal phalanges of fingers 2–5 (but not the thumb).

Innervation.   The thumb, index and middle fingers are activated by the median nerve; the ring and little fingers are activated by the ulnar nerve.

Action.   Flexion of the fingers. The two latter muscles are part of a sophisticated system that controls precise complex movements of the fingers (Fig. 9.49).

Posterior compartment

Extensor carpi radialis (Fig. 9.50)

Origin.   From the lateral epicondyle of the humerus.

Insertion.   Into the bases of the second and third metacarpals.

Innervation.   Radial nerve.

Action.   Extension and abduction of the wrist.

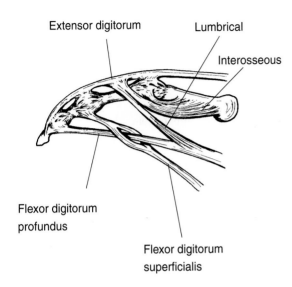

Figure 9.49   Tendons that move the fingers.

Extensor digitorum (Fig. 9.48)

Origin.   From the lateral epicondyle of the humerus.

Insertion.   The body of the muscle splits into four tendons that become bands of connective tissue that are attached to the backs of the phalanges.

Innervation.   Radial nerve.

Action.   Extension of the wrist and fingers.

Extensor carpi ulnaris (Fig. 9.50)

Origin.   From the lateral epicondyle of the humerus.

Insertion.   Into the base of the fifth metacarpal.

Innervation.   Radial nerve.

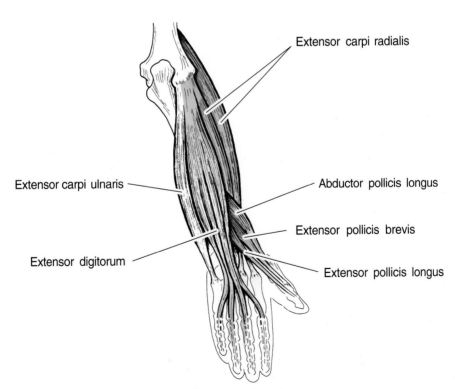

Figure 9.50   Muscles of the forearm – posterior compartment.

Action.   Extension and adduction of the wrist.

MUSCLES OF THE FOREARM THAT MOVE THE THUMB

The thumb is essential in the grasping of objects (it allows a pincer grasp) and it therefore has its own separate system of muscles.

Flexor pollicis longus

Origin.   From the middle of the anterior surface of the radius.
Insertion.   Into the base of the distal phalanx of the thumb.
Innervation.   Median nerve.
Action.   Flexion of the thumb.

Extensor pollicis longus (Figs 9.50 and 9.51)

Origin.   From the lower portion of the posterior surface of the ulna.
Insertion.   Into the base of the distal phalanx of the thumb.
Innervation.   Radial nerve.
Action.   Extension of the thumb.

Extensor pollicis brevis (Figs 9.50 and 9.51)

Origin.   From the lower portion of the posterior surface of the radius.
Insertion.   Into the base of the proximal phalanx of the thumb.
Innervation.   Radial nerve.
Action.   Extension of the thumb.

The tendons of the above two muscles outline the depression at the base of the thumb known as the anatomical **snuff box**.

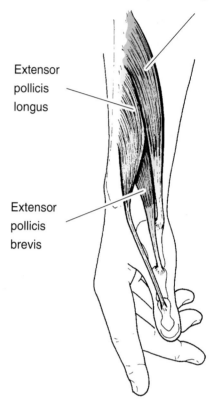

Figure 9.51   Muscles that move the thumb.

Abductor pollicis longus (Figs 9.50 and 9.51)

Origin.   From the posterior surfaces of both the radius and ulna and the membrane between them.
Insertion.   Into the base of the first metacarpal.
Innervation.   Radial nerve.
Action.   Abduction of the thumb.

MUSCLES OF THE HAND

The intrinsic muscles of the hand are on the palmar aspect and can be divided into three groups:

1. the thumb or **thenar muscles**
2. the little finger or **hypothenar muscles**
3. the lumbrical muscles and interosseous muscles.

The intrinsic muscles of the hand act together with the long tendons of the four lateral fingers and the thumb to create the fine and intricate movements of the fingers.

The thenar muscles

Movements of the thumb are critical to the proper function of the hand and account for about 50% of all hand movements.

The three thenar muscles (abductor pollicis brevis, flexor pollicis brevis and opponens pollicis) are chiefly responsible for the most important movement – **opposition** – whereby the tip of the thumb is brought into contact with the palmar surface of other fingers (Fig. 9.52).

Abductor pollicis brevis (Fig. 9.53)

Origin. From the carpal bones and the flexor retinaculum.

Insertion. Lateral side of the base of the proximal phalanx of the thumb.

Innervation. Median nerve.

Action. Abduction of the thumb and assisting the opponens pollicis muscle during the early stages of opposition.

Flexor pollicis brevis (Fig. 9.53)

Origin. From a carpal bone and the flexor retinaculum.

Insertion. Lateral side of the base of the proximal phalanx of the thumb.

Innervation. Median and ulnar nerves.

Action. Flexes thumb and assists in opposition.

Opponens pollicis (Fig. 9.53)

Origin. From the flexor retinaculum.

Insertion. Entire length of the palmar surface of the first metacarpal bone.

Innervation. Median nerve.

Action. Opposes the thumb.

Adductor pollicis (Fig. 9.53)

This muscle is a deep muscle of the palm and is not part of the thenar muscles.

Origin. There are two heads of origin: the oblique head from the bases of the second and third metacarpal bones and from the carpal bones, and the transverse head from the anterior surface of the third metacarpal bone.

Insertion. Medial side of the base of the proximal phalanx of the thumb.

Innervation. Ulnar nerve.

Action. Adducts the thumb and provides power for grasping.

The hypothenar muscles

The hypothenar muscles include the abductor digiti minimi, the flexor digiti minimi brevis and the opponens digiti minimi. These muscles have no major functional rule.

The lumbrical and interosseous muscles

Lumbrical muscles (see Fig. 9.49, Fig. 9.53, Fig. 9.54)

The four slender lumbricals, one for each finger, were named because of their elongated, worm-like form.

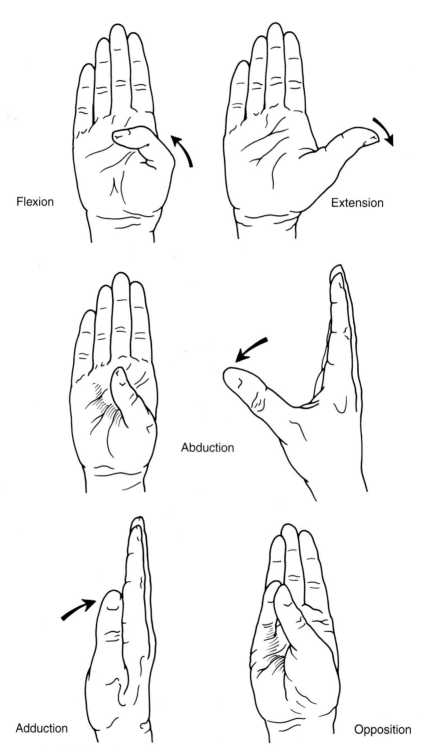

Figure 9.52   Movements of the thumb.

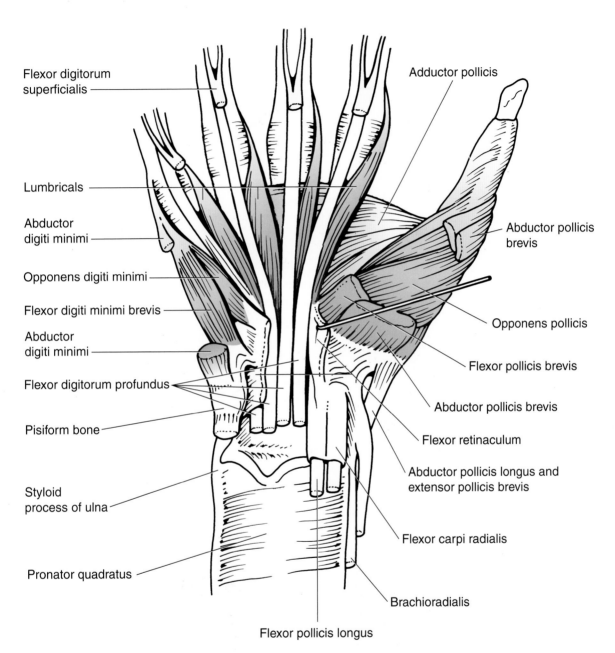

Figure 9.53   Anterior view showing the muscles of the hand.

Origin.   From the tendons of the flexor digitorum profundus muscle.

Insertion.   Lateral sides of the extensor tendons of fingers 2–5.

Innervation.   Ulnar nerve.

Action.   Flexes the fingers at the metacarpophalangeal joints and extends the interphalangeal joints.

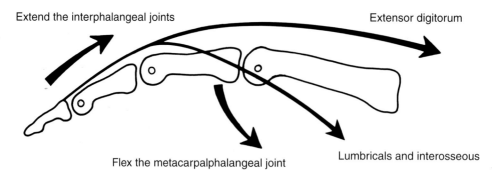

Extend the interphalangeal joints

Extensor digitorum

Flex the metacarpalphalangeal joint

Lumbricals and interosseous

Figure 9.54   The action of the lumbricals and interosseous.

Interosseous muscles (Fig. 9.49, Fig. 9.54, Fig. 9.55)

The seven interosseous muscles (four dorsal and three palmar) occupy the spaces between the metacarpal bones.

Origin.   From the sides of the metacarpal bones.

Insertion.   Bases of proximal phalanges of fingers 2–5.

Innervation.   Ulnar nerve.

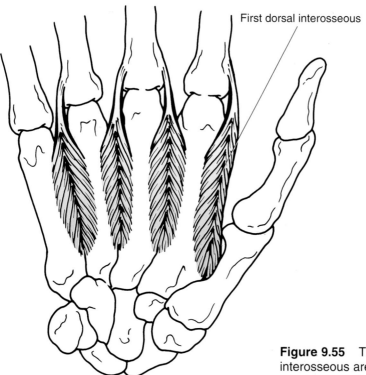

First dorsal interosseous

Dorsal interosseous

Figure 9.55   The interossei. The four dorsal interosseous are shown. The first dorsal interosseous abducts the index finger and is important when holding a key.

Action. Abduct and adduct the fingers, and also assist the lumbricals in flexion of the metacarpophalangeal joints and extension of the interphalangeal joints. These are vital in finely coordinated activities such as writing, typing and playing the piano.

Carpal tunnel

The **carpal tunnel** is located in the anterior aspect of the wrist. The carpal bones form the floor and the lateral walls of the tunnel and the **flexor retinaculum** (also called the volar carpal ligament) forms the roof of the tunnel (see Fig. 9.53). The carpal tunnel contains the long flexor tendons of the fingers and the median nerve. It is a closed compartment and any lesion that significantly raises the pressure in the tunnel (e.g. inflammation of the tendons) can cause compression and dysfunction of the median nerve, called **carpal tunnel syndrome**. The clinical signs include tingling (**paresthesia**) or diminished sensation (**hypoesthesia**) in the fingers. If medical treatment fails to relieve the symptoms, surgical release of the flexor retinaculum is performed.

PELVIC MUSCLES

Gluteus maximus (Fig. 9.56)

Origin. From the outer surface of the ilium, the posterior surface of the sacrum and the coccyx.

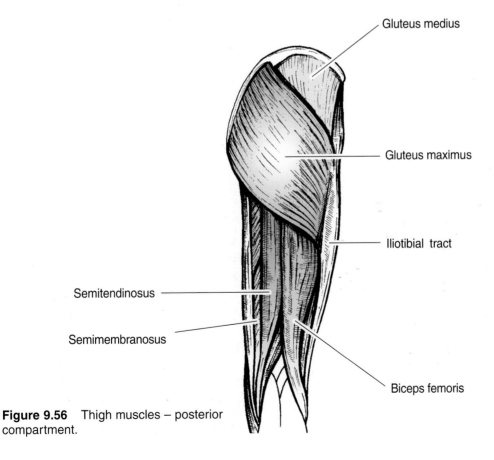

Gluteus medius

Gluteus maximus

Iliotibial tract

Semitendinosus

Semimembranosus

Biceps femoris

Figure 9.56 Thigh muscles – posterior compartment.

Insertion.   Into the lateral surface of the upper femur and the iliotibial tract (see p. 156).

Innervation.   Gluteal nerve.

Action.   Extension and lateral rotation of the thigh. This muscle is important when standing up from a seated position.

Gluteus medius (Fig. 9.56)

Origin.   From the outer surface of the ilium.

Insertion.   Into the greater trochanter of the femur.

Innervation.   Gluteal nerve.

Action.   Abduction of the thigh. This muscle also plays an important role in walking. Because the center of gravity of the body is lateral to the hip joint, lifting a leg while walking would cause the pelvis to drop towards that side, if the gluteus medius muscle on the opposite side did not contract to keep the pelvis level (Fig. 9.57).

Psoas (Fig. 9.58)

(In cattle, this muscle provides beef tenderloin or fillet steak.)

Origin.   From the transverse processes of vertebrae T12–L5.

Insertion.   Into the lesser trochanter of the femur. (This is a deep muscle that cannot be felt.)

Innervation.   Lumbar plexus.

Action.   Flexion of the thigh.

Iliacus (Fig. 9.58)

Origin.   From the internal surface of the ilium.

Insertion.   The tendon of this muscle joins the tendon of the psoas and they share a

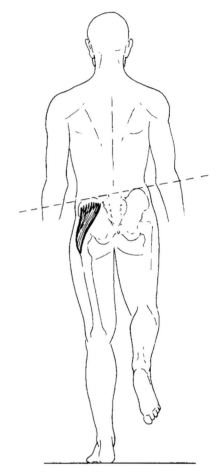

Figure 9.57   The gluteus medius muscle stabilizes the pelvis while the opposite leg is raised.

common insertion. It is a deep muscle that cannot be felt.

Innervation.   Femoral nerve.

Action.   Flexion of the thigh.

THIGH MUSCLES

Anterior compartment

Quadriceps (Figs 9.59 and 9.60)

Origin.   This muscle has four heads (Latin *quad* = four and *caput* = head). Three of the

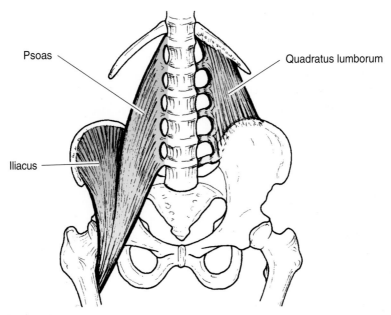

Figure 9.58   Pelvic muscles.

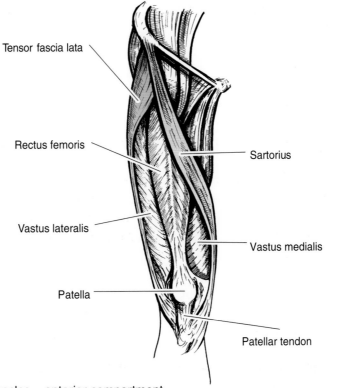

Figure 9.59   Thigh muscles – anterior compartment.

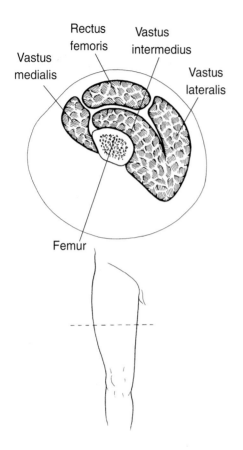

Vastus medialis
Rectus femoris
Vastus intermedius
Vastus lateralis
Femur

Figure 9.60   Transverse section through the quadriceps muscle.

Insertion.   The four heads join to form the **quadriceps tendon**, inserted to the upper pole of the patella (kneecap). From the lower part of the patella arises the short, thick, and strong patellar tendon attached to the tibial tuberosity. The inner surface of the patella is covered by a layer of cartilage, which is in contact with the cartilage on the anterior surface of the bottom of the femur (the femoral condyles). If there were no patella, the quadriceps muscle would end in a tendon that would pass over the front of the knee joint directly to the tibia. Whenever the knee was bent, this tendon would rub against the lower femur. Because of the patella, the contact is not between tendon and joint surface but between two cartilage joint surfaces, lubricated by synovial fluid. Furthermore, the patella increases the lever effect of the quadriceps tendon, and multiplies the strength of the quadriceps muscle.

Innervation.   Femoral nerve.

Action.   The first three heads of the quadriceps extend the knee. The fourth head (the rectus femoris) also passes over the hip joint (its origin is proximal to the hip joint) and also flexes the hip joint when it contracts.

heads arise from the femur and one from the pelvis. Each head is given a separate name:

- **Vastus medialis**: from the medial surface of the femur
- **Vastus lateralis**: from the lateral surface of the femur
- **Vastus intermedius**: from the front of the femur
- **Rectus femoris**: from the anterior surface of the ilium.

Sartorius (Fig. 9.59)

Origin.   From the anterior superior iliac spine.

Insertion.   Into the medial part of the upper tibia.

Innervation.   Femoral nerve.

Action.   Flexion, abduction and lateral rotation of the thigh. This is the traditional cross-legged position of the tailor, hence the name (Latin *sartor* = tailor).

Medial compartment

Adductor magnus (Fig. 9.61)

This is one of a group of muscles in the medial compartment of the thigh, and has been chosen as an example.

Origin. From the inferior portion of the pubis and from the ischial tuberosity.

Insertion. Into the linea aspera of the femur.

Innervation. Obturator nerve.

Action. Adduction of the thigh. Horse riding requires constant use of the medial thigh muscles, so someone who does not ride frequently feels pain in the medial aspect of the thigh after riding (Fig. 9.62).

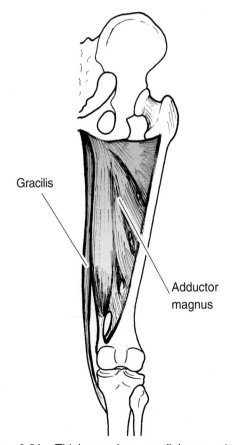

Gracilis

Adductor magnus

Figure 9.61 Thigh muscles – medial compartment.

Gracilis (Fig. 9.61)

Origin. From the inferior part of the pubis and the ischium.

Insertion. Into the medial part of the upper tibia.

Innervation. Obturator nerve.

Action. Adduction of the thigh and flexion of the leg.

Posterior compartment

Biceps femoris (see Fig. 9.56)

Origin. From the ischial tuberosity and from the lower part of the linea aspera of the femur (two heads).

Insertion. Into the head of the fibula. The tendon of biceps femoris can be felt easily behind the knee, on the lateral side.

Innervation. Tibial nerve.

Action. Extension of the thigh and flexion of the knee.

Semitendinosus (see Fig. 9.56)

Origin. From the ischial tuberosity.

Insertion. Into the medial part of the upper tibia. This tendon can easily be felt behind the knee, on the medial side.

Innervation. Tibial nerve.

Action. Extension of the thigh and flexion of the knee.

Semimembranosus (see Fig. 9.56)

Origin. From the ischial tuberosity.

Insertion. Into the medial surface of the upper tibia.

Innervation. Tibial nerve.

Action. Extension of the thigh and flexion of the knee.

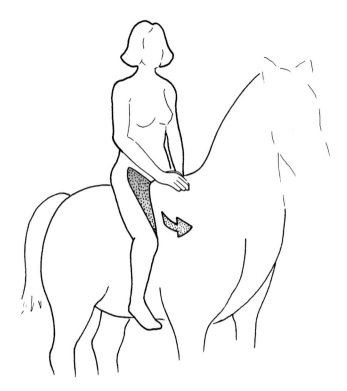

Figure 9.62   The function of the medial thigh muscles.

The latter three muscles, together with a portion of the adductor magnus muscle, are called the **hamstrings**.

Iliotibial tract

The entire thigh is enclosed in a layer of connective tissue called the **fascia lata**. This becomes thicker toward the lateral side of the thigh and develops into a ligament called the iliotibial tract (Fig. 9.63). This sheet of fibrous tissue is attached to the iliac crest, passes downwards on the lateral side of the thigh and is attached to the connective tissue layer that envelops the leg.

The **tensor fascia lata** (Fig. 9.63) is a muscle that arises from the iliac crest and inserts into the connective tissue band – the iliotibial tract. This muscle helps to abduct the thigh.

LEG MUSCLES

Anterior compartment

Tibialis anterior (Fig. 9.64)

Origin.   From the lateral surface of the upper tibia.

Insertion.   Into the base of the first metatarsal.

Innervation.   Deep peroneal nerve.

Action.   Dorsiflexion and inversion of the foot.

Extensor digitorum longus (Fig. 9.64)

Origin.   From the anterior surface of the fibula.

Insertion.   Into the fibrous sheets that enclose the toes (not the great toe).

Innervation. Deep peroneal nerve.

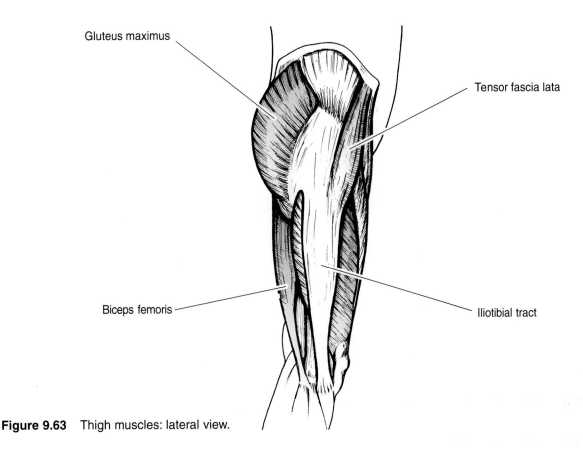

Figure 9.63   Thigh muscles: lateral view.

Action.   Extends the toes and dorsiflexes the foot.

Extensor hallucis longus (Fig. 9.64)

Origin.   From the anterior surface of the fibula.

Insertion.   Into the base of the distal phalanx of the great toe.

Innervation.   Deep peroneal nerve.

Action.   Extension of the big toe and dorsiflexion of the foot.

Lateral compartment

Peroneus longus (Fig. 9.65)

Origin.   From the lateral surface of the upper fibula.

Insertion.   The tendon passes behind the lateral malleolus of the fibula and inserts into the base of the first metatarsal.

Innervation.   Superficial peroneal nerve.

Action.   Flexion and eversion of the foot.

Peroneus brevis (Fig.9.65)

Origin.   From the anterior surface of the fibula.

Insertion.   The tendon passes behind the lateral malleolus of the fibula, and inserts into the base of the fifth metatarsal.

Innervation.   Superficial peroneal nerve.

Action.   Flexion and eversion of the foot.

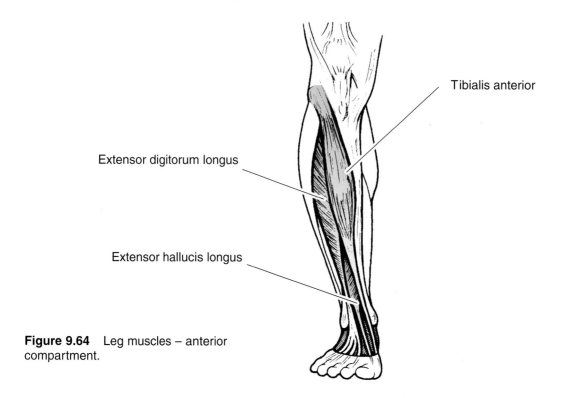

Tibialis anterior

Extensor digitorum longus

Extensor hallucis longus

Figure 9.64   Leg muscles – anterior compartment.

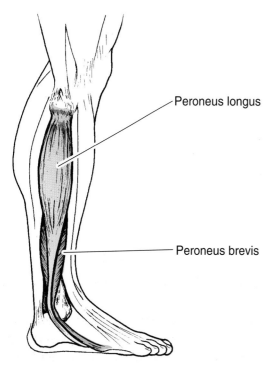

Peroneus longus

Peroneus brevis

Figure 9.65   Leg muscles – lateral compartment.

Posterior compartment

Gastrocnemius (Fig. 9.66)

Origin.   This muscle has two heads. A lateral head originates from the lateral surface of the lower part of the femur and a medial head originates from the medial side of the lower part of the femur.

Insertion.   A large tendon called the tendo calcaneus (**Achilles tendon**) which inserts into the back of the calcaneus.

Innervation.   Tibial nerve.

Action.   Plantarflexion of the foot.

This muscle pushes the body forward during walking.

Soleus (Fig. 9.66)

This muscle lies largely underneath the gastrocnemius.

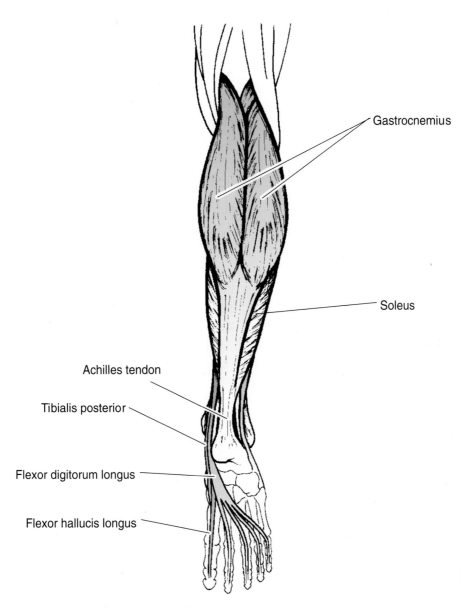

Figure 9.66   Leg muscles – posterior compartment.

Origin.   From the posterior surface of the upper tibia and from the posterior surface of the back of the fibula.

Insertion.   Its tendon joins the tendon of the gastrocnemius and forms the Achilles tendon.

Innervation.   Tibial nerve.

Action.   Plantarflexion of the foot.

Flexor digitorum longus (Fig. 9.66)

Origin.   From the posterior surface of the tibia.

Insertion.   Its tendon passes behind the medial malleolus of the tibia and inserts into the bases of the distal phalanges of toes 2–5.

Innervation.   Tibial nerve.

Action. Plantarflexion and inversion of the foot, flexion of the toes and support for the arch of the foot.

Flexor hallucis longus (Fig. 9.66)

Origin. From the posterior surface of the fibula.

Insertion. The tendon passes behind the medial malleolus, and inserts into the distal phalanx of the great toe.

Innervation. Tibial nerve.

Action. Flexion of the big toe, plantarflexion of the foot and support for the arch of the foot.

Tibialis posterior (Fig. 9.66)

Origin. From the posterior surfaces of both the tibia and the fibula.

Insertion. The tendon passes behind the medial malleolus and inserts mainly into the navicular bone (one of the bones of the midfoot).

Innervation. Tibial nerve.

Action. Plantarflexion and inversion of the foot. The muscle is very important in maintaining the arch of the foot.

MUSCLES OF THE FOOT

Underneath the thick skin of the sole of the foot is the **plantar aponeurosis**, a sheet of strong connective tissue that runs from the calcaneus to the connective tissue sheaths surrounding the toes. It consists of a strong, thick central part and weaker, thinner medial and lateral portions. The plantar aponeurosis helps to support the longitudinal arches of the foot and to hold the structure of the foot together.

There are four layers of muscle in the sole of the foot, which maintain the arches of the foot,

enabling standing on uneven surfaces. Their function is not as delicate as the function of those in the hand.

The first plantar muscle layer contains three muscles: the abductor hallucis, abductor digiti minimi and flexor digitorum brevis, all of which extend from the posterior part of the calcaneus to the phalanges.

Abductor hallucis (Fig. 9.67)

Origin. From the medial side of the calcaneus.

Insertion. Into the medial side of the base of the great toe.

Innervation. Plantar nerve.

Action. Abducts and flexes the great toe. When the foot is bearing weight, it supports the medial longitudinal arch of the foot.

Abductor digiti minimi (Fig. 9.67)

Origin. From the lateral side of the calcaneus.

Insertion. Into the lateral side of the base of the little toe.

Innervation. Plantar nerve.

Action. Abducts and flexes the little toe.

Flexor digitorum brevis (Fig. 9.67)

Origin. From the posterior portion of the calcaneus.

Insertion. The muscle divides into four bellies, each with its own tendon. The tendons then split into two halves and each half inserts on either side of the bases of the middle phalanges of the toes. The tendons of the flexor digitorum longus pass through the split in the brevis tendons and continue to insert into the distal phalanges (similar to the arrangement in the hand).

Innervation.   Plantar nerve.

Action.   Flexes the lateral four toes. When the foot is bearing weight, it supports the medial and lateral longitudinal arches of the foot.

The second layer of plantar muscles, located deep to the first layer, consists of the quadratus plantae and the lumbrical muscles.

Quadratus plantae (Fig. 9.68)

Origin.   From the medial surface of the calcaneus and from the lateral margin of plantar surface of calcaneus.

Insertion.   Into the posterolateral margin of the tendon of the flexor digitorum longus. This muscle insertion is unique because it inserts to another tendon.

Innervation.   Plantar nerve.

Action.   Assists the flexor digitorum longus in flexing the lateral four toes by adjusting the pull of the flexor digitorum longus, bringing the tendon more directly in line with the long axes of the toes.

Lumbrical muscles (Fig. 9.68)

Origin.   From the tendons of the flexor digitorum longus. The origin of these muscles is unique – they are from a tendon.

Insertion.   Medial sides of the bases of proximal phalanges of the lateral four toes and extensor expansions of the tendons of the extensor digitorum longus muscles.

Innervation.   Plantar nerve.

Action.   Flexes the proximal phalanges at the metatarsophalangeal joint and extends the

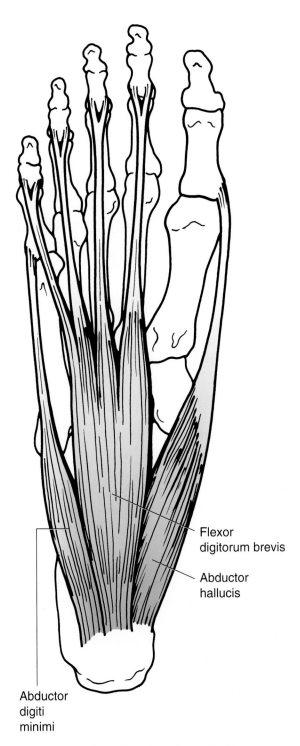

Flexor digitorum brevis

Abductor hallucis

Abductor digiti minimi

Figure 9.67   Muscles of the foot – first layer.

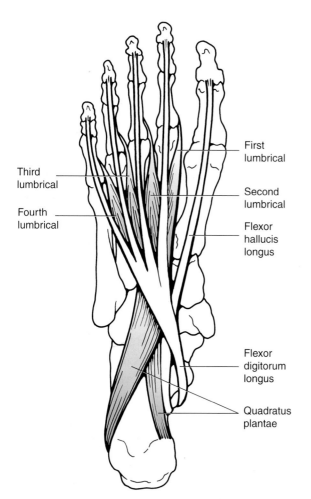

Figure 9.68   Muscles of the foot – second layer.

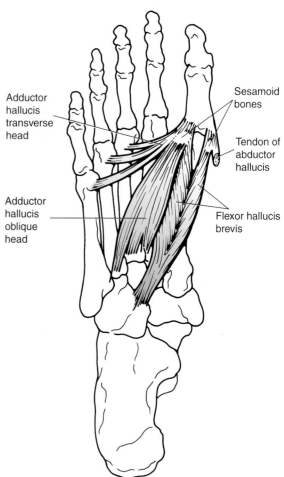

Figure 9.69   Muscles of the foot – third layer.

middle and distal phalanges at the inter-phalangeal joints.

The third layer of plantar muscles consists of the short muscles of the great and little toes.

Flexor hallucis brevis (Fig. 9.69)

Origin.   From the plantar surface of the cuboid and lateral cuneiform bones.

Insertion.   Both sides of the base of the prox-imal phalanx of the great toe by two tendons. A

sesamoid bone adheres to each of these tendons and protects the tendons from pressure from the head of the first metatarsal bone during stand-ing.

Innervation.   Plantar nerve.
Action.   Flexes the great toe.

Adductor hallucis (Fig. 9.69)

Origin.   The adductor of the great toe has two heads of origin: the oblique head from the bases of the second, third and fourth metatarsal bones and the transverse head from the plantar ligaments of the three lateral metatarsophalangeal joints.

Insertion. Into the lateral side of the base of the proximal phalanx of the great toe.

Innervation. Plantar nerve.

Action. Adducts and flexes the great toe.

The fourth layer of the plantar muscles consists of the interosseous muscles and the tendons of the peroneus longus and tibialis posterior muscles, which cross the sole of the foot to reach their insertion points.

Interosseous muscles (Fig. 9.70)

There are three plantar and four dorsal interossei and they occupy the spaces between the metatarsal bones.

Origin. From the sides of the metatarsal bones.

Insertion. Into the sides of the bases of the proximal phalanges of the four lateral toes (not including the great toe).

Innervation. Plantar nerve.

Action. Abduction and adduction of the toes, and flexion of the toes at the metatarsophalangeal joints of the four lateral toes.

NECK MUSCLES

There is a complex array of muscles in the neck. Two of those muscles have been selected as examples – one at the front of the neck and one at the back.

Sternocleidomastoid (Fig. 9.71)

Origin. From the upper part of the sternum (this head is, in fact a tendon) and from the

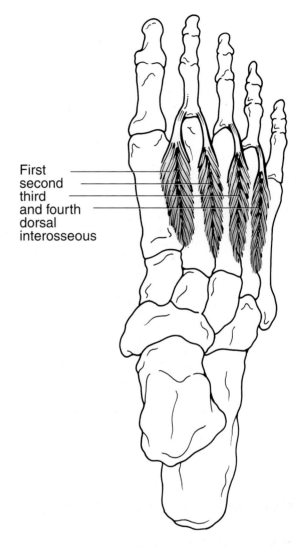

First second third and fourth dorsal interosseous

Figure 9.70 Muscles of the foot – fourth layer.

superior surface of the medial third of the clavicle.

Insertion. Both heads combine into a single muscle and tendon that inserts into the mastoid process, behind the ear.

Innervation. Accessory nerve.

Action. When the sternomastoid contracts, the ear on the side of the muscle is

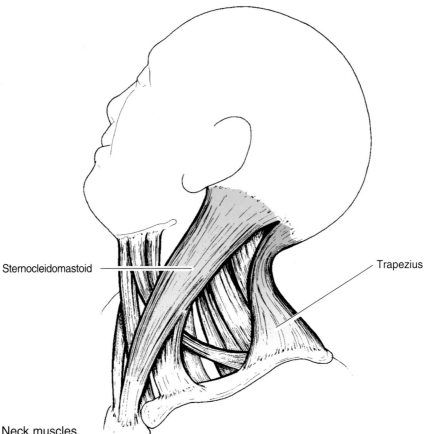

Sternocleidomastoid

Trapezius

Figure 9.71 Neck muscles.

brought closer to the shoulder on that side and the face is turned to the opposite side and upwards.

Splenius capitis

Origin. From the spines of the lower cervical vertebrae and the four upper cervical vertebrae.

Insertion. Into the lateral surface of the occipital bone.

Innervation. Cervical spinal nerves.

Action. Extension and rotation of the head.

FACIAL MUSCLES

Masseter (Fig. 9.72)

Origin. From the zygomatic arch.

Insertion. Into the lower border of the mandible.

Innervation. Mandibular nerve.

Action. This is the powerful muscle that closes the jaw and is involved in chewing (masticating).

Temporalis (Fig. 9.72)

Origin. From the outer surface of the temporal bone.

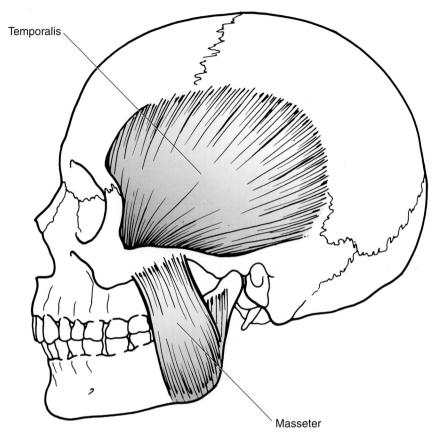

Temporalis

Masseter

Figure 9.72   Muscles of mastication.

Insertion.   The fan-shaped temporalis muscle passes deep to the zygomatic arch and inserts into the upper part of the mandible.

Innervation.   Trigeminal nerve.

Action.   Closes the jaw and retracts the mandible.

Muscles of expression

These muscles control the contours of the face rather than moving actual joints. They also surround the mouth, eyes and nose and act to open and close these orifices.

Their origins are usually from bones of the face or from connective tissue structures in the face, and they usually insert into the skin of the face. All muscles of facial expression are supplied by the facial nerve.

The **depressor anguli oris** depresses the corner of the mouth, as in crying (Fig. 9.73).

The **zygomaticus major** draws the angle of the mouth superolaterally, as in laughing.

The **orbicularis oris** is the sphincter muscle of the mouth, with its fibers lying within the lips and encircling the mouth. The orbicularis oris closes the mouth, purses the lips and plays an important role in articulation and chewing.

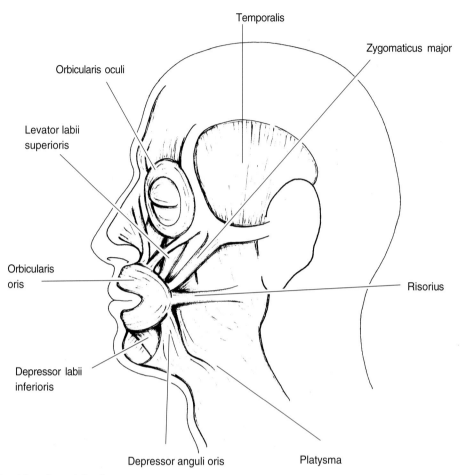

Temporalis

Zygomaticus major

Orbicularis oculi

Levator labii
superioris

Orbicularis
oris

Risorius

Depressor labii
inferioris

Depressor anguli oris

Platysma

Figure 9.73   Muscles of the face.

THE SHOULDER JOINT AND GIRDLE

The clavicle, scapula and humerus form an intercalated complex working in symphony during motion of the shoulder (Fig. 9.74).

The clavicle is S-shaped and serves as a strut that helps to suspend the arm while also providing a site for muscle attachments. The medial aspect of the clavicle articulates with the manubrium at the **sternoclavicular joint**. The clavicle, and therefore the sternoclavicular joint, is normally capable of 30° to 35° of upwards elevation, 35° of combined forwards and backwards movement and 45° to 50° of rotation around its long axis. The sternoclavicular joint is involved in almost all motions of the upper extremity. The lateral aspect of the clavicle articulates with the acromion process of the scapula at the **acromioclavicular joint**. Very little actual motion occurs at the acromioclavicular joint and its main function is to serve as connection between the clavicle and the scapula. The stability of the acromioclavicular joint is maintained by the **acromioclavicular ligaments** which surround the joint, and the **coracoclavicular ligaments**

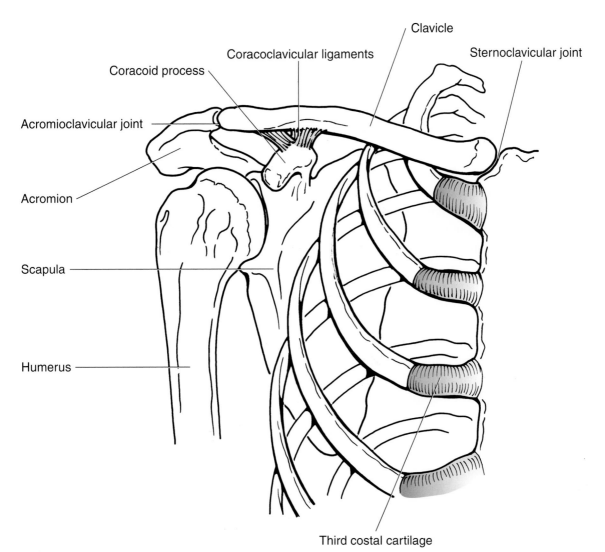

Figure 9.74   The shoulder girdle.

which connect the coracoid process to the clavicle.

The scapula is encased in muscles and therefore has a pseudoarticulation with the chest wall called **scapulothoracic articulation**. A total of 17 muscles arise or insert on the scapula. The lateral aspect of the scapula forms the glenoid, which articulates with the round head of the humerus at the **glenohumeral joint**. Although the glenohumeral joint is the principal joint of the shoulder complex, its motion is highly coordinated with that of the scapulothoracic articulation. Motion essentially involves sliding of the scapula (which floats in a bed of muscles) over the rib cage.

The two most important muscles that move the scapula are the **serratus anterior** (which arises from the upper eight ribs, passes between the scapula and the ribs and inserts into the medial border of the scapula), which pulls the scapula forwards (a movement called **protraction**) and holds it against the thoracic wall, and the **trapezius,** which rotates and elevates the scapula. The glenohumeral joint and the scapulothoracic articulation work in synchrony to provide arm motion. For example, raising the arm above the head (180° of motion) is done by a combination of glenohumeral joint motion (120°) and scapular rotation (60°). The clavicle which is connected to the scapula rotates and elevates during the movement (Figs 9.75 and 9.76).

The glenohumeral joint is the major articulation of the shoulder complex. It is formed by the articulation between the surfaces of the hemispheric humeral head and the smaller shallow glenoid. This geometry allows more motion than that of any other joint in the body, but at the expense of stability. Stability of the joint is provided by surrounding soft-tissue structures, which can be separated into static and dynamic restrains (stabilizers). The static restrains consist of the **glenoid labrum**, joint capsule and glenohumeral ligaments (Fig. 9.77). The labrum is a fibrous structure that forms a rim around the periphery of the glenoid, deepens the glenoid and serves as an anchoring source for the joint capsule, which surrounds the joint. The glenohumeral ligaments are part of the capsule where it is thickened.

The dynamic stabilizers consist of the rotator cuff muscles and the long head of the biceps. These muscles compress the humeral head against the glenoid and keep it centered during motion. Damage to the static or dynamic stabilizers can result in glenohumeral instability with subluxation or dislocation of the joint.

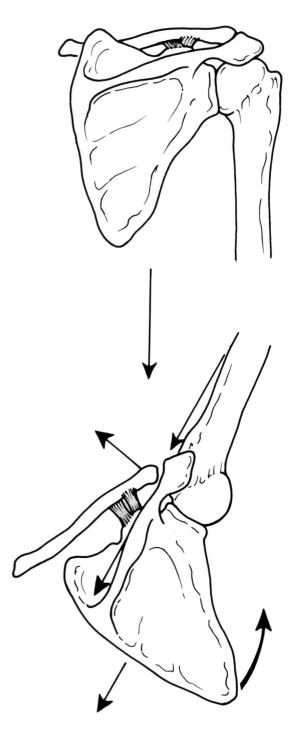

Figure 9.75 Rotation of the scapula during raising of the arm above the head.

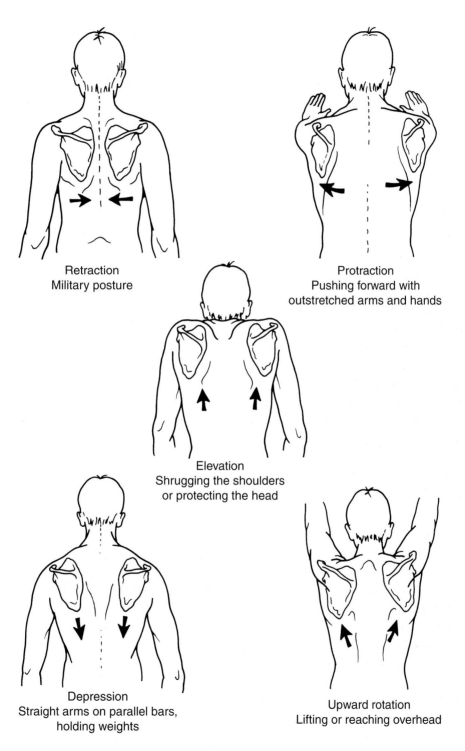

Retraction
Military posture

Protraction
Pushing forward with
outstretched arms and hands

Elevation
Shrugging the shoulders
or protecting the head

Depression
Straight arms on parallel bars,
holding weights

Upward rotation
Lifting or reaching overhead

Figure 9.76 Movements of the scapula.

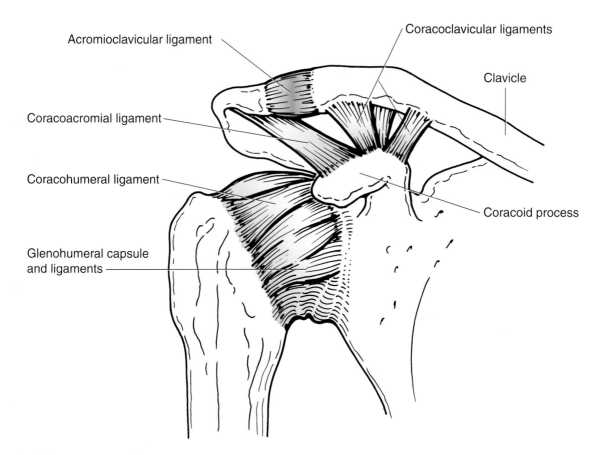

Figure 9.77 The glenohumeral capsule and ligaments

THE ELBOW JOINT

The elbow joint consists of three different articulations:

1. **Humeroulnar articulation:** is between the trochlea of the humerus and the trochlear notch of the ulna. These form a hinge-type of synovial joint, which permits movement in one axis (flexion and extension).

2. **Humeroradial articulation:** is between the capitulum of the humerus and the head of the radius. The capitulum fits into the slightly cupped surface of the round head of the radius. The radial head rotates during movements of pronation and supination of the forearm.

3. **The proximal radioulnar joint:** is between the head of the radius and the radial notch of the proximal ulna. This joint permits rotation of the radius about the ulna while carring out movements of pronation and supination of the forearm.

The elbow joint is stable because of the hinge-like arrangement of the humeroulnar articulation. In addition, the joint is stabilized by the fibrous capsule and the medial and lateral collateral ligaments on both sides of the joint.

The elbow can be flexed or extended. The main flexor is the brachialis muscle and the main extensor is the triceps muscle.

THE HIP JOINT

The hip joint is a ball-and-socket-type of synovial joint between the globular head of the femur and the cup-like acetabulum of the hip bone. The head of the femur is almost completely covered by cartilage. The cartilage of the acetabulum is horseshoe-shaped and part of the acetabulum is not covered with cartilage at all. The depth of the acetabulum is increased by the acetabulum labrum, a fibrous structure attached to the bony rim of the acetabulum.

The movements of the hip joint are flexion and extension, adduction and abduction, external rotation, and internal rotation and circumduction. The hip joint is a very strong and stable joint. The articulating bones are united by a dense thick fibrous capsule strengthened by strong ligaments. The powerful muscles that surround the joint also add to its stability.

THE ANKLE JOINT

The ankle joint is a hinge-type synovial joint between the distal ends of the tibia and fibula and the superior part of the talus. The inferior ends of the tibia and fibula form a deep socket or box-like mortise into which the superior part of the talus fits.

The fibula has an articular surface on the medial aspect of the malleolus, which articu-lates with the lateral surface of the talus. The tibia has its articular surface on the inferior surface and the lateral aspect of the malleolus, which articulates with the superior and medial surfaces of the talus. The movements of the ankle joint are dorsiflexion and plantarflexion (see Fig 9.37).

The stability of the ankle joint is due to its bony arrangement and strong collateral ligaments. The **deltoid ligament** attaches the medial malleolus to the tarsal bones (Fig. 9.78). The **lateral ligaments** attach the lateral malleo-slus to the talus and calcaneus. The distal fibula and tibia are united by strong ligaments. A sprained ankle results from twisting the weight-bearing foot and results in damage to the lateral ligaments (Fig. 9.79).

THE KNEE JOINT

The knee joint consists of two different articulations:

1. the **tibiofemoral articulation** between the large curved condyles of the femur and the superior surface of the tibial condyles.
2. the **patellofemoral articulation** between the patella and the inferior anterior surface of the femur.

On the superior surface of each, the tibial condyle is an articular area for the correspond-ing femoral condyle. These articular areas are called medial and lateral **tibial plateaus**.

The medial and lateral menisci are cresentic plates of cartilage that lie on the articular surface of the tibia (Fig 9.80). The menisci serve several functions, all of which play important roles in maintaining a properly functioning knee joint. These include weight

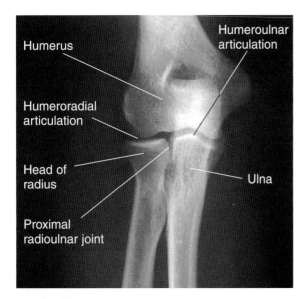

Humerus

Humeroulnar articulation

Humeroradial articulation

Head of radius

Ulna

Proximal radioulnar joint

X-ray of the elbow: anterior view

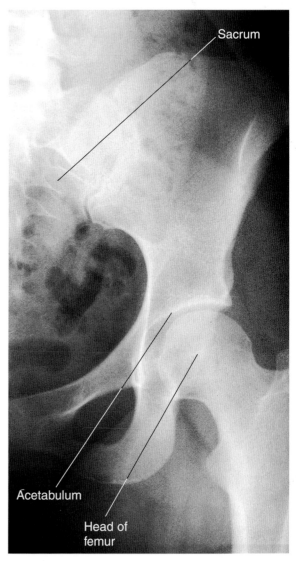

Sacrum

Acetabulum

Head of femur

X-ray of the hip: anterior view

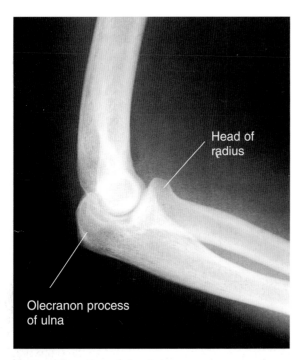

Head of radius

Olecranon process of ulna

X-ray of the elbow: lateral view

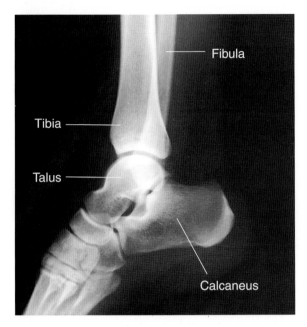

X-ray of the ankle: lateral view

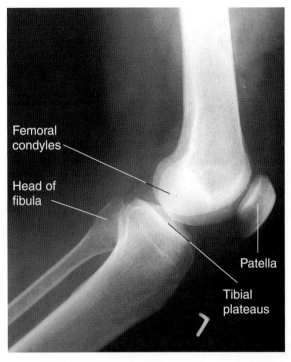

X-ray of the knee: lateral view

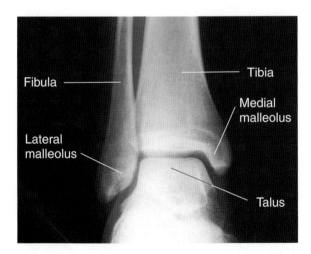

X-ray of the ankle: anterior view

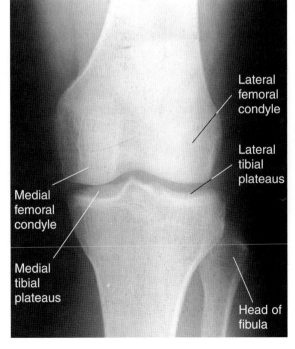

X-ray of the knee: anterior view

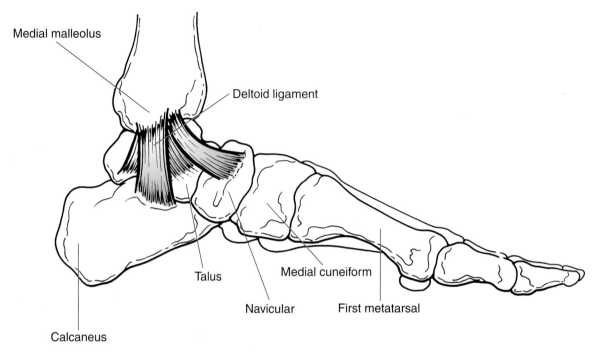

Medial malleolus

Deltoid ligament

Talus

Medial cuneiform

Navicular

First metatarsal

Calcaneus

Figure 9.78   Medial view of the ankle showing the deltoid ligament.

bearing and load distribution, shock absorption and maintenance of joint stability.

The patella is a sesamoid bone. The quadriceps tendon inserts into its superior pole and the patellar tendon emerges from its inferior pole and inserts into the tibial tuberosity (Fig. 9.81). The patella slides on the patellar surface of the distal femur during flexion and extension of the knee. The patellar surface is created by the medial and lateral femoral condyles, which blend with each other anteriorly. The patella plays a major role facilitating the function of the quadriceps muscle by increasing the moment arm, thus increasing quadriceps muscle force by 50%. Furthermore, the patella allows the extensor mechanism to glide smoothly due to the minimal friction between the articular surfaces of the patella and the patellar surface of the femur. The patella also protects the knee joint.

Stability of the knee joint is provided by surrounding soft tissue structures, which can be separated to static and dynamic restrains. The static restrains consist of the fibrous capsule and four major ligaments. The **fibular collateral ligament** extends from the lateral femoral condyle to the head of the fibula, and prevents the tibia from moving to the medial side (see Fig. 9.81). The **medial collateral ligament** extends from the medial femoral condyle to the medial tibial condyle, and prevents the tibia from moving laterally (see Fig. 9.82). Within the knee joint are two ligaments that run from the superior surface of

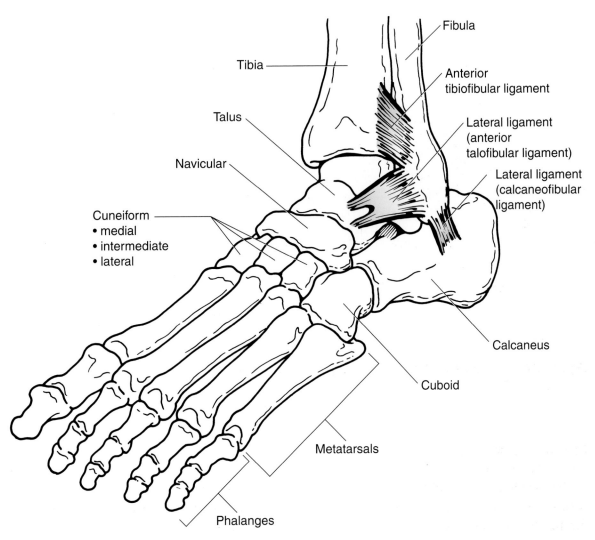

Figure 9.79 Lateral view of the ankle showing the lateral ligaments (anterior talofibular and calcaneofibular) and the anterior distal tibiofibular ligament.

the tibia to the inferior surface of the femur. These two ligaments cross over each other and are therefore called cruciate ligaments. The **anterior cruciate ligament** arises from the anterior part of the superior surface of the tibia and extends superiorly and posteriorly to attach to the posterior aspect of the lateral femoral condyle (Figs 9.82 and 9.83). The anterior cruciate ligament prevents the tibia from moving anteriorly. The **posterior cruciate ligament** arises from the posterior superior aspect of the tibia and extends superiorly and anteriorly to attach to the anterior aspect of the medial femoral condyle (Fig. 9.84). The

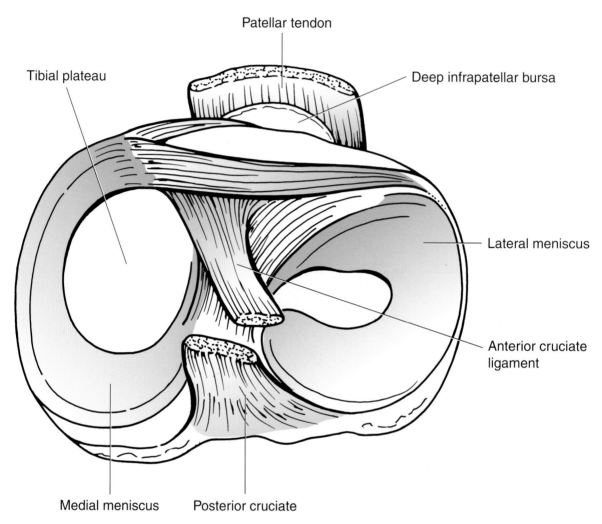

Patellar tendon

Tibial plateau

Deep infrapatellar bursa

Lateral meniscus

Anterior cruciate ligament

Medial meniscus

Posterior cruciate

Figure 9.80 Superior view of the tibial plateaus showing the menisci and the cruciate ligaments.

posterior cruciate ligament prevents the tibia from moving posteriorly. The dynamic stabilizers consist of the surrounding muscles, especially the quadriceps. The knee permits flexion and extension and some degree of rotation. The soft tissues that surrounds the knee prevent it from hyperextension above 180°.

BLOOD VESSELS AND NERVES OF THE LIMBS

Arteries of the upper limb

The **subclavian artery** arises from the arch of the aorta, passes betrween the first rib and the clavicle, and enters the axilla. From the lower

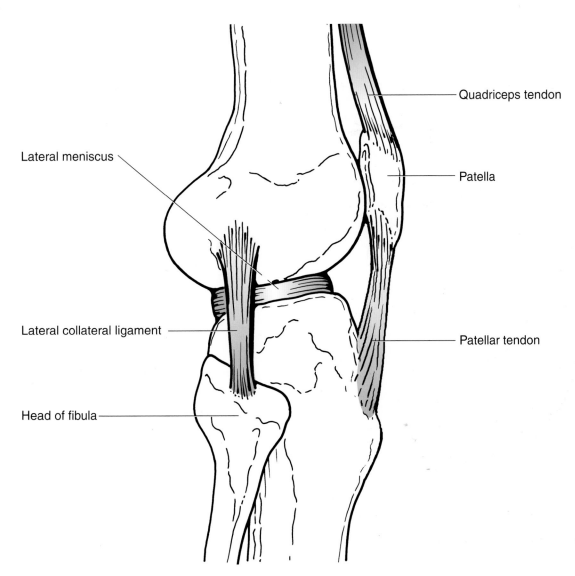

Figure 9.81   Lateral view of the knee.

border of the first rib, it becomes the **axillary artery** (Fig. 9.85).

The axillary artery runs through the axilla towards the arm and, in turn, becomes the **brachial artery** when it passes the lower border of the teres major muscle.

The brachial artery passes down the upper arm, along its medial side, to the lower end of the arm across the front of the elbow joint, where it divides into two vessels – the **radial artery** and the **ulnar artery**.

The **ulnar artery** passes down the medial side of the forearm underneath the flexor digitorum superficialis muscle and reaches the hand on the medial side of the wrist.

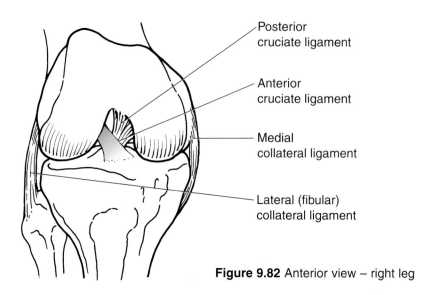

Posterior cruciate ligament

Anterior cruciate ligament

Medial collateral ligament

Lateral (fibular) collateral ligament

Figure 9.82 Anterior view – right leg

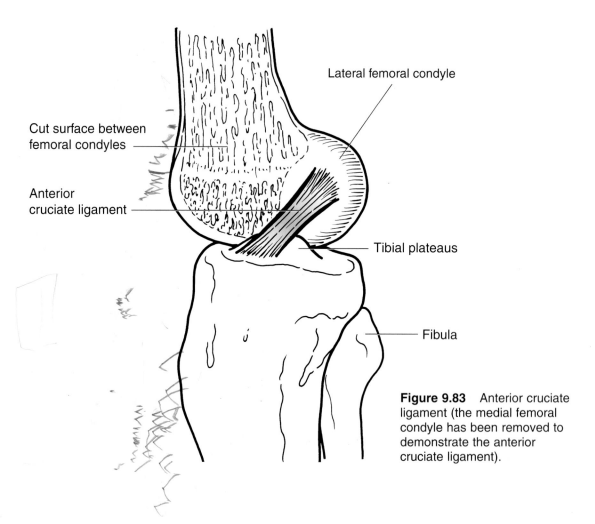

Lateral femoral condyle

Cut surface between femoral condyles

Anterior cruciate ligament

Tibial plateaus

Fibula

Figure 9.83 Anterior cruciate ligament (the medial femoral condyle has been removed to demonstrate the anterior cruciate ligament).

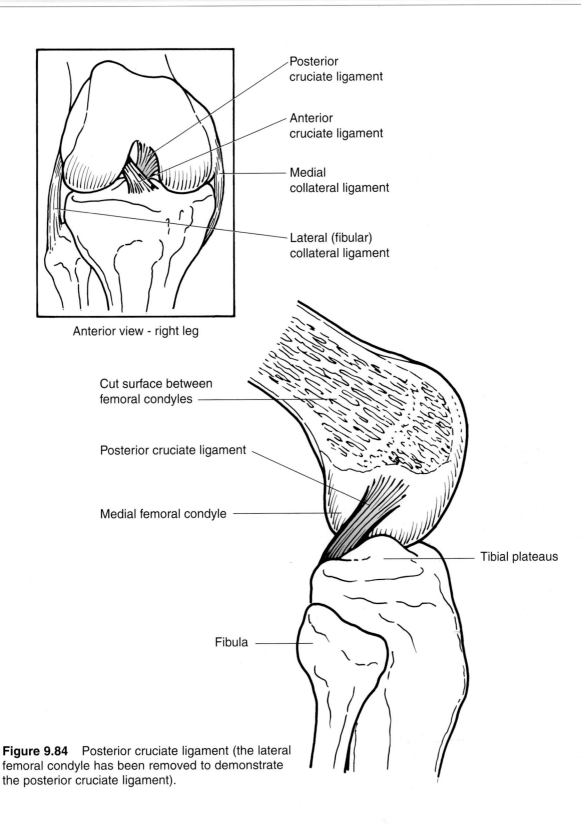

Posterior
cruciate ligament

Anterior
cruciate ligament

Medial
collateral ligament

Lateral (fibular)
collateral ligament

Anterior view - right leg

Cut surface between
femoral condyles

Posterior cruciate ligament

Medial femoral condyle

Tibial plateaus

Fibula

Figure 9.84 Posterior cruciate ligament (the lateral femoral condyle has been removed to demonstrate the posterior cruciate ligament).

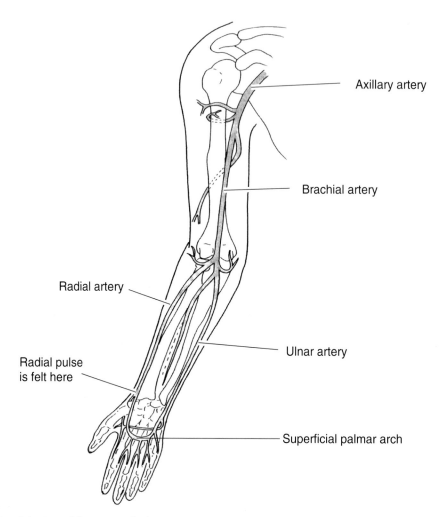

Figure 9.85 Arteries of the upper limb.

The **radial artery** passes down the lateral side of the forearm underneath the brachioradialis muscle and reaches the hand on the lateral side of the wrist. In the hand, the radial and ulnar arteries join to form two arterial arches – the **deep palmar arch** and the **superficial palmar arch**.

The arteries described above are the major trunks, but all along their route they send off branches to provide blood to the tissues of the arm.

The brachial artery pulse can be felt at the medial side of the upper arm, and in the front of the elbow. The radial artery pulse can be felt at the lateral side of the wrist and, to a lesser extent, the ulnar artery pulse can be felt on the medial side of the wrist.

Veins of the upper limb

The blood drains from the upper limb by a series of deep veins that run alongside the arteries described above, and by a series of superficial veins. The superficial veins can be quite easily seen and felt under the skin, and these are the veins that are usually punctured to provide blood samples.

Arteries of the lower limb

The abdominal aorta at the level of the fourth lumbar vertebra divides into two large arteries called the left and right **common iliac arteries**. Each common iliac artery becomes the **external iliac artery**, which passes down toward the groin and, as it enters the thigh, it becomes the **femoral artery** (Fig. 9.86).

The femoral artery passes down the thigh medial to the femur, anterior to the adductor longus muscle. At the lower end of the thigh, it passes behind the knee and becomes the **popliteal artery**. At the upper part of the thigh, the femoral artery gives off a large branch called the **profunda femoris artery**, which supplies blood to the thigh muscles.

The popliteal artery divides below the knee into three arteries: the **posterior tibial artery**, the **anterior tibial artery** and the **peroneal artery**. The posterior tibial artery descends between the soleus and tibialis posterior muscles, passes behind the medial malleolus at the lower end of the tibia and then divides into two arteries that supply the foot – the **medial** and **lateral plantar arteries**.

The anterior tibial artery descends in the anterior muscle compartment of the leg, anterior to the interosseous membrane (the ligamentous sheet that connects the tibia and fibula). At the ankle, it becomes the **dorsalis pedis artery** which runs along the medial side of the dorsum (back) of the foot.

The pulses in various arteries can be felt: the femoral artery in the groin, the popliteal artery at the back of the knee, the posterior tibial artery behind the medial malleolus, and the dorsalis pedis artery on the top (dorsum) of the foot.

Nerves of the upper limb

The spinal nerves C5, C6, C7, C8 and T1 interconnect to form a complex 'interchange' called the **brachial plexus** (Fig. 9.87). The brachial plexus is situated in the neck and axilla, and from it emerge the nerves to the chest wall, the back, the shoulder and the arm. These nerves contain motor axons that activate the skeletal muscles, sensory axons that transmit sensations from the skin and other organs (e.g. muscles, joints) and axons of the autonomic system, which activate smooth muscle in the blood vessel walls and the sweat glands.

The four major nerves in the arm are the median nerve, the ulnar nerve, the radial nerve and the musculocutaneous nerve.

The **median nerve** passes down the medial side of the arm, and at the distal end of the upper arm, passes across the front of the elbow. It then passes down the center of the forearm between the flexor digitorum superficialis and the flexor digitorum profundus muscles to reach the hand. At the wrist, it passes underneath a band of connective tissue in the front of the wrist, called the **flexor retinaculum**, underneath which the flexor tendons heading toward the fingers also pass. In the palm of the hand, the median nerve divides into a number of branches called the **digital nerves**, which innervate the fingers.

In general, the median nerve innervates the flexor muscles of the hand and fingers, and

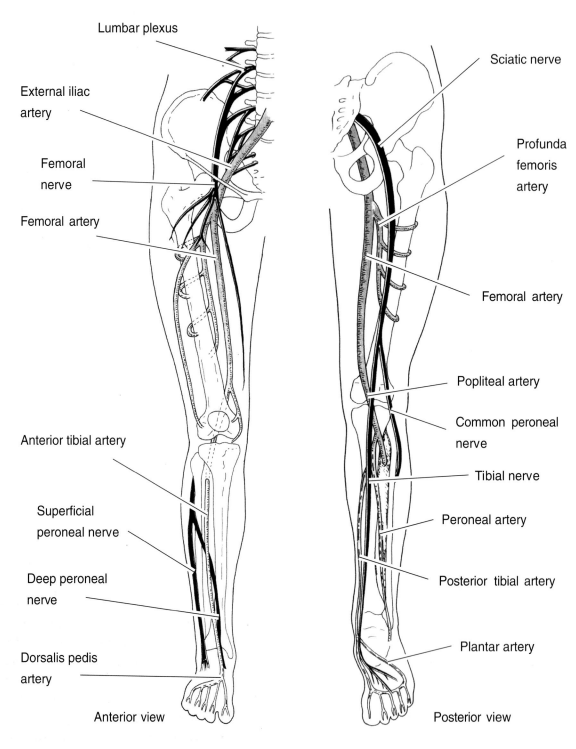

Lumbar plexus

External iliac artery

Femoral nerve

Femoral artery

Anterior tibial artery

Superficial peroneal nerve

Deep peroneal nerve

Dorsalis pedis artery

Anterior view

Sciatic nerve

Profunda femoris artery

Femoral artery

Popliteal artery

Common peroneal nerve

Tibial nerve

Peroneal artery

Posterior tibial artery

Plantar artery

Posterior view

Figure 9.86   Arteries and nerves of the lower limb.

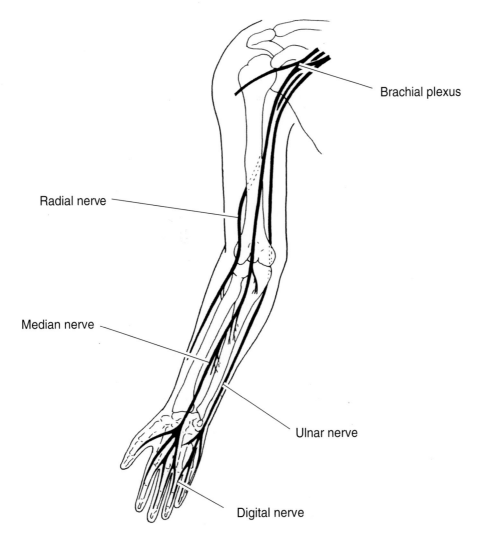

Figure 9.87   Nerves of the upper limb.

transmits sensation from the skin of the thumb, index, middle and the lateral half of the ring finger.

The **ulnar nerve** passes down the medial side of the upper arm and behind the medial epicondyle of the elbow, where it is immediately underneath the skin and can be felt. A blow at this point (the 'funny bone') causes a tingling sensation and is quite painful. In the forearm, the ulnar nerve passes down the medial side between the flexor digitorum superficialis and flexor digitorum profundus muscles, and enters the hand on its medial side. In the hand, it divides into a number of branches called the **digital nerves**, which innervate the fingers.

The ulnar nerve innervates the portions of the flexor carpi ulnaris and flexor digitorum profundus related to the ring and little fingers, as well as the internal muscles of the hand. It transmits sensation from the skin of the little finger and the medial half of the ring finger. Injury to the ulnar nerve will affect sensation, and cause tingling in those areas.

The **radial nerve** passes down the back of the upper arm between the lateral and medial heads of the triceps muscle. At the elbow, it passes in front of the lateral epicondyle and splits into two branches. One sensory branch passes underneath the brachioradialis muscle and, in the lower third of the forearm, it passes into the posterior compartment of the forearm muscles and continues on to the back of the hand. The second motor branch passes into the posterior compartment of the forearm muscles, immediately below the elbow, and continues down to the wrist. The radial nerve innervates the triceps muscle and the extensor muscles of the hand and fingers, and transmits sensation from the skin of the back and lateral side of the hand.

The **musculocutaneous nerve** passes between the biceps and brachialis muscles in the upper arm. At the elbow, it is lateral to the biceps tendon and, in the forearm, it becomes a superficial sensory nerve that runs under the skin on the lateral side of the forearm to the base of the thumb.

The musculocutaneous nerve supplies the biceps and brachialis muscles and transmits sensation from the skin of the lateral side of the forearm.

Nerves of the lower limb

The major nerves in the lower limb are the **sciatic nerve** (which is made up of the **tibial nerve** and the **common peroneal nerve**), the **femoral nerve** and the **obturator nerve** (see Fig. 9.86).

As the spinal nerves emerge from the vertebral column, they interconnect to form a series of complex 'interchanges' called the **lumbar plexus** and the **sacral plexus**, similar to the brachial plexus in the upper limb. The sciatic nerve is the largest nerve in the body and is formed in the pelvis by nerve fibers that originate in the spinal nerves L4, L5, S1, S2 and S3.

The sciatic nerve emerges from the back of the pelvis, passes down the buttock, underneath the gluteus maximus muscle, and down the back of the thigh between the adductor magnus and biceps femoris muscles. In the lower third of the thigh, the sciatic nerve divides into two major branches – the **tibial nerve** and the **common peroneal nerve**.

The tibial nerve runs behind the knee next to the popliteal artery, passes down the leg in the posterior muscle compartment, behind the medial malleolus of the tibia and finally divides into the **plantar nerves** of the foot. The tibial nerve innervates the muscles of the posterior compartment of the thigh (the hamstring muscles) and the calf muscles. Injury to the tibial nerve affects flexion of the knee and plantarflexion of the foot.

The common peroneal nerve, once it has branched off from the sciatic nerve (halfway down the thigh), passes down the lower third of the thigh to the lateral side of the knee, where it divides into two branches – the **deep peroneal nerve** and the **superficial peroneal nerve**. The deep peroneal nerve passes down the lower leg in the anterior compartment and reaches the dorsum (top) of the foot. The superficial peroneal nerve descends in the lateral compartment of the calf muscles and reaches the dorsum of the foot, where it is very superficial and can be felt beneath the skin.

The superficial peroneal nerve innervates the peroneal muscles and transmits sensation from the dorsum of the foot. Injury to the superficial peroneal nerve affects eversion of the foot. The deep peroneal nerve innervates the muscles of the anterior compartment of the lower leg and injury affects dorsiflexion of the foot.

The **femoral nerve** is formed by nerve fibers that originate in the spinal nerves L2, L3 and L4. It passes through the pelvis lateral to the psoas muscle and enters the groin on the lateral side of the femoral artery. Approximately 4 cm below the groin it divides into a number of motor and sensory branches. The femoral nerve innervates the muscles of the anterior compartment of the thigh. Injury to it affects extension of the knee.

The **obturator nerve** is formed by nerve fibers originating in the spinal nerves L2, L3 and L4. It emerges from the pelvis, passes through the obturator foramen and innervates the muscles in the medial compartment of the thigh. It also transmits sensation from the hip joint and knee. Injury to the obturator nerve affects adduction of the thigh.

Diseases of the locomotor system

LOW BACK PAIN

Low back pain is one of the most common medical problems in the Western world. Approximately 80% of the population suffers from it at least once during their life. In the United States, low back pain is the most common cause of time off work in people under the age of 45 and costs the American economy $16 billion annually.

In most cases, low back pain originates in the intervertebral joints and the back muscles. In only a minority of cases can an actual anatomic abnormality be demonstrated.

Low back pain tends to resolve on its own without treatment. In 50% of cases it resolves within a week; in 90% of cases it resolves within a month; and in only 10% of cases does it become chronic. These statistics show that low back pain is usually self-limiting and probably does not require treatment! These facts should be kept in mind when assessing the degree of effectiveness of various treatments for low back pain.

Certain occupations have an increased risk of developing low back pain. (e.g. baggage porters, secretaries, nurses and drivers). Porters and nurses put considerable pressure on the spinal column and back muscles by carrying heavy loads; secretaries exert pressure on the spine by prolonged sitting. Drivers sit for prolonged periods of time and engine vibrations can jar and damage the spinal column. Interestingly, smoking is a risk factor for the development of back pain, probably bacause of a decrease in the supply of oxygen to the intervertebral discs.

Causes of low back pain

Degeneration of the discs and intervertebral joints

Over time, the intervertebral disc undergoes a process of aging: the fluid content diminishes (the disc dries out) and the disc becomes thinner. As the thickness of the intervertebral discs contributes approximately one-quarter of the height of the spinal column, this degeneration causes a significant loss of height.

Disc degeneration produces back pain in several ways. It affects the ability of the disc to absorb shocks and, as a result, the intervertebral joints and the spinal column itself become unstable. Although this process is not limited to the lower back area, this is where the pain is usually felt, as most of the body weight is borne by the lower spine.

Instability of the spine leads to inflammation of the joints and the appearance of tiny bony outgrowths, called **osteophytes**, around the joints. These osteophytes can press on adjacent nerves and cause pain. Inflammation of the joints in itself also causes pain, probably due to nerve irritation.

Narrowing of the discs brings the vertebrae nearer together, resulting in narrowing of the openings between them (the intervertebral foramina), which, in turn, produces compression (pinching) of the nerves that emerge from the foramina.

The general term for the degenerative processes in the spine is **spondylosis**. It is important to note that in many cases severe degenerative changes can be seen in spinal X-rays of someone who has no low back pain at all. Conversely, a person with severe low back pain might have normal spinal X-rays. In such cases, presumably there are anatomic changes that are too small to show up in X-ray, but can cause pain.

Disc herniation

The intervertebral disc is composed of a peripheral fibrous ring and a central gel (see p. 114 and Fig. 9.13). As a result of weakening caused by aging or by extreme pressure on the disc in a young person (e.g. when lifting a heavy weight or carrying out some stressful movement), the fibrous ring can rupture. The most common site of such rupture is the intervertebral disc between the fourth and fifth lumbar vertebrae, or between the fifth lumbar vertebra and the sacrum.

As a result of the rupture, the gel 'escapes' from the disc, usually in a posterior or lateral direction, and might press on a spinal nerve nearby. It might also cause a chemical irritation of the nerve. The end result is that the patient feels pain in the lower back; this pain radiates down the leg on the side of the rupture (herniation). The leg pain results from irritation of the nerve that innervates the leg. The actual site of the disc rupture determines the area of the leg where the pain is felt.

The patient will usually limp and will tend to lean the body towards the side opposite to that of the disc herniation in an attempt to

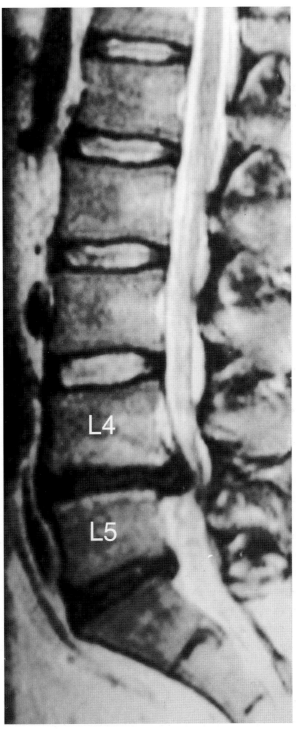

MRI image of lumbar spine showing herniation of L4–L5 disc.

relieve the pressure on the nerve. There could also be some muscular weakness of the painful leg, reduced skin sensation or a feeling of 'pins and needles'. The pain of a disc herniation ranges from relatively mild discomfort, which allows the patient to continue normal activities, to extremely severe pain, confining the patient to bed and causing much distress.

If the gel escapes in a posterior direction it will press directly on the spinal cord. In this case, the low back pain will be associated with a sensation of 'pins and needles' in the groin as well as loss of control over the bladder and bowel. This constitutes a medical emergency known as the **cauda equina syndrome**, which requires immediate surgery to relieve the pressure on the spinal cord. Any delay in treatment could result in the patient being paralyzed downwards from the level of the herniation.

The diagnosis of disc herniation is based on the history, the physical examination and imaging techniques such as CT or MRI.

Disc herniation is treated surgically by removal of the ruptured disc. Although this relieves the symptoms in the short term, it is a dangerous procedure, with significant potential risks, and does not guarantee long-term recovery. It is performed only on patients who are in severe pain, who have not responded to other forms of treatment for at least 6 weeks and in whom progressive neurologic signs appear, such as muscle weakness. The alternatives to surgery are physiotherapy, analgesic and anti-inflammatory medications, and bed rest.

Pain arising from the back muscles

The back muscles form a complex anatomic structure. In most cases, we do not know the precise mechanisms that cause pain arising from these muscles. The back muscles are intimately related, both anatomically and functionally, to the system of the vertebrae, the intervertebral joints and the ligaments of the back. It is quite possible that a problem in one of those components can cause problems in the others.

There are several known situations that are related to the pain in the lower back muscles:

Obesity, pregnancy and weakness of the abdominal muscles. As the back muscles are the antagonists of the abdominal muscles (the deep back muscles cause extension of the spine and the abdominal muscles cause flexion), weakness of the abdominal muscles could place an extra burden on the back muscles, resulting in pain. In obesity and in pregnancy, the extra weight in the front of the abdomen creates lordosis of the spine, again placing an extra burden on the back muscles.

Physical exertion, sudden movements, or lifting a heavy weight. All these can cause small, painful tears in the back muscles.

Trigger points. Sometimes one can feel tender, tense areas in the back muscles (**'trigger points'**). The exact reason for this phenomenon is not known but it could perhaps be associated with psychological stress.

Pain arising from a vertebral body

Osteoporotic fractures. Fractures of vertebral bodies are seen mainly in post-menopausal women as a result of **osteoporosis**. Osteoporosis, which occurs with increasing frequency after the menopause, causes the bone density to diminish, and the bone to become weaker. The weight of the body pressing on the weakened vertebral bodies compresses them, causing a crush fracture. If this occurs suddenly, such as following the lifting of a heavy weight, there is an instant severe pain, as well as loss of height. An X-ray will clearly show the collapsed vertebra. This does not usually, incapacitate the patient for very long and the pain will subside following a period of rest.

Cancer.   Many types of cancer metastasize (seed cancerous cells) to the vertebrae, such as cancer of the prostate in men, and breast cancer in women. Metastases destroy the vertebral body and cause chronic, unremitting pain. In fact, back pain can sometimes be the first symptom of such cancer.

Bacterial infection of the vertebrae. This is a process known as **osteomyelitis**, in which bacteria invade the body of the vertebra and cause severe back pain, accompanied by fever and weakness.

Pain arising from internal organs. Inflammation in the ovaries, a kidney tumor, and other such diseases of abdominal or pelvic organs can present as backache.

Psychological   causes.   There   is significant correlation between anxiety or depression and the presence of backache, although the underlying mechanism is unknown.

There are often support facilities, financial provision and compensation for people suffering back pain. To some extent, these provide a disincentive for complete rehabilitation. Such 'secondary gain' can have a very significant effect (whether conscious or subconscious) on the severity and duration of the pain, as well as on compliance with treatment.

Treatment of back pain

Rest

Lying in bed decreases the pressure on the nerves, in the case of a disc prolapse, and also provides rest for the back muscles. Remember that back pain arising from a disc or from the muscles usually resolves on its own with time. In practice, most people who have severe back pain do rest in bed, simply because they are unable to walk.

Surgery for disc herniation

In an operation known as a **discectomy**, the herniated disc is removed. The operation is carried out in those cases where the patient is suffering severely and does not respond to other treatment, or where there are signs of progressive neurologic deficit (see p. 188).

Medications

The commonly used medications are analgesics (pain killers), anti-inflammatory medications, muscle relaxants and antidepressants.

Injections

Analgesics   and   corticosteroids   (anti-inflammatory) drugs can be injected directly into the painful back muscles or to the epidural space of the spine.

Brace

This treatment is not recommended because it weakens the back muscles and the pain becomes worse once the brace is removed.

Other treatments

These include chiropractic, shiatsu, reflexology, physiotherapy and treatment by application of heat and cold to the back.

The fact that there are so many types of treatment for low back pain (and not all of them have been listed above) is understandable if one remembers the episodic nature of the problem. The pain occurs in attacks, which in most cases last for less than 1 month even without any treatment at all. Thus a treatment might be seen as being effective when, in fact, improvement would have occurred on its own anyway.

OSTEOPOROSIS

Bone is constantly undergoing a process of destruction and rebuilding. The cells that are responsible for the breakdown of bone are called **osteoclasts**, which 'drill' microscopic channels in the bone. The production of new bone is carried out by special cells called **osteoblasts**, which burrow into these channels and refill them with bone.

In childhood, the rate of bone production is greater than the rate of destruction, so the bones grow. At about the age of 30, the bone mass (amount of bone) in the body is at its maximum (**peak bone mass**). After 30, the rate of destruction exceeds that of production and the bone gradually starts to lose mass at a rate of 0.7% per year.

Bone density is defined as the bone mass per unit of bone volume. The strength of a bone depends on its density, such that the denser a bone, the stronger it is. The natural process of decreasing bone mass leads to a decrease in bone density and to weakening of the bone. **Osteoporosis** refers to a decrease in bone density that causes weakening of the bone and increases its risk of fracture. The common lay term 'calcium loss' is not accurate because in osteoporosis, the calcium content of the bone is not affected.

The greater the peak bone mass (around age 30), the lower the chance that, over the years, the bones will become weak to the point of fracture.

The peak bone mass depends on various factors such as heredity, nutrition and physical exercise. Patients with osteoporosis can be divided into three groups:

1. women in the first decade of their menopause
2. the elderly
3. people with diseases that result in osteoporosis.

Women in the first decade of their menopause

During this period there is a marked acceleration of loss of bone density. The precise reason for this is unclear but it is thought to involve a decrease in levels of the hormone **estrogen**. The main component of the bone that is affected is the spongy bone.

The actual bones that are most affected are the vertebral bodies. As the vertebral bodies carry most of the body weight, microscopic fractures often appear, which can lead to collapse. Clinically, the patient feels a severe pain in the back following some movement or after lifting a heavy weight, followed by a loss of height of 1–2 cm.

Elderly men and women

It is in old age that the process of osteoporosis becomes most clinically manifest. Women are affected more than men because they lose more bone mass due to the menopause. In the elderly, it is mainly compact bone that is affected and the common fracture sites are the neck and the trochanteric area of the femur (Fig. 10.1), the distal radius (called a **Colles' fracture**) and the proximal humerus. These fractures can take a long time to heal and cause ongoing problems. In the past, a fracture of the proximal femur was treated by putting the patient in bed until healing occurred. However, patients often died as a result of the prolonged immobilization or from complications such as pneumonia, or pulmonary embolus. Today, this fracture is treated by immediate surgery and prompt mobilization, sometimes on the following day.

Osteoporosis that is secondary to other illnesses or due to medications

Certain diseases produce accelerated bone density loss: hyperparathyroidism (excessive secretion of parathyroid hormone), hyperthyroidism (excessive secretion of thyroid hormone), hypothyroidism (inadequate secretion of thyroid hormone) and diabetes. Some medications, notably corticosteroids, or substances such as alcohol, can also accelerate the process of bone density loss.

Prevention

Administration of the female sex hormone, estrogen, to postmenopausal women has been shown to be an effective preventive treatment for postmenopausal loss of bone density. The treatment does not interfere with the natural, constant turnover of bone that occurs in both men and women.

Physical exercise (weight-bearing exercise – not swimming) slows down the process of loss of bone density, and is also recommended for other reasons, such as prevention of cardiovascular disease. Various medications, such as calcium, Vitamin D and especially drugs that inhibit osteoclasts, appear to have some effect, particularly when combined.

OSTEOMALACIA AND RICKETS

Osteomalacia is a disease involving the mineralization of bones. Mineralization refers to the

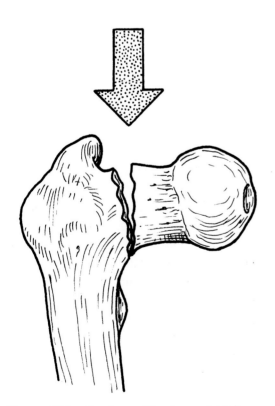

Figure 10.1   Fracture of the femoral neck.

incorporation of mineral (calcium and phosphorus) into the intercellular matrix of bone.

In a growing child, new bone is formed mainly in the area of the growth plate (a sheet of cartilage). Mineralization occurs some time after as bone growth. In adults, there is a constant process of destruction and rebuilding of bone (by the osteoclasts and the osteoblasts). In this process, the mineralization of the new bone also occurs a short time after it has been laid down.

The process of mineralization requires **vitamin D**, a lipid substance present in certain foodstuffs such as fish and grains, as well as in vitamin D-enriched milk products. In addition, the body also itself manufactures vitamin D from cholesterol. The first step in the production of vitamin D takes place in the skin and requires sunlight. In the skin, cholesterol is converted into a substance that enters the bloodstream and is carried to the liver, where it undergoes a further chemical change. From there, it circulates in the bloodstream until it reaches the kidney, where it is converted to the final substance – active vitamin D. Vitamin D is required in the absorption of calcium and phosphorus in the intestine and for the mineralization of bone.

A deficiency of vitamin D can arise if nutritional deficiency is combined with inadequate exposure to sunlight. In this way, both sources of vitamin D – the nutritional and the intrinsic production within the body – are affected. Various diseases, such as certain kidney diseases, can also interfere with the production of vitamin D.

A lack of vitamin D in children gives rise to the disease known as **rickets**. In rickets, the bone that is formed remains soft because it is not mineralized. The clinical features include bowing of the legs (because they are unable to support the body weight), widening of the costochondral junctions of the ribs ('the rachitic rosary'), and the occurrence of soft areas in the skull, with delay in closure of the fontanelles.

In adults, vitamin D deficiency results in a condition known as **osteomalacia** (from the Greek *osteo* = bone and *malakia* = softness), in which pathologic fractures occur because of the weak bone. The treatment involves the administration of vitamin D.

BONE INFECTION

Infection of bone is called **osteomyelitis** and is nearly always caused by bacteria (in most cases by staphylococci). There are several ways in which bacteria can invade bones:

- via the bloodstream
- during an operation on a bone or following an open fracture
- from neighboring infected soft tissue.

Via the bloodstream ('hematogenous spread'). The blood flow in bones is slow, mainly in the region between the ends and the shaft of long bones (metaphysis). This means that bacteria that do happen to be in the blood tend to become 'trapped' in the bone and cause infection. Osteomyelitis resulting from hematogenous spread (in the bloodstream) usually occurs in the long bones in children and in the vertebral bodies in adults. The bacteria that invade the bone from the blood destroy the bone and produce necrotic areas in the bone.

Direct introduction during an operation or following a fracture. During orthopedic surgery, extreme caution must be taken to maintain a sterile environment in order to prevent infection.

An open fracture (a fracture open to the exterior) must be irrigated copiously, removing any necrotic tissue, and treated with antibiotics to prevent the development of infection. Yet, despite such precautions, osteomyelitis may occasionally occur.

Direct spread from infected soft tissues near a bone.   A deep and infected skin ulcer can contaminate bone and cause osteomyelitis.

The clinical features of osteomyelitis include a rise in body temperature, weakness, and pain and warmth in the infected area.

Treatment involves intravenous antibiotics for prolonged periods and sometimes, if the infection results in necrotic bone, an operation to remove the dead bone tissue.

Inadequate treatment of osteomyelitis can lead to the development of chronic infection. This type of infection is very difficult to treat and can continue for years. In such cases, antibiotic treatment does not help because there is a large necrotic area in the bone that does not receive any blood supply, so that the antibiotic cannot reach its target. Surgical treatment is also problematic because, in some cases, excision of all of the necrotic bone would involve removing a large amount of bone.

FOOT PAIN

Pain in the foot is a much less common complaint than low back pain.

The structure of the foot is such that in most cases it stands up remarkably well to the stresses applied to it. Nevertheless, there are some foot conditions that can result in significant pain.

Flat foot

This is also known as **pes planus**. In most cases, the medial arch of the foot flattens only when there is weight on it, and the basic structure of the foot is normal. In a small minority of cases, the flat foot is rigid rather than flexible, as a result of an abnormality of the bony structure itself. In infants, there is a fat pad in the area of the medial arch, so that all babies look as if they have flat feet, although the skeletal structure is, in fact, normal.

In some cases, the flat arch causes pain. However, it must be stressed that there are many people with strikingly flat feet who suffer no foot pain.

The treatment is by means of appropriately shaped arch supports that support the medial arch of the foot. In rare cases where the flat foot is caused by an actual bony abnormality (rigid flat foot), surgery might be needed to correct it.

High arch

This situation in which the medial arch is excessively high is called **pes cavus**. In most cases it is seen in healthy people, symmetrically in both feet, and with no anatomic abnormality. Not everybody with pes cavus has pain in the foot. Those cases that are painful can be treated by a medial arch support.

Occasionally, a high arch is the result of a neurologic abnormality, such as cerebral palsy or polio, which affects the muscles of the foot. These situations may require surgery.

Metatarsalgia

The weight of the body is supported at the end of the calcaneus (heelbone) and the distal end of the metatarsal bones. If for some reason, more weight is transferred to one or more of the metatarsal heads (usually the second and third metatarsals) painful calluses form over them. This is referred to as **metatarsalgia**. An appropriate arch support can be used to lessen the pressure on the painful areas.

Heel spur

A heel spur usually occurs in people who are overweight, in sprinters or in people who stand for long periods. The pain is in the plantar (sole) surface of the foot, in the area of the heel. It usually occurs when getting out of bed in the morning, or after resting for a long time.

The pain is due to inflammation in the ligament known as the **plantar fascia** (or **plantar aponeurosis**). This ligament is connected posteriorly to the plantar surface of the back of the calcaneus and anteriorly to the bases of the toes. It plays an important role in maintaining the medial arch of the foot. If this ligament becomes stretched because of trauma or prolonged physical exertion, small tears and inflammation occur at its point of attachment to the calcaneus. As a result, a tiny bony spur grows out of the calcaneus, hence the name 'heel spur'. Applying weight to the foot after a period of rest irritates the inflamed area and causes pain. The condition can be treated by an appropriate arch support or by injecting steroids into the area. As a last resort, surgery can be performed.

Hallux valgus

This condition is particularly common in women and is related to wearing narrow shoes that press at the sides of the front of the foot, as well as having a hereditary component. As the condition develops, the bones of the great toe tend to become angled laterally and the first metatarsal becomes angled medially. In the region of the joint between the first metatarsal and the proximal phalanx (the first metatarsophalangeal joint), a bony protuberance called a **bunion** develops. Narrow shoes press on this protuberance, causing it to become red and painful.

Treatment consists of changing to a wider shoe and, in severe cases, surgery might be needed to correct the deformity.

Hallux rigidus

Several joint disorders affect the first metatarsophalangeal joint (the joint between the first metatarsal and the proximal phalanx). These can affect extension of the joint and walking becomes painful, because, as the heel is raised during walking, the big toe must extend (bend upwards).

Treatment consists of appropriate shoes with a rigid sole that prevents extension of the big toe. Surgery can also be used.

OSTEOARTHRITIS

Osteoarthritis is a disease of the joints caused by damage to the articular cartilage. In most cases, it occurs in older patients and the cause of the damage to the cartilage is not known. In a minority of cases the cartilage is affected as a result of some other process such as trauma to the joint, infection of the joint or autoimmune joint diseases (in which the body produces antibodies that attack its own cartilage). In these patients it can appear at a younger age.

Damage to the articular cartilage leads to limitation of movement of the joint and to pain upon movement. The pain is due to the fact that the contact between the joint surfaces is now between two mismatched cartilage surfaces, or in advanced cases· where there has been considerable damage or loss of cartilage, movement between two bony surfaces without intervening cartilage.

The joints most commonly affected by osteoarthritis are the joints between the wrist bones (carpals) and the first metacarpal, the interphalangeal joints of the fingers, the weight-bearing joints (such as the knee and hip), and the synovial joints in the spine. The pain occurs when moving the affected joint and is relieved by rest. As the disease progresses, pain can also appear at rest (pain in the hip at night is a well-known symptom). Sometimes, one can hear or feel a scraping sensation when the joint is moved (crepitus).

Small spicules of bone called **osteophytes** grow around the edges of the joint. As the disease progresses, deformity of the affected joint may appear. The most common place for osteoarthritis to appear is in the distal joints of the fingers. Small bony lumps called **Heberden's nodes** are found around the affected joints. Damage to the articular cartilage of the hip or knee causes severe limitations of mobility. At a more advanced stage of the disease, the joint becomes very deformed and almost completely unable to move; walking becomes extremely painful and difficult.

Treatment of osteoarthritis consists of symptomatic treatment, such as with analgesic and anti-inflammatory medications, avoiding stress to the joints and physiotherapy to prevent degeneration of the joint. There are surgical treatments for more advanced disease and these include operations to repair the damaged joints or replacement of the joint with an artificial (prosthetic) joint. Joint replacement provides an excellent solution to the problem but it does involve major surgery, with its attendant risks and potential complications (particularly as most of the patients are elderly and might have cardiovascular or other diseases). Furthermore, the 'lifespan' of an artificial joint is about 10–20 years. Thus, joint replacement is not recommended in a young patient because of the relatively short life of the artificial joint. For those patients, it might be more appropriate to permanently fix the joint so that it cannot move and cause pain.

ORTHOPEDIC INJURIES

Dislocation

Dislocation is a separation of the cartilage surfaces of a joint. In most cases, dislocation occurs as a result of external force being applied to the joint, such as can occur in a fall or a car accident. When a joint is dislocated it cannot move and any attempt to move it proves extremely painful.

A dislocation is usually associated with rupture of the joint ligaments. Normally, the ligaments hold the joint in place and prevent dislocation.

In people who are extremely supple (i.e. with very elastic ligaments), even a normal movement can dislocate a joint. Such people are usually able to relocate the joint themselves.

The joint most often dislocated is the shoulder but dislocations can also occur in the elbow, thigh, ankle and other joints.

A joint that has been dislocated, should be immobilized in the most comfortable position and the person should be sent to hospital. There the joint will be X-rayed to ensure that a fracture has not occurred and then the joint can usually be relocated by specific techniques.

Subluxation is defined as a situation in which the cartilage joint surfaces are partially separated, that is, there is still some contact between the joint surfaces over a certain area.

Sprain

A sprain is defined as a partial or complete tear of joint ligaments as a result of excessive stretching. A sprain usually occurs following forceful movement of a joint beyond its normal range of movement. This temporarily pulls the joint surfaces apart and tears the ligaments. At the end of the movement, the joint surfaces return to their normal position but the ligaments are damaged. The tear in the ligaments leads to localized bleeding, swelling and pain.

The most common site for a sprain is the ankle. In most cases, this follows sudden inversion and plantar flexion of the ankle during a fall (the body weight suddenly falls on the dorsum (top) of the foot). The treatment of a sprained ankle consists of reducing the swelling, by elevating the leg, and applying cold compresses. A pressure bandage is applied and active movement of the ankle should be started as soon as possible.

Strain

Strain is defined as stretching or tearing of a muscle. When this happens, the area becomes painful to move and tender.

Fracture

A fracture is defined as disruption to the continuity of a bone and results from the exertion of excessive force on a bone. The type of force exerted determines the type of fracture. For example, a rotary force exerted on a long bone causes a spiral fracture (common in skiing accidents); a direct blow to the surface of a long bone can cause a comminuted fracture (more than one fracture line – the bone is broken into several pieces).

The force needed to fracture a bone is usually quite considerable because a normal healthy bone is an extremely strong structure. However, if there is some disease that weakens the bone, a **pathologic fracture** can occur. This type of fracture follows relatively minor force to weakened, abnormal bone.

The signs of a fracture are pain, local tenderness, swelling, a blue color of the overlying skin, limitation of movement and visible deformity of the bone. Not all these signs are found in every fracture and sometimes a fracture has minimal local signs.

An **open fracture** is one associated with a tear in the skin, with direct exposure of the broken bone to the exterior. Sometimes the broken ends of the bone actually protrude through the skin wound, or the broken bone can remain in the wound and not be visible externally (this is still defined as an open fracture because the broken bone is in contact with the external enviroment). In an open fracture, there is a serious risk of infection in the bone.

A fracture within a joint can disrupt the close fit of the opposing joint surfaces and eventually lead to destruction of the articular cartilage and impaired function of the joint.

A fracture in itself is not a life-threatening injury but there are potentially fatal complications arising from it. For example, fractures of the femur or the pelvis can tear large blood vessels, leading to severe internal hemorrhage. A fracture can also endanger a limb if, for example, the fragments of bone cause damage to an artery or nerves in the limb.

Treatment of a fracture includes immobilization (splinting) of the fracture at the accident site and then transfer of the patient to a medical facility. Splinting and immobilizing a fracture lessens the pain and prevents complications that may arise from movement of the broken bone, such as laceration (tearing) of blood vessels or nerves. In hospital, an X-ray is performed to confirm the diagnosis of a fracture and to define its anatomy precisely, and only then is a decision made regarding the appropriate form of treatment. In most frac-tures the bones can be returned approximately to their normal anatomic position by external force on the limb, followed by immobilization in a plaster cast. Usually, the cast is extended to include a joint above and a joint below the fracture site. This prevents movement of the bone ends and allows them to heal. Some fractures require surgery to return the bone ends to their normal position and to splint the bone using internal fixation (plates, nails, screws, etc.).

The process of repair of a fracture involves cells derived from the periosteum, which multiply and produce new tissue that fills the gap at the fracture line. This new tissue then becomes mineralized and turns into new bone that fills the fracture site. The mass of new bone is called **callus**. The primary bone that makes up the callus is eventually remodeled and the original shape and structure of the original bone are usually restored.

The nervous system

The nervous system regulates the activity of all body systems; it also has its own internal activity that is unrelated to other organs.

Today, death is defined as cessation of function of the brain stem, which is a vital part of the nervous system. It is possible for a person to be defined as dead, because brain stem functions have ceased, while the heart is still beating. Under these circumstances, organs for transplantation can be removed from the patient.

The nervous system basically works on the same principle as a computer. It receives information (**input**), processes the information (**data processing**), and produces some result (**output**).

$$\text{Input} \rightarrow \text{Data processing} \rightarrow \text{Output}$$

The input is information that reaches the brain from the senses and the internal organs; this information is 'processed' within the brain. The output is the activation of various organs in the body, such as muscles or glands, by the nerves leading to them. Functions that determine the personality of the individual, such as thought, emotions, memory and others are termed 'higher functions' of the nervous system.

We know that the nervous system is responsible for the higher functions but, despite enormous amounts of information that have accumulated about the structure and function of the nervous system, we still are very far from understanding how thought processes work in the brain. This chapter will deal with the structure and basic functions of the nervous system. Some of the processes involved will be presented schematically for simplicity. Although they are very important, highly complex processes of the nervous system are beyond the scope of this text.

THE NERVE CELL

Nervous tissue comprises several different types of cell but the cell that is responsible for carrying out the basic functions of the system is the **neuron**. Neurons form connections with each other and with various organs in the body; it is these connections that determine the function of the nervous system.

A person is born with the maximum number of neurons that will be present (some 10 billion). Throughout life, the number of neurons progressively decreases. The main development of the nervous system takes place in the first year of life, during which time the weight of the brain increases from 300 g to 1 kg! This increase is due mainly to the formation of new connections between neurons.

Neurons are unable to divide or replicate, so that when a neuron dies it is not replaced by a new one. However, under certain circumstances, when neurons are damaged the nervous system can create new connections between the remaining neurons and, in this way, the impaired function can be partially restored.

A neuron is a cell that has become specialized to receive stimuli from other neurons or from sensory organs in the body, to process those stimuli and to transmit changes in electrical charge (by means of a long fiber, called an **axon**, arising from the cell body) to other neurons or to organs in the body.

Structure of a neuron

There are different types of neuron within the nervous system. These differ from each other in their size and shape but they all have certain features in common (Fig. 11.1).

Cell body. The body of the neuron is no different in its features from other cell bodies in other systems and organs, and contains the same organelles as other cells. Some neurons are elliptical in shape, some are round, and some are triangular. Neurons vary in size from 0.15 mm to 0.004 mm.

Axon. This is a long fiber-like extension of the cell body. If an axon is detached from the cell body it dies. Some neurons have axons of up to 1 m in length (the longest cells in the body) and others have an axon that is merely a fraction of a millimeter long, depending on the particular neuron's specific task. The axon transmits changes in electrical charge – called the **action potential** – along its length. The action potential moves along the axon at a speed of between 1 and 100 m per second, depending on the type of neuron.

Dendrites. These are short, branch-like processes attached to the cell body. Some neurons have many dendrites and others have only one. In some neurons the dendrites branch repeatedly to form what is termed the dendritic tree.

Neurons are connected to one another. The connection is formed between the end of one

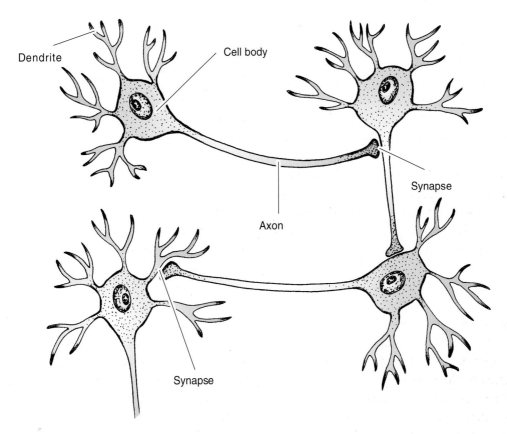

Dendrite

Cell body

Synapse

Axon

Synapse

Figure 11.1 Structure of a neuron and interneuronal connections.

neuron's axon and a dendrite or the cell body of another neuron. One neuron can establish connections with hundreds, or even thousands, of other neurons.

A chemical substance (**a transmitter substance**) passes across from the end of the axon of one neuron to the dendrite or cell body of another neuron. This stimulates the second neuron, which alters the electrical charge in its axon.

THE SYNAPSE

A **synapse** is the area between the end of one neuron's axon and another neuron's cell body or dendrite (Fig. 11.2). At its end, the axon splits into tiny branches, with a little bulge at the tips (the **end bulb**). Within the end bulb of the axons are vesicles (sacs) that contain a chemical substance called a **transmitter**. Within the nervous system there are several different transmitter substances, the two main ones being **acetylcholine** and **noradrenaline**.

The synaptic end bulb is very close to the area of the second neuron that contains **receptors**, which bind the transmitter substance. The synaptic end bulb belongs to one neuron and the receptors are in the other neuron. Between them there is a microscopic gap called the **synaptic space**. A change in electrical potential

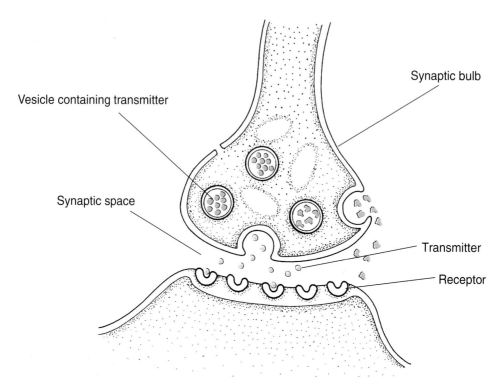

Figure 11.2   Synapse.

(the action potential) travels down the axon of the first neuron, reaches the synaptic end bulb at the end of the axon, and causes the vesicles to burst open and release the transmitter within them. This passes into the synaptic space, moves across the space, reaches the receptors in the other neuron and binds to them.

As the transmitter binds to the receptors it causes a change in the electrical potential of the axon of that neuron. As long as the transmitter is bound to the receptors, action potentials keep occurring within the axon. Therefore, to stop the effect of the transmitter, a special enzyme within the synaptic space breaks down the transmitter substance. Where the transmitter is acetylcholine, the enzyme that breaks it down and halts its effect is called **acetylcholinesterase**.

In addition to synapses between one nerve and another, there are synapses between nerves and muscles, and between nerves and glands. When the transmitter binds to the receptors within the muscle or the glands, it results in contraction of the muscle or secretion by the gland.

Nerve gas.   This gas contains an organophosphate compound, similar to substances used in some pesticides. The organophosphate acts at the synapse. It binds to the enzyme that breaks down the transmitter (acetylcholinesterase), and neutralizes it. As a result, the effect of the transmitter that binds to the receptors continues unabated and the organs innervated by the nerves (other nerves, muscles, glands, etc.) keep on functioning uncontrollably. The muscles contract repeatedly and continuously and the glands (sweat glands, salivary glands, mucus glands, etc.) continue to secrete their secretions incessantly. Ultimately, the muscles become 'exhausted', and the victim dies because the respiratory muscles stop working.

Muscle paralysis in the operating room. During certain operations under general anesthesia, a substance that acts on the synaptic space and prevents the transmitter from binding to the receptor can be administered to the patient. The result is total paralysis of the muscles, which makes it easier for the surgeon to perform certain procedures. This substance (**curare**) was originally discovered by the South American Indians, who used it on the tips of poison darts and arrows to hunt birds and small animals.

THE REFLEX ARC

A muscle reflex is a very rapid, involuntary response of a muscle to a specific stimulus. For example, if you touch a hot object, you withdraw your hand automatically (reflexly).

The knee jerk is a relatively straightforward reflex. A blow to the tendon under the kneecap causes the thigh muscle to contract reflexly and the leg jerks forwards. This reflex is a simple example of how the nervous system works – a stimulus occurs (input), the 'data' are processed, and there is a response (output).

Structure of the reflex arc

The reflex arc that is responsible for the knee jerk reflex involves two neurons, which are connected at a synapse. One is called a **sensory neuron**, and transmits the stimulus from the kneecap; the other is a **motor neuron**, which transmits the response to the thigh muscle (Fig. 11.3). The particular sensory neuron involved in this arc is unusual in that it does not have any dendrites but only a very long axon, with one end within the tendon of the thigh muscle and the other end near the spinal cord. A short connection joins the cell body to the axon. The motor neuron is a typical neuron, with a cell body with many dendrites, within the spinal cord and a long axon that reaches from there to the thigh muscle.

Action of the reflex arc

The end of the axon of the sensory neuron is connected to a special sensory organ called a stretch receptor, located within the tendon below the kneecap. Tapping the tendon stretches it slightly and the stretch receptors send a message via the axon that is connected to them. An action potential moves quickly along the axon until it reaches the synapse with the motor neuron in the spinal cord.

When the action potential reaches the end of the axon of the sensory neuron (at the synapse), it causes the release of the transmitter, which crosses the synaptic gap and is taken up by the receptors in the dendrites of the motor cell. This results in an action potential that travels down the axon of the motor neuron. When the action potential reaches the end of the axon (at the synapse with the muscle), it causes the release of transmitter at that synapse. Once it has crossed the synaptic gap the transmitter binds to the receptors in the muscle cell, and triggers a contraction of the muscle. In this case, the 'data processing' takes place within the spinal cord, so the entire process is called a simple reflex arc (see Fig. 11.3).

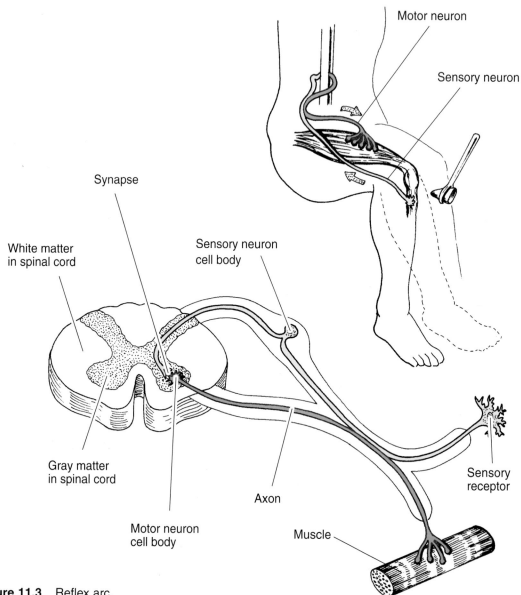

Figure 11.3   Reflex arc.

STRUCTURE OF THE NERVOUS SYSTEM

The central nervous system (CNS) is defined as that nervous tissue that is found in the brain and the spinal cord.

The peripheral nervous system (PNS) is defined as that nervous tissue that is outside the brain and the spinal cord. The peripheral nerves and ganglia are part of the peripheral nervous system.

It is possible for a single neuron to be partly within the central nervous system and partly within the peripheral nervous system. For example, a cell body might be within the spinal cord and the axon that arises from it might pass out of the spinal cord and reach a target organ elsewhere in the body.

Within the central nervous system, the nervous tissue is comprised of neurons and supporting cells, called **glial cells**. There are approximately 10 glial cells for each neuron, and their task is to support, protect and nourish the neuron.

Examination of the nervous tissue in the central nervous system shows it to be made up of **white matter**, which consists of axons and supporting cells, and **gray matter**, which contains the neuronal cell bodies, axons that are attached to the cell body and supporting cells. It is the cell bodies of the neurons that give the gray matter its characteristic color.

The peripheral nervous system consists of peripheral nerves and ganglia. A **peripheral nerve** is a tube-like structure that contains axons (Fig. 11.4). The nerve looks like a white

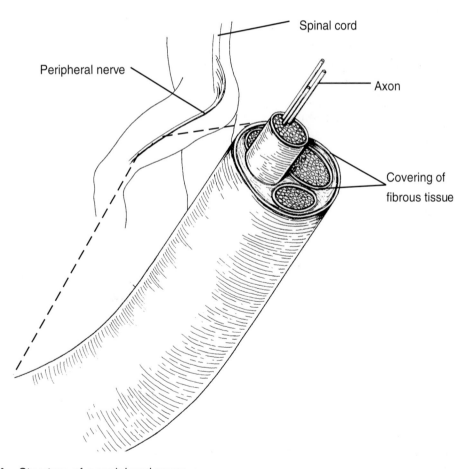

Figure 11.4 Structure of a peripheral nerve.

thread. The thickness of the peripheral nerves varies, depending on how many axons they contain.

Those peripheral nerves that emerge from the skull are called **cranial nerves**; those that emerge from one of the openings in the sides of the spinal column are called **spinal nerves**.

Under the microscope, a peripheral nerve can be seen to be made of a connective tissue wrapping, which contains chains of cells called **Schwann cells**. The axons pass through these Schwann cells (which look like a string of sausages). Some of the axons that pass through the Schwann cells are covered in a layer of a fatty substance called **myelin**. This substance speeds up the transmission of action potentials along the axon.

Ganglia (singular = ganglion) are groups of neuronal cell bodies lying outside the central nervous system, such as alongside the spinal column or attached to various organs within the body.

NERVE TRACTS

A nerve tract is a series of neurons that are connected via synapses, and which carry out a specific function. Motor tracts control skeletal muscles, sensory tracts transmit sensation and the autonomic tracts are involved in regulating the activity of internal organs.

Motor tracts

The brain is made up of two halves. The right side of the brain controls the muscles on the left side of the body, and the left side controls the muscles on the right half of the body.

The cell body of the first neuron in a motor tract (or pathway) is situated in a specific area of the gray matter of the outer layer of the brain known as the **motor cortex** (Fig. 11.5).

The axon of this first neuron in the motor tract passes through a region of white matter, which contains only axons from the motor tracts, crosses over to the opposite side within the brain, leaves the skull and passes down the spinal cord in the white matter.

The next neuron in the motor tract is situated in the gray matter of the spinal cord. It connects (via a synapse) with the axon of the first neuron and its axon then passes out of the central nervous system and enters a peripheral nerve, through which it reaches its target muscle. The axon of the final neuron ends in a synapse at the muscle and, when that synapse is activated by an action potential, the muscle contracts.

Each muscle in the body has specific neurons that activate it. A **motor unit** is defined as a single neuron together with the muscle cells that it activates. The motor units in the muscles of the back are enormous, with each neuron activating hundreds of muscle cells. By way of contrast, in very fine muscles involved in delicate, precise movements, such as those of the eyeball, the motor units are much smaller: each neuron is 'in charge' of only a few muscle cells (see Fig. 9.29).

Sensory tracts

The end of the axon of the first neuron in a sensory tract is connected to a sensory organ called a sensory receptor. There are many types of sensory receptors: **photoreceptors** react to light (the sense of sight), **chemoreceptors** react to chemical substances (e.g. the sense of taste), **thermoreceptors** react to changes in temperature and **mechanoreceptors** react to mechanical

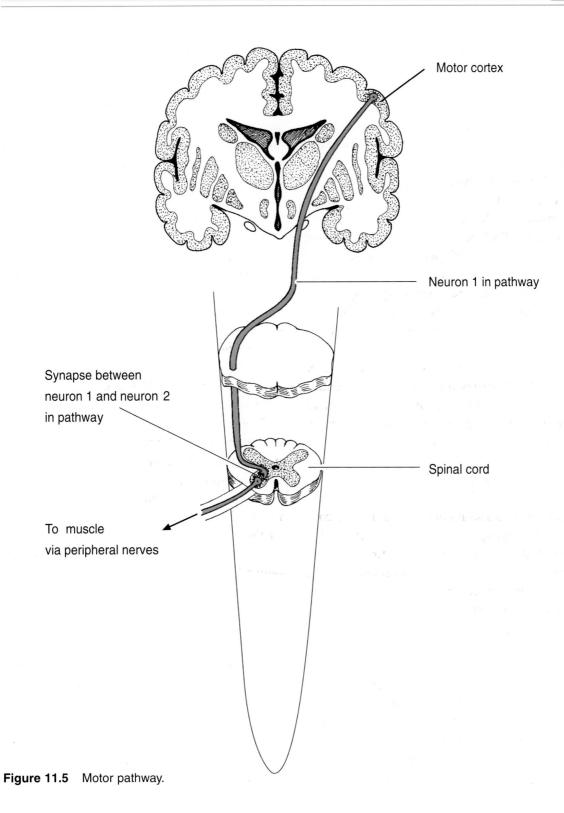

Figure 11.5   Motor pathway.

pressure (e.g. the sense of touch, the sense of hearing). When a receptor is stimulated it initiates an action potential in its attached axon. A sensory receptor will only react to its specific stimulus: a photoreceptor will react only to light and a mechanical pressure receptor reacts only to mechanical pressure.

Note that the traditional division of the sensory system into the five senses is not accurate because the sense of hearing and the sense of touch both involve mechanoreceptors that respond to pressure exerted upon them. A more accurate classification defines each sense on the basis of the type of receptor involved.

The concept of a sensory tract (or pathway) will be illustrated using the example of the sense of temperature in the skin (Fig. 11.6).

The end of the first neuron in the sensory tract is connected to a thermoreceptor in the skin. When that receptor is stimulated by the appropriate stimulus (heat), an action potential is generated and moves along the axon. This axon reaches the spinal cord via a peripheral nerve.

The cell body of the first neuron is in a ganglion alongside the spinal cord, and is connected to the axon. The particular type of sensory neuron that is described in this example does not actually have any dendrites, but only one long axon from its cell body.

Within the gray matter of the spinal cord, this first axon synapses with a dendrite of the second neuron in the pathway. The axon of this second neuron crosses over to the other side of the spinal cord and then heads upwards within the white matter of the spinal cord, together with other sensory axons, to reach the brain. In the brain, the second neuron synapses with the cell body of the third neuron in the pathway. The axon of this third neuron travels through the white matter of the brain to the sensory center within the brain, which is situated in a strip of the cortex (the **sensory cortex**), where it synapses with the last neuron in the sensory pathway.

Sensations arising from, for example, the left leg, reach the spinal cord via the peripheral nerves from the lower limbs and ultimately arrive at the sensory cortex on the right (opposite) side of the brain.

Every part of the body is represented by a specific area of the sensory cortex: signals from the leg are transmitted to the upper part of the sensory cortex strip; signals from the trunk are received in the central part of the strip; and signals from the upper limbs and head arrive at the lower part of the cortical strip. In fact, it is possible to draw a 'map' of the body on the sensory cortex. The result is an upside down representation of one half of the body, called a **homunculus** (from the Latin word meaning–'Little man') (Fig. 11.7).

The regions of the homunculus that represent the head, palms and soles of the feet are very large. This is because these areas are innervated by a large number of sensory nerves and thus their representation in the sensory cortex is also large. This is in contrast to regions such as the back, where there are fewer sensory nerves.

The area of skin innervated by a single axon is called the **receptive field** of that neuron. Hence, on the back, the receptive fields are very large (several square centimeters), so that it is difficult, for example, to distinguish between two separate points that are being touched if they are within the same receptive field (they feel like a single point). This is because both points stimulate the same axon. In contrast, on the lips or fingertips, the receptive fields are

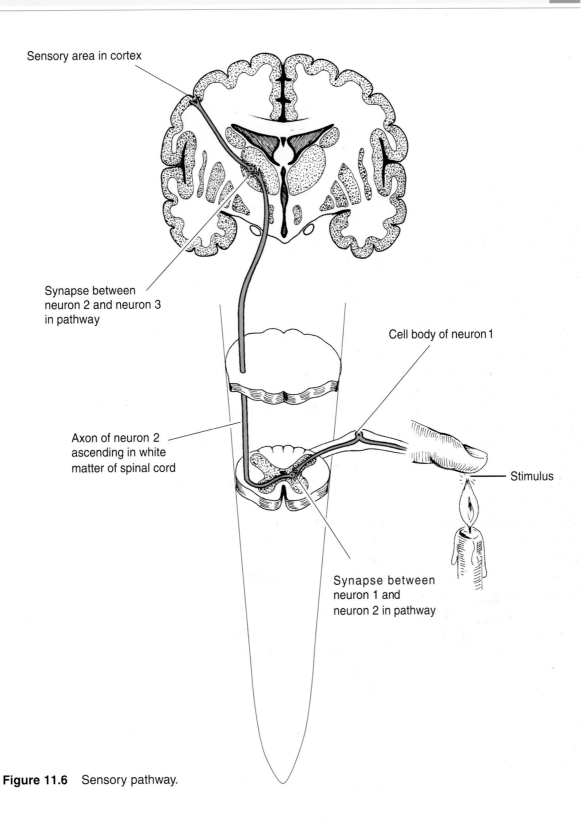

Sensory area in cortex

Synapse between
neuron 2 and neuron 3
in pathway

Cell body of neuron 1

Axon of neuron 2
ascending in white
matter of spinal cord

Stimulus

Synapse between
neuron 1 and
neuron 2 in pathway

Figure 11.6   Sensory pathway.

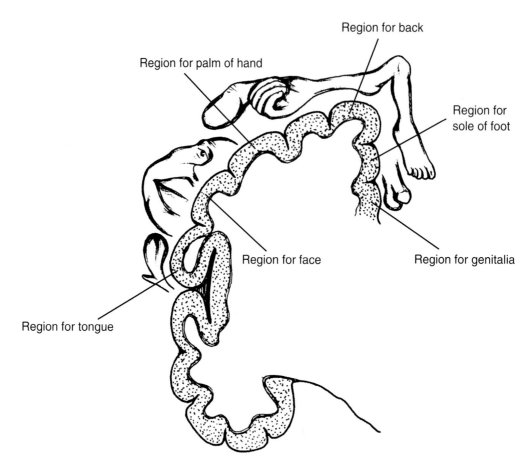

Figure 11.7   Homunculus – sensations arising from the tongue, face, palm, sole and the genitalia are represented by large areas in the sensory cortex. The back is represented by a small area in the cortex, despite covering a large area of skin.

very small (less than a square millimeter), so that one can detect two separate points being touched even if they are only a millimeter apart.

Dermatomes

A dermatome is an area of skin from which sensation reaches the spinal cord via a single spinal nerve. For example, the sensation from the dermatome of L1 (the first lumbar nerve) is in the area of the groin (Fig. 11.8). Sensations from this particular area pass via axons that reach the spinal cord in the spinal nerve L1, which enters between the first and second lumbar spinal vertebrae (L1 and L2). There is some overlap between adjacent dermatomes. In other words, the same area of skin might contain sensory organs that transmit sensations via axons that reach the spinal cord in different spinal nerves. Despite this rather confusing situation, in general it can be said that the sensory axons from any given area of skin enter the spinal cord within a single spinal nerve. On this basis, a 'map' of skin

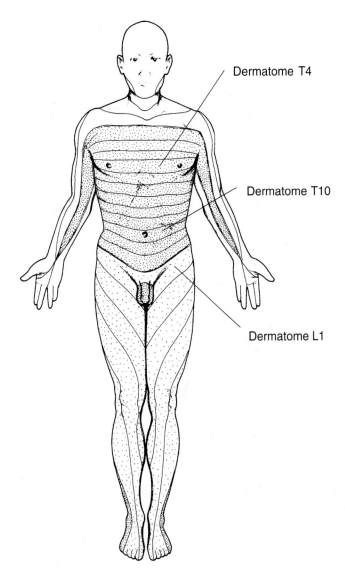

Dermatome T4

Dermatome T10

Dermatome L1

Figure 11.8   Dermatomes.

dermatomes can be drawn, showing which spinal nerve is associated with which area of skin.

AUTONOMIC NERVOUS SYSTEM

The autonomic nervous system is that part of the peripheral nervous system that controls the function of the internal organs of the body. Although there is an obvious connection between the nervous system's higher functions (thought, emotion, etc.) and the autonomic nervous system, some of the autonomic nervous system functions are totally involuntary and unconscious. For example, we are unaware when our gall bladder contracts or when a peristaltic wave passes along our colon – functions that are controlled by the autonomic nervous system. Nevertheless, it is well known that there is a close association between one's emotional state and the function of many internal organs, for example pre-exam diarrhea or constipation during a long hike.

The autonomic nervous system has sensory incoming pathways that transmit information from the internal organs to the brain, and outgoing pathways from the brain back to the body, which transmit signals that control and regulate the function of internal organs.

These outgoing pathways are divided into **sympathetic** and **parasympathetic** pathways. Both lead in parallel to the body's internal organs. In other words, the internal organs are innervated by both sympathetic and parasympathetic nerves.

In general, the sympathetic nerves activate the organs during periods of stress, and the parasympathetic nerves act during periods of quiescence. Stress can occur with danger and the body systems have to prepare for a state of 'battle', injury or retreat (the so-called 'fight or flight' reaction). 'Relaxation' in this context is when the body is calm and quiescent, and engaged in resting, eating, digesting food and conserving energy.

An example from the animal kingdom will be used to illustrate the difference between the states of stress and relaxation, and the different effects of the sympathetic and parasympathetic systems. Let us consider a zebra resting quietly after a meal. Its body is in a state of relaxation as a result of the actions of the parasympathetic pathways: the heart rate is slow, the cardiac output is low, the respiratory rate is slow, the diameter of the airways is relatively narrow and the blood flow to the

muscles is decreased. On the other hand, the salivary glands are secreting large amounts of salivary juices, the stomach is contracting and secreting gastric juices, the duodenum and gall bladder are secreting various secretory products and the bowel is active. The blood-flow to the entire digestive system is increased. All of those functions result from parasympathetic stimulation.

Should a lion suddenly appear, the zebra has to flee and its internal organ systems must function appropriately. At the precise moment the zebra sees the lion, the sympathetic nervous system swings into action: the heart rate and cardiac output increase, the respiratory rate and the depth of respiration increase, the airways dilate, blood-flow to the muscles increases and the skin is covered with sweat. All these changes are the result of sympathetic stimulation. At the same time, secretion of saliva stops, the activity of the digestive organs decreases and less blood flows to the digestive organs. These changes enable the zebra's body to switch quickly from a state of rest and digestion to a state of flight that requires powerful muscle movements.

The sympathetic and parasympathetic systems have opposite effects. Body organs are generally innervated by axons from both systems. When the sympathetic pathway is activated, the organs involved function to deal with a stress situation and, when the parasympathetic system is activated, the organs' activities are appropriate for the resting state.

Parasympathetic pathways

The parasympathetic pathways run via the cranial nerves (which emerge from various openings in the skull) and via spinal nerves in the region of the sacrum (the lowest portion of the spinal cord).

The **vagus** nerve is the cranial nerve that emerges through a large opening in the skull and contains parasympathetic fibers that reach all the internal organs other than the genitalia, the urinary system and the last part of the digestive tract (these organs receive their parasympathetic innervation via the nerves that emerge from the sacrum).

There are ganglia along the way in the parasympathetic pathway; these are groups of cell bodies outside the central nervous system. The ganglia generally lie alongside various organs.

The cell body of the first neuron in the pathway is either in the brain or in the spinal cord. Its axon emerges from the brain or spinal cord and enters a peripheral nerve, in which it travels until it has nearly reached the organ that it innervates. Near the organ, the axon reaches a ganglion, where it forms a synapse with the cell of the second neuron in the pathway, which is inside the ganglion. The axon of the second neuron emerges from the ganglion and reaches the organ.

Sympathetic pathways

The sympathetic pathways pass along certain spinal nerves. This system also includes ganglia, which lie alongside the spinal column, where they form a chain known as the **sympathetic chain**. The body of the first neuron in the pathway is in the spinal cord. Its axon emerges within the spinal nerve and, near the spine, it leaves the spinal nerve and enters the ganglion. Inside the ganglion, the first axon synapses with the body of the second neuron in the pathway. The axon of that neuron then leaves the ganglion, re-enters the spinal nerve, and in this way reaches its target organ, where it forms another synapse. When the sympathetic system is activated, transmitter substance is released from the end of that axon, is taken up by the end organ and stimulates its function.

PERIPHERAL NERVES

A peripheral nerve is a structure that looks like a white thread; it contains many axons (see Fig. 11.4).

The cell body that gives rise to these axons is situated within the brain, the spinal cord or within a ganglion.

SPINAL NERVES

The spinal nerves, of which there are 31 pairs, pass through openings in the sides of the spinal column, between the vertebrae. Just before the nerve reaches those openings, it divides into two **roots** (Fig. 11.9). The front (anterior) root, which joins the anterior portion of the spinal cord, contains mainly axons of motor nerves, while the posterior (back) root, which enters the posterior portion of the spinal cord, contains mainly axons from sensory nerves. In the shoulder and lumbar regions, the spinal nerves are joined to each other and axons run through these connections from one spinal nerve to another. The interconnections between the spinal nerves in these areas form a complex network of nerves called a **plexus**.

The peripheral nerves that are derived from the spinal nerves reach various parts of the body. A nerve that reaches the hand, for example, will contain axons from motor nerves that control the muscles of the hand, axons from

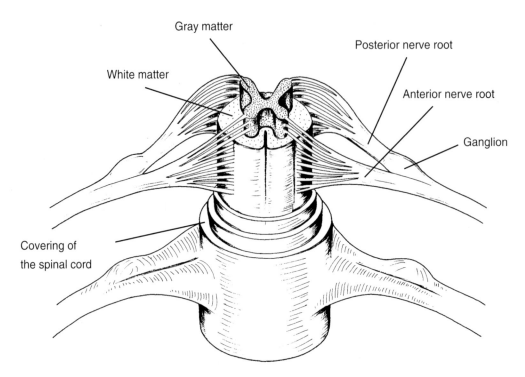

Figure 11.9   Spinal nerves and the spinal cord.

sensory nerves that transmit sensations from the hand to the spinal cord and brain, and axons from the autonomic nervous system that innervate the smooth muscle in the blood vessels walls and the sweat glands in the skin.

CRANIAL NERVES

The cranial nerves emerge from openings within the skull and innervate mainly the head and neck region. There are 12 pairs of cranial nerves, numbered 1 to 12.

The first cranial nerve is called the **olfactory** nerve, which contains only axons that transmit the sense of smell from receptors in the roof of the nasal passages.

The second cranial nerve is the **optic** nerve. This contains only axons that transmit vision

impulses from receptors in the retina of the eye.

The third cranial nerve is called the **oculomotor** nerve because it contains mainly axons that innervate the muscles which move the eyeball.

The fourth cranial nerve is the **trochlear** nerve and contains only axons that innervate one specific muscle involved in movement of the eyeball.

The fifth cranial nerve is the **trigeminal** nerve, which contains axons that transmit sensations from the face and axons that innervate the chewing muscles. The trigeminal nerve has three branches (hence its name): a branch that reaches the region of the eye and nose, a branch that reaches the upper jaw and a branch that reaches the lower jaw.

The sixth cranial nerve is the **abducens** nerve, which contains axons that innervate one specific muscle involved in movement of the eyeball.

The seventh cranial nerve is the **facial** nerve. This contains axons that innervate the muscles of expression, axons that transmit the sensation of taste from the anterior (front) two-thirds of the tongue and axons that innervate the salivary and tear glands.

The eighth cranial nerve is the **vestibulo-cochlear (acoustic)** nerve, which contains axons that transmit the sensations of sound and balance from the inner ear.

The ninth cranial nerve is called the **glos-sopharyngeal** nerve and contains axons that innervate the salivary glands, axons that transmit taste from the posterior third of the tongue, and others.

The tenth cranial nerve is the **vagus** nerve, which contains parasympathetic axons from the autonomic nervous system that innervate the internal organs of the chest and abdomen, axons that innervate muscles in the pharynx and throat, and axons that transmit sensation from the pharynx and throat.

The eleventh cranial nerve is called the **accessory** nerve. It contains axons that innervate muscles in the neck and upper back.

The twelfth cranial nerve is called the **hypoglossal** nerve and contains only axons that innervate the tongue muscles.

THE BRAIN

The term **brain** refers to the nervous tissue within the skull. In fact, the spinal cord, which is a direct continuation of the structures within the skull, can be considered an extension of the brain. The two together form the central nervous system (Fig. 11.10). The actual compo-nents of the central nervous system are the spinal cord, the brain stem, the hypothalamus, the thalamus, cerebellum and the cerebrum.

The spinal cord. This is the continuation of the brain stem, and contains both white and gray matter. The gray matter lies in the center of the cord, and is butterfly-shaped. It contains the cell bodies of the motor tracts, the sensory tracts, and the autonomic nerves. The white matter serves as a pathway for nerve tracts passing to and from the brain. The gray matter in the spinal cord ends at the level of the L1 vertebra; below this level are the roots of spinal nerves that emerge below the level of L1 – this collection of nerve roots is called the **cauda equina** ('horse's tail').

31 pairs of nerves, called the **spinal nerves**, emerge from the spinal cord. They include axons that innervate voluntary muscles, axons that transmit sensory impulses from the body and axons of the autonomic nervous system.

The brain stem. This is situated immedi-ately above the foramen magnum, which is the largest opening in the base of the skull. It is continuous with the spinal cord and con-tains vital centers, such as the respiratory center and the centers responsible for con-trolling pulse and blood pressure. All of the nervous pathways from the body to the brain pass through the brain stem. A severe injury to the brain stem usually results in immediate death.

The hypothalamus. This part of the brain is situated above the brain stem and is the center of the autonomic system, the control center for the endocrine system, and the center for feelings of hunger, the sexual drive and aggression. Hunger, sex and aggression form the basis of the survival drive. The hypophyseal

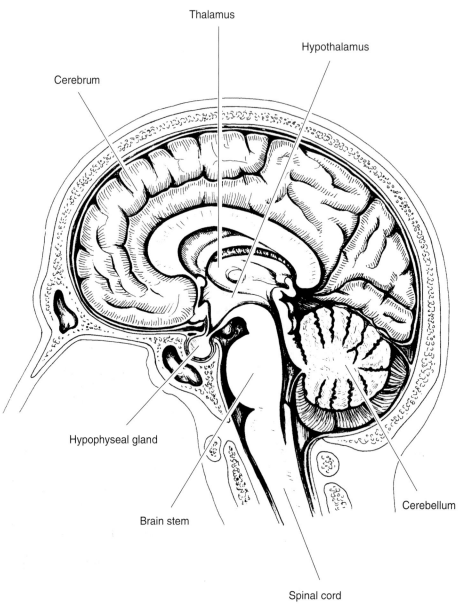

Figure 11.10 The brain.

gland is located below the hypothalamus and directly connected to it.

The thalamus. This part of the brain acts mainly as a transit station for sensory data from the skin.

The cerebellum ('small brain'). This is situated in the posterior part of the skull and is made up of two lobes, each involved in functions of one half of the body. The cerebellum is responsible for balance, muscle coordination and muscle tone. An injury to the cerebellum affects those functions.

The cerebrum. This is the largest part of the brain. It is made up of two halves, called **hemispheres**. Each hemisphere is divided into a number of **lobes**. The lobes are named according to the skull bones adjacent to them.

Thus there are four: the **frontal, parietal, temporal,** and **occipital lobes** (Fig. 11.11).

The gray matter of the cerebrum lies in the outer layers of the brain known as the **cortex**, as well as in 'islands' of gray matter ('nuclei') within the white matter. The cortex of the brain has many ridges and grooves, known as **gyri**

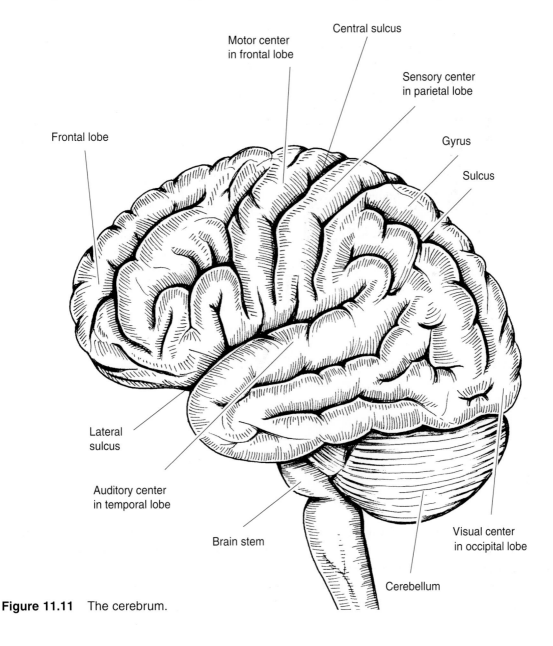

Figure 11.11 The cerebrum.

(singular = gyrus) and **sulci** (singular = sulcus), which considerably increase the total surface area of the gray matter. The **central sulcus** separates the frontal lobe, which is located anterior to the central sulcus, and the parietal lobe, which is located posterior to the central sulcus. The **lateral sulcus** separates the temporal lobe, which is located inferior to the lateral sulcus, and the frontal and parietal lobes, which are located superior to the lateral sulcus. The cortex of each hemisphere controls the opposite side of the body and contains various centers, such as the motor center that controls the voluntary muscles, the sensory center for receiving skin sensations, the visual center that processes stimuli arriving from the eye and the hearing center. Each such center is situated in a specific area of the cortex and injury to an area of the cortex will affect the specific centers in that area. The various centers within the brain are interconnected by nerve tracts. Most of the volume of the cerebrum consists of white matter, which largely comprises axons that connect the various centers within the brain.

The speech center (which is responsible for the understanding and generation of speech, the interpretation of written words, etc.) is present in only one hemisphere, which is called the dominant hemisphere (the left in most people). The dominant hemisphere is more adept at controlling muscles, hence in about 90% of right-handed people the left hemisphere is the dominant one. Among left-handed people, the dominant hemisphere is the right in 50% of cases and the left in the other 50%.

In the non-dominant hemisphere, those anatomic areas corresponding to the speech centers in the dominant hemisphere contain the centers for intuition, i.e. the ability to interpret the emotional aspects of speech, body language, and so on. The centers for musical ability, artistic talent and spatial orientation lie mainly in the non-dominant hemisphere.

Thought processes and personality are largely based in the frontal lobes of the cerebrum. This region of the brain is more highly developed in humans than in other animals. There is much to be learned about the higher cerebral functions because of the extreme complexity of the billions of anatomic connections among millions of neurons involved in even simple thought processes.

THE VENTRICLES OF THE BRAIN

The cerebral ventricles are fluid-filled spaces within the various lobes of the brain (Fig. 11.12).

In the embryo, the nervous system develops from a hollow tube. The anterior (front) part of the tube expands considerably and develops into the two cerebral hemispheres; the rest of the tube develops into the other parts of the central nervous system (including the spinal cord). The original cavity around which the brain has developed remains to form the ventricles of the brain.

There are four ventricles within the brain, which are all connected to each other and are continuous with the central canal within the spinal cord. They all contain cerebrospinal fluid (CSF).

MENINGES

The tissue making up the central nervous system is covered by three membranes called meninges. The outermost and thickest layer is called the **dura mater**. This is made up of tough fibrous tissue and is adherent to the inside of the skull bones. The dural sheath is

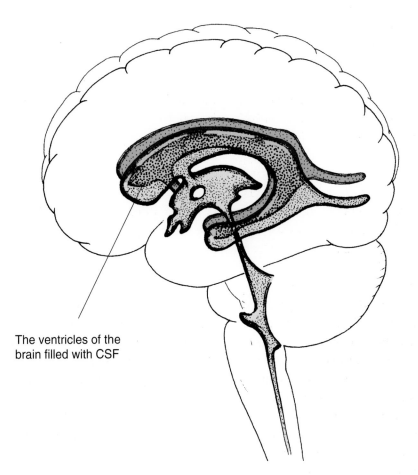

The ventricles of the
brain filled with CSF

Figure 11.12 The ventricles of the brain.

separated from the walls of the vertebral canal by the **extradural space** which contains loose connective tissue. The second layer is called the **arachnoid mater**. This is much thinner than the dura mater and is adherent to the inside of the dura. The innermost layer is the **pia mater**, which is a very thin layer that is adherent to the brain tissue and which follows its complex contours closely.

Between the arachnoid mater and the pia mater is a space called the **subarachnoid space**. This is filled with a clear fluid called the **cerebrospinal fluid (CSF)**. This fluid is pro-

duced within the ventricles of the brain, filling them and the central spinal canal, and flows out through special openings into the subarachnoid space. This fluid acts as a shock absorber for the brain within the skull, and nourishes the meninges.

Below the level of L1 no spinal cord exists, but only the roots of the lower spinal nerves. At this point, the subarachnoid space is relatively large, which allows for the insertion of a needle to withdraw a sample of CSF for examination – a procedure called a **lumbar puncture** (or spinal tap).

12 Diseases of the nervous system

PAIN

Pain is one of the most important sensations transmitted from the body to the brain. The body perceives pain when the pain pathway is activated, which serves to warn the brain of damage to tissues somewhere in the body.

The pain pathway

Pain receptors are called **nociceptors**, and are present in various sites, such as the skin, the covering of bones (periosteum), joints and the internal organs.

Pain receptors are connected to special axons that belong to the pain pathway. This pathway is similar in its organization to the sensory pathway described on p. 208 of Chapter 11. The pain pathways that transmit sensation from the right half of the body end in the pain center in the left half of the brain; those from the left side of the body reach the pain center in the right half of the brain.

Different types of stimuli can stimulate pain receptors. Some stimuli originate outside the body, such as when an object is pressing on tissues. Other stimuli originate from internal processes within the body.

Some of the pain stimuli cause actual tissue damage. Damaged tissue secretes various chemical substances that activate the pain receptors. The activation of these receptors results in a change in electrical charge, which then moves along the neural pathways of the pain tracts until it reaches the pain center in the brain. **Pain is experienced within the brain.**

Pain-associated phenomena

Measurement of pain

Pain cannot be objectively measured because **pain is a subjective sensation!** A given stimulus might cause one person to feel excruciating pain while the same stimulus in another person might result in only a mild bearable pain.

It is common to assess the degree of pain by the extent to which it interferes with daily activities. For example, a stomach ache that keeps the patient confined to bed is not equal in magnitude to pain that allows the patient to continue working.

Pain threshold

The pain threshold is the minimal stimulus that activates the pain receptors. Light pressure on the periosteum will first activate the pressure receptors (these are not pain receptors). Only when the pressure reaches a certain level (the 'threshold') will the pain receptors be activated and warn the brain of impending danger to the bone.

The pain threshold differs from person to person and there is a definite association between the level of the pain threshold and the person's cultural background.

Absent pain sensation

In certain diseases, the pain pathway functions only partially or not at all. Patients suffering

from one of those diseases are potentially at risk of serious bodily harm. They can suffer burns from touching hot objects, or injure the soles of their feet without being aware of it. Because the injury to the foot does not hurt, the patient continues walking on the injured tissue and can cause the wound to enlarge or even develop into a large ischemic area.

Lack of pain adaptation

Adaptation is a process whereby one 'gets used' to a stimulus arriving at the brain repeatedly via the sensory pathways. For example, prolonged exposure to a certain smell eventually leads to decreased awareness of the smell. The sensation of pain does not involve this process of adaptation; in other words, one does not 'get used' to pain. This is obviously a useful and desirable situation, because the purpose of pain is to warn the brain of impending or actual damage to body tissues.

'Slow' and 'fast' pain

Some pain receptors are connected to axons that transmit the electrical action potential very quickly, and others are connected to axons that transmit it more slowly. The faster pathway causes an immediate, sharp feeling of pain, which only later changes to a duller, more prolonged pain as that signal arrives at the pain center in the brain along the 'slow' pain fibers. For example, if you hit your shin on a chair, instantly there is a sharp, acute pain and then, a few seconds later, a dull, persistent pain.

Referred pain

Referred pain denotes pain that is felt in an area other than where the tissue damage actually occurs. For example, the pain of a myocardial infarct is referred to the left arm; inflammation or injury to the diaphragm can cause pain that is referred to the shoulder; a kidney stone causes pain that is felt in the groin. The reason for this phenomenon is beyond the scope of this discussion.

Phantom limb pain

Phantom limb pain is pain felt in a limb that has been amputated. This phenomenon is particularly common in the foot of an amputee. Phantom pain usually appears within the first few days of losing the limb. In the region of the stump, the severed ends of the axons of the sensory nerves that had transmitted sensation from the foot continue to send action potentials to the brain via the sensory pathway. Thus the pathway that transmits sensation from the foot to the sensory center in the brain is activated, although there is no foot! This phenomenon demonstrates that pain sensation occurs in the brain.

Pain modulation

In a life-threatening emergency situation, the brain is capable of suppressing the activity of the pain pathways. Under such circumstances, the brain secretes substances known as **enkephalins** that suppress the pain pathways. The purpose of this suppression is to ensure that the pain will not interfere with the animal's ability to flee or fight. For example, it is well documented that in a battle situation soldiers can sustain extremely painful injuries of which they are totally unaware until the danger has passed, and sportsmen can sustain injuries in the heat of the competition that they only 'feel' at a later time.

Medications such as morphine act chemically to suppress the function of the pain pathways and can thus significantly reduce pain. Local analgesics work by blocking the transmission of the action potential at a certain point, thereby totally suppressing the pain sensation from that area of the body.

Visceral pain

Visceral pain is pain that arises from the internal organs of the body. As opposed to pain arising from the skin or the periosteum, visceral pain is not localized to a specific point. In many cases, the pain is referred to another part of the body. Because the pain is not localized (such as in abdominal pain or chest pain), it is difficult to be sure which organ is the source of the pain. Various methods, such as imaging investigations (X-rays, ultrasound, CT scans, etc.) or direct inspection of the internal organs during surgery, can enable the localization of the source of the pain to a particular organ.

HEADACHE

Most people suffer from headache at some time in their lives. The pain arises as a result of stimulation of nerve endings by various stimuli. Nerves that respond to pain are found in the skin of the scalp, the sinuses, the arteries and the periosteum of the skull bones.

The brain itself has no pain-sensitive nerves, so that headache is always due to stimulation of nerves in one of the structures listed above and not from the brain itself.

There are many causes of headache, some trivial and others serious and even potentially fatal.

Tension headache and non-specific headache

Most people suffer from time to time from non-specific headache. This is the headache that occurs when a person is tired, tense, has a fever or is dehydrated. The headache that occurs under these circumstances varies from person to person in its intensity, quality (e.g. variable or constant), location in the head, and duration.

Migraine

This is a type of headache with certain characteristic features. Migraine is quite common among children and young adults and tends to disappear after the age of 50. In most cases, there is a family history of migraine and it is more common in females than in males. In women, migraine is often related to pregnancy or to the menstrual cycle. It is known that the pain itself is caused by initial constriction followed by dilatation of blood vessels in the base of the skull, but what is still unknown is why those changes occur in the first place.

Migraines occur in attacks, the frequency of which vary from person to person, ranging from several attacks per week to an attack every few months. Each episode can last from 2 hours to 3 days. Certain trigger factors can provoke a migraine attack, such as bright lights, a loud noise, some odors, chocolate or cheese, stress and the menstrual period.

The following is a description of the typical symptoms of 'classic migraine'. It is important to note that only 10% of migraine sufferers have this type of migraine. Before the actual headache begins, there are warning signs, called an **aura**, which may involve alterations in mood, a feeling of pins and needles in the hands, disturbances of vision including flashing lights and geometric shapes or, rarely, weakness or paralysis of one side of the body. These symptoms are related to constriction of the cerebral blood vessels. The actual pain of the headache itself occurs as the blood vessels dilate. The headache is a pounding, pulsating pain, usually on one side in the region of the temple, and is accompanied by nausea and sensitivity to light, noise or smell. It typically increases with physical exertion. The patient usually prefers to rest in a quiet, dark room and wait for the attack to subside.

As mentioned above, most migraine attacks are not classic migraines and consist of headache associated with nausea, light and noise sensitivity, but without the preceding aura. This is called 'common migraine'.

Cluster headache

This is a relatively rare type of headache, which occurs in adults due to unknown causes. The pain is very severe but not pounding, and occurs on one side of the head behind the eye and cheek.

On the affected side of the face, the eye waters, the nose runs and the upper eyelid may droop. Each attack lasts between 20 minutes and an hour and can recur several times within a day.

Headache related to chemical substances

Alcohol, lead and certain medications such as morphine can cause headache. Sometimes, laboratory workers or people working in chemical factories suffer headache as a result of exposure to various substances during the course of their work.

Headache caused by high blood pressure

High blood pressure (hypertension) is a dangerous cause of headache and it is important to exclude it in a patient with headache.

Headache secondary to problems in the eyes, ears, teeth or sinuses

Various eye disorders, such as incorrectly prescribed glasses, or increased pressure within the eye can cause headache. An ear infection or infection in the teeth or sinuses can also result in headache.

Raised intracranial pressure

There are several serious medical conditions in which the pressure within the skull is increased, and headache is one of the important symptoms. For example, a brain tumor might cause headache as well as vomiting, which occurs typically upon arising in the morning (often without associated nausea). Severe headache with nausea, vomiting and fever can be a sign of intracranial infection with bacteria, a virus or other infection.

Bleeding within the skull raises the intracranial pressure and can produce a severe headache, usually together with other signs such as a decrease in consciousness.

CEREBRAL INFARCT

A **cerebrovascular accident (CVA)** is defined as an infarct of the brain tissue due to lack of blood supply (ischemia). It can appear at any age, although it is more common in later life, and is the third leading cause of death in the Western world, after heart disease and cancer.

Most CVAs are caused by a process similar to that causing heart attacks – a blood clot that blocks an artery. The area of brain that receives its blood supply from that artery becomes ischemic and necrotic. Sometimes a CVA is caused by rupture of a blood vessel, which results in bleeding into the brain tissue or into the ventricles. High blood pressure is an important risk factor for cerebrovascular accidents. Other risk factors are high blood cholesterol level and smoking.

The term **stroke** usually refers to the clinical features that appear following a CVA. It is common for the CVA to occur at night and for the patient to awake in the morning with some neurologic deficit, depending on the location and size of the cerebral infarct. Some examples are described below:

- An infarct in the motor cortex of the right hemisphere will result in weakness or paralysis of the left half of the body. Paralysis of one side of the body is called **hemiplegia**, and weakness is called **hemiparesis**.
- Damage to the sensory cortex of the left cerebral hemisphere will result in loss of feeling on the right side of the body.
- Damage to the cerebellum will affect coordination and balance, resulting in a characteristic wide-based, unsteady gait called **ataxia**.
- An infarct in the speech center of the brain, usually in the left cerebral hemisphere, will affect speech – a condition known as **aphasia**. There are two main types of aphasia. In **motor aphasia**, the patient partially or totally

loses the ability to speak but has no trouble understanding the written or spoken word. In the other type of aphasia – **sensory aphasia** – the patient cannot understand what is said, with resulting severe speech and communication difficulties. (Note: The subject of aphasia is very complex and the above is only a very simplified description.)

One-third of patients will recover the lost function(s) completely; in one-third there will be partial recovery; in the remaininig one-third the neurologic deficit is permanent. In many cases physiotherapy and speech therapy can be of considerable benefit in helping the patient recover lost functions. However, it is impossible to accurately predict the degree and rate of recovery following CVA. Such recovery occurs as a result of the formation of new connections among neurons. (Recall that damaged or destroyed neurons are themselves not replaced.)

DEMENTIA

Dementia is defined as a loss of intellectual abilities (e.g. memory, analysis of sensory input, alertness, awareness of surroundings) to such a degree that the patient's social and work functions are affected

The incidence of dementia increases with increasing age and occurs in 20% of males over the age of 80. It is the leading cause of incapacity in the elderly. The disease can also occur under the age of 65. The signs of dementia are the same regardless of age.

There are few causes of dementia. In a small percentage of cases, when there is a specific and defined cause, treatment of that cause may actually cure the dementia. This can be seen, for example, when the dementia is caused by a brain tumor, by lack of thyroid hormone or by lack of vitamin B12, which are all examples of potentially reversible conditions. It is therefore extremely important to exclude such treatable causes in any demented patient. However, in most cases, dementia is progressive and incurable. The two major causes of dementia are Alzheimer's disease and multiple cerebral infarcts.

Alzheimer's disease

This is the most common cause of dementia. The gene responsible for the disease has now been discovered.

Alzheimer's disease causes progressive death of cells in the cerebral cortex. As a result, the brain mass decreases and the grooves (sulci) in the cortex become wider as the brain tissue shrinks. Microscopic examination of brain tissue from Alzheimer's patients reveals the accumulation of a specific protein substance in the spaces between the brain cells.

The initial symptoms appear very slowly and subtly, and it is difficult to pinpoint the actual onset. At first, the patient loses interest in pastimes, hobbies and social interactions. It becomes hard to learn new information, and short and medium term memory decreases. Subsequently, the patient becomes progressively apathetic, lacks initiative, and makes mistakes in everyday tasks such as dressing and personal hygiene.

In the final stages of the disease, the patient becomes withdrawn and confused, and does not recognize others. The gait becomes unstable, bladder and bowel control is lost and attacks of aggressive behavior or restlessness may occur.

In the early stages of the illness, the patient is aware of the changes in function but, with time, this insight disappears and is replaced by social withdrawal into a private closed world. The family and significant others around the patient also suffer greatly as the patient's condition degenerates.

There is no treatment for Alzheimer's disease, and the average patient usually dies about 8 years after the onset of the disease. However, some promising treatments are being studied and used in selected patients.

Multiple cerebral infarcts dementia

Individuals who have had several strokes can develop chronic cognitive defects, commonly called multiple cerebral infarcts dementia. The strokes can be small or large and the occurrence of dementia seems to depend partly on the total volume of damaged cortex. Most of these patients have hypertension – an important risk factor for stroke.

SPINAL INJURIES

Injury to the spinal cord usually results from a fracture of the spinal column, with contusion of the spinal cord by bone fragments. Other causes of spinal cord damage include tumors, infections and chronic neurologic disorders. Total tearing of the spinal cord (spinal cord transection) cuts off all the neurologic pathways from the level of the transection downwards. Transection that results in total muscle paralysis of the legs (**paraplegia**), is usually associated with total lack of sensation below the level of the injury and lack of control over the bladder or bowel, because of disruption of the autonomic pathways. Paralysis of all four limbs is called **quadriplegia**, and is usually the result of transection of the spinal cord at a high level (neck), such as may occur in a diving accident.

If the spinal cord is only partially transected, the neurologic damage will depend on the particular nerve pathways that are damaged.

Complete transection of the spinal cord is irreversible because there is no regeneration of the damaged neural tissue. The neurologic deficit does not improve with time. This is in contrast to damage to the brain, where a certain degree of neurologic improvement can occur as a result of the formation of new neural connections.

In any situation that might involve spinal cord damage (a fall from a height, a traffic accident, etc.), it is extremely important not to move the person, as there might be damage to the spinal column that might not be causing any damage to the spinal cord itself. Moving the person could drive a fragment of fractured bone into the cord, causing avoidable neural damage.

PERIPHERAL NERVE DAMAGE

Peripheral nerves can be damaged as the result of being accidentally cut or by any of the diseases that involve peripheral nerves (e.g. diabetes, alcoholism).

Complete transection of a peripheral nerve usually occurs in a limb and results in total paralysis of the muscles innervated by the nerve, as well as in loss of sensation in the area of skin innervated by that nerve. Such denervated muscles quickly become thin and weak, and 'shrivel up' within weeks, a process known as 'atrophy'. The axons on the near (proximal) side of the injury, that is between the spinal cord and the injury, do not die because they are still attached to their cell bodies. However, the axons distal to the injury die off and eventually disappear.

If the two cut ends of the axons are very close to each other, the axons from the proximal end may grow into the distal end of the cut nerve, at a rate of up to 1 mm a day, until they reach the target organ (muscle, for example) and innervate it once again. This phenomenon is known as **peripheral nerve regeneration**, and allows for recovery of the neurologic deficit in the affected area.

EPILEPSY

Epilepsy is caused by a disturbance of the electrical activity of the brain. This disturbance can appear in an area of the brain damaged by various diseases, such as a tumor, trauma or infection. However, it more commonly appears in the absence of such underlying disease.

Epilepsy occurs in attacks characterized by a decrease in consciousness, involuntary movements of various parts of the body, abnormal sensations or changes in behavior.

There are various types of epilepsy. In the type known as **grand mal**, the patient loses consciousness and falls, occasionally while emitting a cry. The muscles then become stiff, breathing might stop momentarily and the limbs might twitch for several minutes.

Finally, the muscles relax and the patient lies limply, often with some salivation. During the attack, the patient can bite the tongue and lose control of the bladder and bowel. Following the attack, the patient is usually confused for several hours.

Another type of epilepsy, which commonly occurs in children, is called **petit mal**. Petit mal attacks are extremely brief (several seconds), during which time the person is momentarily out of touch with the surroundings. The patient exhibits a glassy stare and occasionally blinking movements or other minimal facial twitches. Up to several hundred attacks can occur in a single day and, if the epilepsy is not diagnosed, the patient might be labeled as a 'daydreamer'.

Some other types of epilepsy involve only one part of the body and are called **focal epilepsy**, as opposed to the above two examples, which are **generalized** forms of epilepsy involving the entire body.

The diagnosis of epilepsy is based on the clinical features together with abnormalities of the recorded electrical activity of the brain, such recording being called an **electroencephalogram (EEG)**. Between attacks, the EEG of an epileptic patient is often normal.

The disease is treated by medications that prevent the attacks or, in the case of an underlying treatable disease (e.g. a tumor), treatment of that disease (e.g., surgical excision).

13 The urinary system

Homeostasis literally means 'remaining the same' (from the Greek word *Homeo* = the same and *Stasis* = standing). Despite changes in the environment and surroundings, certain body functions and states, such as temperature and the composition of blood, are strictly maintained within a narrow range of values. Any deviation from these normal values, such as a rise in body temperature of 5°C, can be fatal.

Several complex mechanisms in the body maintain homeostasis in the face of changes in the external environment. The kidneys play a crucial role in maintaining the homeostasis of water and electrolytes in the body.

The urinary system consists of the kidneys, which produce urine, the ureters that conduct the urine to the urinary bladder and the urethra, through which urine passes from the bladder to the exterior (Fig. 13.1).

KIDNEYS

The kidneys are situated behind the abdominal organs against the posterior (back) wall of the abdominal cavity, beside the bodies of the spinal vertebrae at the level of T12 to L3. The right kidney is a little lower than the left.

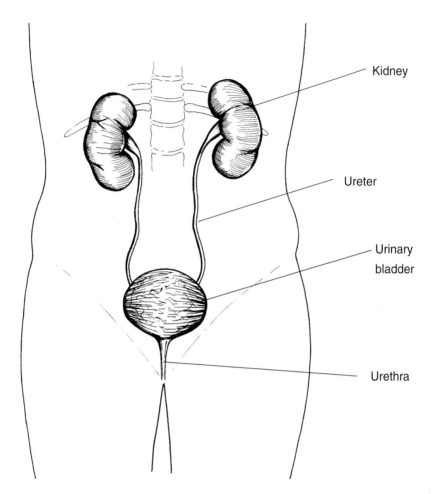

Figure 13.1   The urinary system.

When a person breathes in, the diaphragm flattens and the kidneys are pushed down about 2.5 cm.

Functions of the kidneys

Water, salt (electrolyte) and blood pressure homeostasis

The amount of water in the body, and in particular the volume of water in the circulatory system, is kept constant, despite often extreme variations in the amount of water taken in. If the water balance is positive, such as after drinking a large amount, the kidneys will excrete large amounts of water (and the urine looks pale and dilute); if the water balance is negative, such as on a hot day when insufficient liquids are drunk, the kidneys excrete less water and the urine looks darker and more concentrated.

The concentration of electrolytes within the blood is kept within extremely rigid limits because even a minor deviation from the normal range can have dire consequences.

The kidneys play a vital role in maintaining the normal blood concentrations of electrolytes. They excrete larger or smaller amounts of the various substances in the urine, depending on their concentration in the blood.

Excretion of waste products

The body gets rid of waste products through the kidneys, for example, a substance called **urea**, which gives urine its characteristic odor. Urea contains nitrogen and is produced as a result of the breakdown of proteins.

The concentration of urea in the blood is kept quite low because it is constantly being excreted through the kidneys. If the kidneys are not working properly, urea and other substances will accumulate in the blood, and this can have serious effects on the body. Many medications are also excreted in the urine. Again, if the kidneys are malfunctioning, the blood levels of these medications may rise, which could lead to overdose.

Hormone production

A hormone is a protein or lipid that is produced by a specific organ in the body and secreted into the bloodstream. It then circulates in the blood, becomes bound to some specific target organ and exerts some effect on that organ. The hormones produced by the kidney are listed below.

Vitamin D.   The body can obtain vitamin D from dietary sources or it can manufacture its own vitamin D. The 'production line' for vitamin D involves a 'production site' in the skin (a process that requires sunlight), a 'site' in the liver and a final 'site' in the kidney. Vitamin D is involved in the regulation of calcium and phosphorus stores: it stimulates the absorption of calcium and phosphorus from the digestive system and their subsequent incorporation into bone (in other words it is important in the **mineralization of bones**).

Erythropoietin.   This hormone is needed for the production of red blood cells in the bone marrow; a deficiency of erythropoietin could cause anemia.

Renin.   This hormone is involved in the regulation of blood pressure. If the blood pressure falls (e.g. because of dehydration due to inadequate fluid intake), the blood pressure in the renal artery (the artery supplying blood to the kidney) will also fall. In response to this drop, the kidney secretes renin. This hormone stimulates the production of other hormones that cause vasoconstriction and thereby raise the blood pressure. One of the hormones produced as a result of increased production of renin is called **aldosterone**. This acts on the kidney to decrease water and electrolyte losses in the urine, which also helps to raise the blood pressure.

Structure of the kidney

The kidney is a bean-shaped organ, about 12 cm long, covered by a capsule of fibrous and fatty tissue. The medial side of the kidney (the side nearer the center of the body) is the area known as the **hilum**, through which the blood vessels, lymphatic vessels, and nerves enter and leave the kidney.

A cross-section of a kidney shows it to be divided into several areas. The outermost area is called the **cortex** and the inner area is the **medulla** (Fig. 13.2). Most of the urine is produced in the cortex. It then passes into a system of **calyces** (from the Greek word

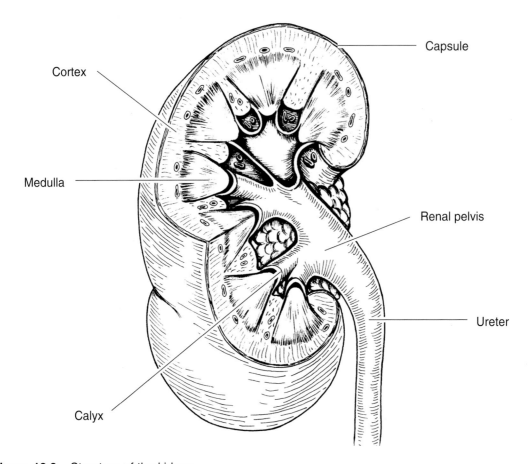

Cortex

Capsule

Medulla

Renal pelvis

Calyx

Ureter

Figure 13.2   Structure of the kidney.

Calyx = cup of flower) in the medulla, from where it passes into the **renal pelvis**, and leaves the kidney via the ureter.

Nephrons

The part of the kidney that produces urine is a microscopic structure called the **nephron**. Each kidney contains approximately 1 million nephrons. A nephron comprises a capsule that contains blood vessels and from which a tubule emerges. An arteriole enters the capsule, where it becomes very coiled and

twisted; it then emerges from the capsule. The capsule together with its arteriole is known as a **glomerulus** (Fig. 13.3).

The arteriole is semipermeable, that is, only certain molecules from the blood can pass out through its wall and enter the space within the glomerular capsule. The tiny openings in the arteriolar wall are too small to allow blood cells to pass through but are large enough to allow the passage of small molecules such as water, electrolytes or urea, into the glomerular space. Furthermore, within the capsule are cells that have extensions, which wrap around

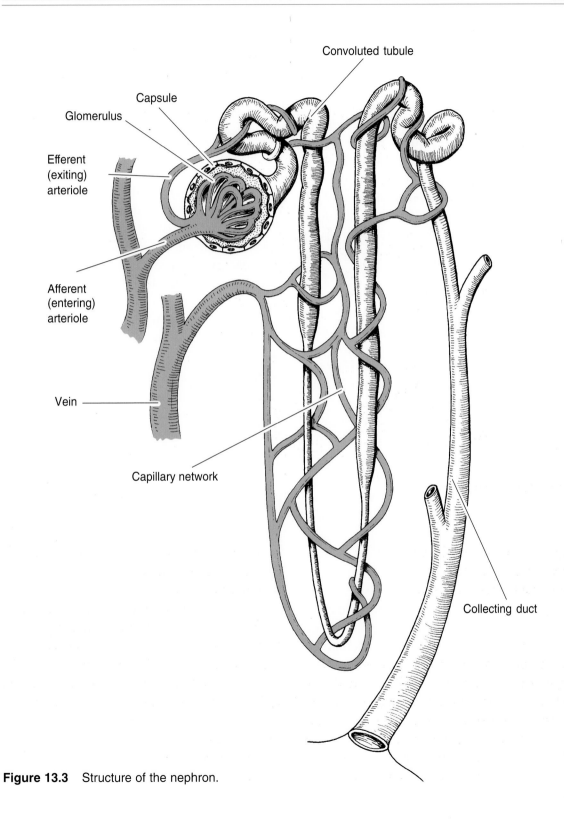

Figure 13.3   Structure of the nephron.

the arteriole and play an important role in maintaining the semipermeability of the arterioles.

From the glomerulus, the fluid that passes out of the arteriole into the glomerular space enters a tubule called the **convoluted tubule**. From there it drains into a larger tubule (**collecting duct**), which in turn drains into the calyces and eventually into the pelvis of the kidney.

In one day, approximately 150 liters of fluid are filtered through the 2 million nephrons in both kidneys, and yet the average volume of urine per day is about 1.5 liters. This indicates that some 99% of the liquid filtered in the glomeruli is reabsorbed and returned to the blood. The same arteriole that enters and leaves the glomerulus runs alongside the tubule that drains the glomerular filtrate. Thus, most of the water, salts and other substances (such as glucose and proteins) that passed out of the arteriole during the filtration process in the glomerulus, now pass out of the convoluted tubule and re-enter the bloodstream. At the end of the tubule a small volume of liquid remains, which is urine. Urine contains water, electrolytes and waste products such as urea.

URETERS

The ureters are narrow tubes, approximately 2.5 mm in diameter and 25 cm long. They drain the urine from the pelvis of the kidney into the urinary bladder. The urine does not pass down the ureters by gravity, but by means of peristaltic waves generated by the smooth muscle in the walls of the ureters.

URINARY BLADDER

The urinary bladder is in the pelvis, immediately behind the **pubis** (one of the major bones of the pelvis). The empty bladder is shaped like an inverted pyramid and, when it fills, it rises up out of the pelvic cavity. The bladder is essentially a muscular sac, which stores urine and passes it out. When it is filled with about 150 ml of urine, an urge to void is experienced: if it is filled with more than 300 ml this urge becomes desperate. In an adult, if the social circumstances are appropriate for **micturition** (passing urine), the bladder neck relaxes, the bladder contracts and urine passes out of it into the urethra. Although the muscle in the bladder is smooth (involuntary) muscle, the 'command' to activate it is voluntary. By contracting the (voluntary) muscles of the abdominal wall and increasing the intra-abdominal pressure, the urine stream can be made more forceful. Conversely, the urine flow can be halted by contracting the muscles of the pelvic floor.

URETHRA

The urethra is the tube through which urine passes from the bladder to the exterior. The male urethra is approximately 15 cm long while in the female it is much shorter – approximately 4 cm.

The urethra passes through a voluntary muscle in the pelvis, which allows one to stop micturition in 'mid-stream'. In the male, the beginning of the urethra passes through the **prostate gland** and changes in the shape or size of the prostate can therefore affect micturition.

Diseases of the urinary system

RENAL FAILURE

Malfunction of the kidneys leads to serious disruptions in bodily function, and eventually to death. There are many causes of renal failure. Some causes (e.g. certain medications, a significant drop in blood pressure) lead to **acute renal failure** that develops over a matter of days, while other causes (e.g. diabetes) result in **chronic renal failure** that develops over months or years. Some of the features of renal failure include:

- Accumulation of fluid and electrolytes in the body, which results in edema and high blood pressure.
- An imbalance in the concentration of electrolytes in the blood.
- A rise in the level of toxic waste products in the blood (mainly nitrogenous products), which affect various body systems.
- Lack of production of the hormones vitamin D and erythropoietin, leading to bone disorders and anemia.

An increase in the blood levels of nitrogenous products leads to a condition called **uremia**, which is characterized by weakness, lack of appetite, nausea and vomiting, shortness of breath, itching, and cardiac and cerebral (brain) malfunction. Most of these phenomena are reversible if kidney function improves.

There are different degrees of renal failure and the treatment depends on its severity. In severe cases, the treatment can involve **dialysis** or renal transplantation. A **dialysis** machine is an apparatus that carries out most of the functions of the kidney artificially.

BENIGN PROSTATIC HYPERTROPHY

Benign prostatic hypertrophy (BPH) is an extremely common condition that occurs in most older males. The prostate gland increases in volume throughout life, presses on the urethra and causes a partial blockage of urine flow. This condition is called benign prostatic hypertrophy to distinguish it from cancer of the prostate gland, a less common but more serious condition with virtually identical initial symptoms. The urethral obstruction causes the patient to suffer from hesitancy – difficulty in starting micturation – a weak urine stream, dribbling at the end of micturition and an urge to pass urine frequently. In some cases, there is also stinging during micturition. The treatment of BPH is by means of either medications or surgery.

URINARY TRACT INFECTION (UTI)

Infection of the urinary tract is usually caused by stool bacteria such as *Escherichia coli*. The bacteria enter the bladder via the urethra, multiply within it and cause infection.

UTI is quite common in women due to, among other reasons, the close proximity of the anal opening (the source of the bacteria) to the opening of the urethra, as well as to the short female urethra. The symptoms of UTI include a burning or stinging sensation when passing urine, urgency (the need to 'run' to the toilet urgently) and frequency (the need to pass urine frequently). Sometimes, the urine also becomes cloudy and foul smelling.

Most UTIs are confined to the bladder (lower urinary tract infection) but sometimes the bacteria ascend the ureters and multiply within the kidney – a condition known as **pyelonephritis** (infection of the kidney). The symptoms of pyelonephritis include high fever, shaking chills (rigors), generalized weakness, and pain or tenderness in the flank area, in addition to the symptoms of bladder infection described above.

The treatment of UTI includes antibiotics and drinking large amounts of fluids. If pyelonephritis is not treated, it can lead to generalized bacterial infection throughout the body and even death.

UROLITHIASIS (KIDNEY STONES)

Most kidney stones are made up of compounds of calcium. The precise reasons behind kidney stone formation are not known but there is an association between their formation and excess calcium in the urine.

Small stones (several millimeters in diameter) pass out of the renal pelvis and into the ureters and the bladder, from where they are excreted out of the body in the urine. As stones pass down the ureter, they cause severe crampy pain known as **renal colic**. The pain comes in waves and radiates from the back towards the groin. Occasionally, there is also blood in the urine, as the ureter is injured by the stone(s) passing through it. In most cases the stone passes down the ureter, reaches the bladder and the pain disappears.

Larger stones (several centimeters in diameter) remain trapped in the pelvis of the kidney, either not causing any symptoms or, in the worst case, causing complete obstruction and ultimately destruction of the kidney.

The treatment of stones larger than 4 mm is by a machine that uses sound waves to break them up into tiny particles, or by surgery. It is prudent to drink large volumes of fluid to prevent the recurrence of kidney stones.

URINARY INCONTINENCE

Normally, as the intra-abdominal pressure rises, urine tends to be 'squeezed out' of the bladder.

However, urine does not escape from the full bladder unless it is passed voluntarily, due to a special anatomic arrangement of the muscles of the pelvic floor. In women after menopause or following pregnancy, there tends to be some weakness of these muscles. As a result, when the intra-abdominal pressure rises, (such as during coughing, laughing or lifting a heavy weight), some urine can 'leak out' involuntarily. Specific pelvic muscle exercises are often helpful in such cases, although in other cases surgery is required.

15

The endocrine system and its diseases

HORMONES

A **hormone** is a substance that is secreted into the bloodstream by a secretory gland and acts on a target organ elsewhere in the body. The endocrine system is a system of internal glands that secrete hormones.

The brain controls the secretion of most of the endocrine glands in the body, and in this way regulates the function of internal organs. This is an alternative way, besides the nervous system, by which the brain controls bodily functions.

The endocrine glands of the body include the pituitary gland (hypophysis), which is situated inside the brain (see Fig. 11.10 and Fig. 15.1); the pancreas, behind the stomach (see Fig. 7.20); the thyroid gland, in the neck; the parathyroid glands, next to the thyroid; the adrenal glands, on top of the kidneys; the testes in the male (in the scrotum) and ovaries in the female (in the pelvic cavity).

In addition to the above endocrine glands, other organs in the body secrete hormones into the bloodstream, including the kidneys, the small bowel and the heart. Hormones secreted by those organs have similar structures and functions to the hormones secreted by the endocrine glands.

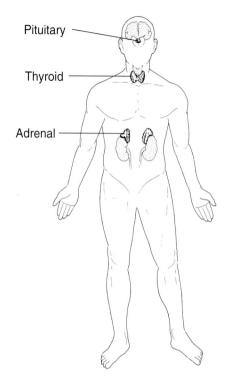

Pituitary

Thyroid

Adrenal

Figure 15.1   Position of the pituitary, thyroid and adrenal glands.

An important principle of hormonal activity is **feedback**. The degree to which a hormone will affect its target cells depends on the concentration of that hormone in the blood and, conversely, the secretion of a hormone depends on the function of its target cells. In this way, the system receives feedback that regulates its processes and therefore the levels of hormone in the blood. In other words, the amount of hormone secreted depends on the function of its target cells or organ.

As an example of feedback, consider the parathyroid hormone, which regulates the level of calcium in the blood. The parathyroid hormone is secreted by the parathyroid glands, usually four in number, measuring about 5 mm in diameter and located on the

posterior border of the thyroid gland. It controls the concentration of calcium in the blood within narrow limits. Any deviation from this range has serious effects on the body and can even be fatal. An increase in the level of parathyroid hormone in the blood affects the kidneys and the bones (the target organs for that hormone), and results in a rise in the level of calcium in the blood; a drop in the concentration of parathyroid hormone in the blood leads to a drop in the blood calcium concentration. However, the rate of production and secretion of the hormone from the glands, and consequently the level of hormone in the blood, are affected by the concentration of calcium in the blood. As the level of calcium in the blood falls, the parathyroid glands secrete more hormone, so that the level of calcium then rises. A rise in blood calcium concentration in turn causes the gland to secrete less hormone, so that the level of hormone in the blood falls. Thus the secretion of parathyroid hormone is controlled by a relatively simple feedback mechanism in which the end result of the hormone's activity affects its secretion. However, the secretion of other hormones, such as thyroid hormone or the sex hormones, is controlled in a more complex way by the brain.

The center for the control of hormone secretion is in a part of the brain called the **hypothalamus**. This organ secretes **releasing factors**, which, in turn, control the secretion of hormones from the pituitary gland.

The **pituitary gland** is situated in a small cave-like depression within the base of the skull, and is closely attached to the hypothalamus. It secretes **stimulatory hormones** that control the secretory activity of the endocrine glands of the body, such as the thyroid gland, the adrenal glands, the testes and the ovaries. In other words, the hormone secretion of some of the endocrine glands is, in fact, controlled by the brain via the pituitary hormones.

The feedback acts via the end-product of the endocrine gland. A rise in the blood concentration of the hormone suppresses the secretion of the hypothalamic releasing factors or the pituitary stimulatory hormones, thereby reducing the amount of hormone secreted. A reduction in the concentration of hormone in the blood stimulates the production of more stimulatory hormones, which, in turn, increases the amount of hormone secreted into the blood by the gland.

Damage to or disease of the hypothalamus or pituitary affects the secretion of those hormones that are under their control.

PITUITARY GLAND

The pituitary gland (also known as the **hypophysis**) weighs about 0.5 g, and is approximately 6 × 13 × 10 mm in size. It lies in a depression in one of the bones of the base of the skull called the **sella turcica ('Turkish saddle')**.

The pituitary gland is made up of a body with a stalk, and looks like a tiny fig. The **stalk** connects the body of the pituitary gland to the hypothalamus above it (Fig. 15.2). The pituitary gland itself is made up of two parts. The front (anterior) lobe is called the **pars distalis**, and contains cells that produce six major hormones which are secreted into the bloodstream. The posterior lobe, called the **pars nervosa**, stores two of the hormones produced in the hypothalamus (these hormones are not produced in the pituitary itself), and subsequently releases them into the bloodstream.

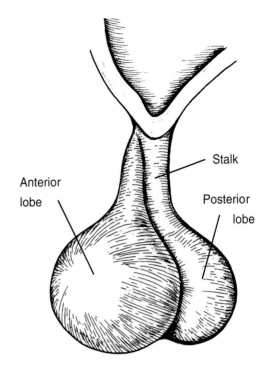

Figure 15.2   Pituitary gland.

Posterior pituitary

The two posterior pituitary hormones are actually produced by specialized neurons within the hypothalamus, and not in the pituitary itself. The axons of these neurons pass down through the pituitary stalk and reach the posterior part of the pituitary. The hormones pass within the axons from the hypothalamus to the posterior pituitary, where they are stored until released into the bloodstream. These hormones are **antidiuretic hormone (ADH)** and **oxytocin**.

Antidiuretic hormone, as its name suggests, acts on the kidneys to regulate the amount of water excreted in the urine. After drinking large amounts of water, less ADH is secreted, so that the water excreted in the urine increases and thus the excess is eliminated.

When the body is dehydrated (excessive water loss due to, for example, sweating on a very hot day, or diarrhea), more antidiuretic hormone is secreted, less water is excreted in the urine and thus water is retained to correct the dehydration.

Disease or injury to the hypothalamus or posterior pituitary, leads to a deficiency of ADH, and results in a disease called **diabetes insipidus**. (Note that this is not to be confused with the more common diabetes mellitus, or 'sugar diabetes', to be discussed on p. 252. Apart from the similar names, there is no connection between the two diseases). In diabetes insipidus, there is a deficiency or total absence of ADH in the blood and consequently the kidneys excrete excessive amounts of water. In an attempt to restore the lost water to the body, the patient drinks huge amounts (up to 20 liters a day!).

The second hormone stored in the posterior pituitary is **oxytocin**. This is produced in very large quantities during childbirth and causes contractions of the muscles of the uterus. Oxytocin is also involved in the secretion of milk from the breast during lactation. Its role in the male is unknown.

Anterior pituitary

The anterior lobe of the pituitary contains cells that produce six major hormones. Some of these are 'stimulatory' hormones, which control the secretion of hormones from other glands, and some are hormones that act directly on various target organs. All of the hormones secreted from the anterior pituitary are under the control of 'releasing factors', (which are other hormones), secreted by the hypothalamus.

Thyroid stimulating hormone (TSH)

This stimulatory hormone controls the secretion of thyroid hormone from the thyroid gland. The secretion of TSH itself is controlled by **thyrotrophin releasing factor (TRF)** – a hormone secreted by the hypothalamus. This is illustrated below:

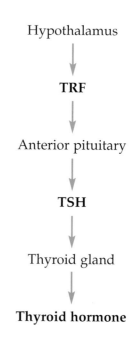

Hypothalamus

↓

TRF

↓

Anterior pituitary

↓

TSH

↓

Thyroid gland

↓

Thyroid hormone

Adrenocorticotrophic hormone (ACTH)

ACTH is the stimulating hormone that controls the secretion of a hormone called **cortisol** from the adrenal gland. The secretion of ACTH itself is regulated by **corticotrophin releasing hormone (CRH)**, a hormone secreted by the hypothalamus.

Luteinizing hormone (LH) and follicle stimulating hormone (FSH)

These are also stimulating hormones that control the secretion of sex hormones from the ovary in the female and the testis in the male. The secretion of both LH and FSH is controlled by **gonadotrophin releasing hormone (GnRH)**, a hormone secreted by the hypothalamus.

Growth hormone (GH)

Unlike the hormones described above, growth hormone is not a stimulating hormone but acts directly on its target organs. The secretion of growth hormone is controlled by **growth hormone releasing hormone (GHRH)**, a hormone secreted by the hypothalamus. Growth hormone is essential for the growth of the bones in children; a lack of growth hormone results in **dwarfism**. Growth hormone can now be manufactured synthetically and administered to children lacking it.

An excess of growth hormone during a child's growth period causes **gigantism**. Excessive growth hormone usually results from a tumor of the pituitary gland, the gland that secretes the hormone. This is an extremely rare condition, which usually causes fatal cardiac problems at a young age. If the excess growth hormone occurs after the growth period, it causes a disease known as **acromegaly** (Fig. 15.3). In this condition, the patient's features gradually 'thicken', with overgrowth of the lower jaw, the nose, the forehead, the hands and the feet. Other problems result from effects on internal organs, joints, nerves and other systems. The treatment of excessive growth hormone involves removal of the growth-hormone-secreting tumor in the pituitary gland.

After the growth period, growth hormone is involved in regulation of the levels of glucose and fatty acids in the blood.

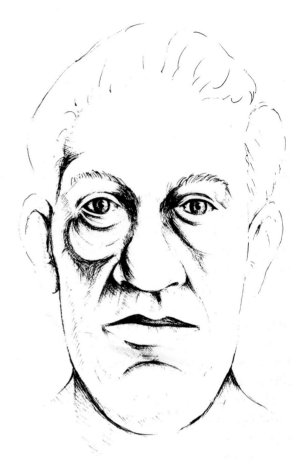

Figure 15.3   Acromegaly: the typical facial appearance of an acromegalic patient

Prolactin (PRL)

This hormone is essential for the secretion of milk in the lactating female. Its secretion is controlled by an inhibitory hormone called **prolactin inhibitory hormone (PIH)**, secreted by the hypothalamus. PIH normally inhibits the secretion of prolactin, except for the period when the woman is lactating. Note that this mechanism is the reverse of the more common situation, in which the secretion of the anterior pituitary hormones is stimulated by the secretion of stimulatory hormones from the hypothalamus. Hypothalamic disease or injury affects the secretion of PIH, so that the level of prolactin in the blood rises (hyperprolactinemia). The role of prolactin in the male is largely unknown.

Hyperprolactinemia is the most common endocrine abnormality of the pituitary gland. It can be due to several causes, the major being a pituitary tumor that secretes prolactin. It results in unexpected milk secretion from the breasts and disturbances of the menstrual cycle. In the male, hyperprolactinemia can cause impotence.

THYROID GLAND

The **thyroid gland** is located in the front of the neck and is composed of two lobes joined by a segment called the **isthmus** (Fig. 15.4).

Normally, the thyroid gland cannot be seen in the neck unless it is enlarged. Histologically, the thyroid contains **follicles**, each consisting of a layer of epithelial cells surrounding a cavity filled with a substance called **colloid**, which is a large storage depot for thyroid hormone. The thyroid is the only endocrine gland in the body that contains stored supply of its hormone, usually sufficient for the body's needs for 3 months.

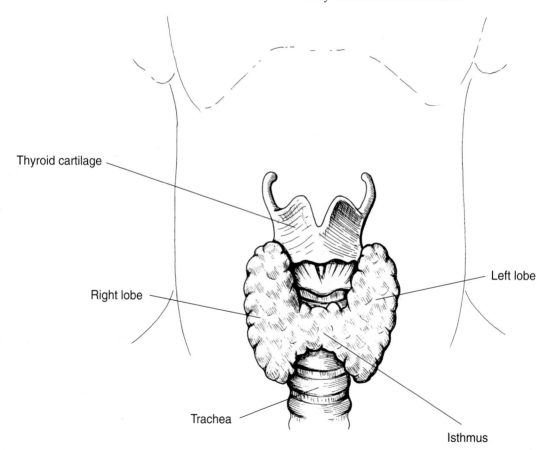

Thyroid cartilage

Right lobe

Left lobe

Trachea

Isthmus

Figure 15.4   Thyroid gland.

Thyroid hormone (TH) is a protein containing iodine, and actually comprises two hormones, known by the abbreviations **T3** and **T4**. The production of thyroid hormone is controlled by the brain through the hypothalamus, which secretes the releasing factor called **thyroid releasing factor (TRF)**, which, in turn, stimulates the (anterior) pituitary to secrete the stimulatory hormone called **thyroid stimulating hormone (TSH)**, which stimulates the thyroid gland to produce thyroid hormone. A decrease in the blood level of thyroid hormone stimulates the secretion of the stimulatory hormones and a rise in the blood level of thyroid hormone inhibits the secretion of the stimulatory hormones.

Thyroid hormone is important for the development of the brain and the bones in the fetus and infant. A lack of thyroid hormone at birth results in mental retardation and abnormalities of the development of the skeletal system – a condition known as **congenital hypothyroidism**. This condition can be prevented if the hormone deficiency is diagnosed soon after birth and the missing hormone is administered. In most countries, the blood level of thyroid hormone is tested routinely in every newborn infant.

In an adult, thyroid hormone determines the 'level of activity' of the body (like the mixture adjustment screw of a carburetor). At the cellular level, thyroid hormone increases oxygen consumption and protein synthesis within cells.

Hyperthyroidism

This occurs when there is an abnormally high level of thyroid hormone in the blood. The disease has many clinical symptoms and signs, which include irritability, restlessness and agitation, fever, inability to tolerate heat, diarrhea, rapid pulse, warm, sweaty skin, tremor, fatigue and difficulty sleeping, increased appetite and weight loss. The overall picture is of a person who is 'hyperactive' (Greek *hyper* = above, over), or on a 'high'. The most common cause of hyperthyroidism is a disease called **Graves' disease**. In this condition, which occurs mainly in women, the patient's own immune system produces antibodies that bind to the thyroid gland and stimulate the secretion of excessive amounts of thyroid hormone. The thyroid gland swells (a condition called **goiter**), and can be seen prominently in the front of the patient's neck. Apart from the various phenomena resulting from an excess of thyroid hormone in the blood, the patient also has bulging eyes (Fig. 15.5).

Hyperthyroidism can be treated by administering medications that interfere with the production of thyroid hormone, by administering radioactive iodide (which destroys part of the thyroid gland) or by surgically removing part of the gland. The risk of the latter two forms of treatment is subsequent hypothyroidism.

Hypothyroidism

This occurs when the blood level of thyroid hormone is too low. The clinical features of hypothyroidism include depression, sluggishness, poor mental functioning, weakness, a slow pulse, constipation, low body temperature and intolerance to cold, dry, coarse skin, thin, brittle hair, hoarseness, and swelling around the eyes. The overall picture is of someone who is 'hypoactive' (Greek *hypo* = under). Ultimately, severe lack of

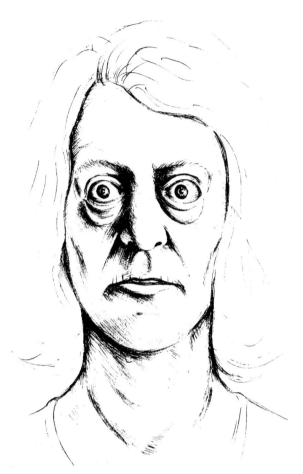

Figure 15.5 Graves' disease: the typical facial appearance of a patient with Graves' disease.

thyroid hormone leads to loss of consciousness and death.

The most common causes of hypothyroidism are treatment of hyperthyroidism by radioactive iodine or surgery, and an autoimmune disease (a disease in which the patient's own immune system attacks his/her gland and destroys it) called **Hashimoto's disease**.

In addition to thyroid hormone, the thyroid gland also secretes a hormone called **calci-**

tonin. This hormone is produced by special cells present between the thyroid follicles. It is important in the control of the level of calcium in the blood. When levels of calcium in the blood rise, the level of calcitonin also rises, which acts to lower the calcium.

ADRENAL GLANDS

The **adrenal glands** are attached to the upper poles of the kidneys (Fig. 15.6). Each gland is a flat, crescentic organ 4–6 cm long, 1–2 cm wide, 4–6 mm thick and weighing approximately 4 g.

The glands are surrounded by a covering of connective tissue. Within the gland are two layers: an outer layer – the **adrenal cortex**, which secretes steroid hormones – and an inner layer called the **adrenal medulla**, which secretes the hormone adrenaline (see p. 254). The adrenal cortex is itself made up of three layers, each of which produces a different hormone.

Aldosterone

Aldosterone is a type of hormone known as a **mineralocorticoid**, and is secreted by the outermost layer of the adrenal cortex. It is involved in control of blood pressure through its effect on the kidneys. Aldosterone acts on the distal tubules of the nephron to increase salt and water retention in the body.

The mechanism that regulates aldosterone secretion is complex. The initial trigger is a fall in blood pressure in the kidney (e.g. following bleeding or dehydration) which causes special cells in the kidney to secrete a hormone called **renin**. The function of renin is to convert another substance in the blood, called **angio-**

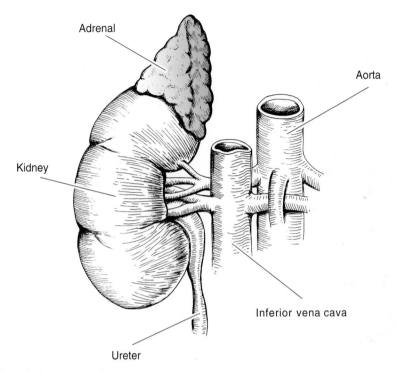

Figure 15.6   Adrenal gland.

tensinogen, into a compound called **angio-tensin I**. Angiotensin I, in turn, when it reaches the lungs via the bloodstream, is converted to **angiotensin II** by an enzyme called **angiotensin converting enzyme (ACE)**. It is angiotensin II that stimulates the secretion of aldosterone from the adrenal gland. In addition, angiotensin II itself has a direct constrictive effect on blood vessels, which also raises the blood pressure.

In summary, the purpose of these complex hormonal processes is to maintain normal blood pressure in the face of fluid losses. The entire hormonal system described here is known as the **renin – angiotensin – aldosterone system**, and it is one of several hormonal systems which control blood pressure:

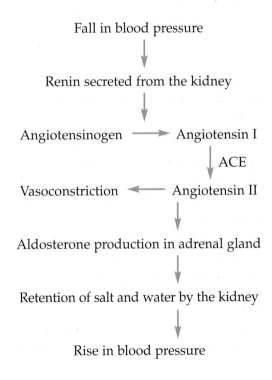

Cortisol

Cortisol is secreted by the middle layer of the adrenal cortex and plays a very important role at times of injury, stress or acute illness. Cortisol increases the levels of nutrient substances in the blood (glucose, amino acids and fatty acids), thereby enabling the body to cope more effectively with the stress situation.

Substances that have similar chemical compositions and similar effects to cortisol (e.g. hydrocortisone, prednisone) are used as medications in certain illnesses. These substances are known collectively as **steroids** and, although they are extremely effective in many situations, they do have serious side-effects and should be used only under strict medical supervision. Steroids are used in many illnesses, including cancer, autoimmune diseases, inflammatory bowel diseases, severe allergy and asthma. The side-effects of steroids tend to appear after taking the medication for about 1 month, and include changes in the appearance of the face (the face becomes round and is referred to as a 'moon face'), a rise in blood pressure, excessive hair growth, decreased bone density, cataracts of the eyes (clouding of the lens), muscle wasting, acne-like skin rashes, defects in the immune system, a tendency to infections and stunting of growth (in children).

Dehydroepiandrosterone (DHEA)

DHEA is secreted by the third layer of the adrenal cortex. This hormone stimulates the appearance of male secondary sexual characteristics, for example, increased muscle mass and body hair growth. The amount of DHEA secreted by the adrenal gland is relatively small, and its actual effect in both males and females is small. However, there are certain diseases in which there is excessive secretion of adrenal male sex hormones. These diseases can affect the development of the external genitalia in a female fetus in the uterus, so she will be born with, among other things, a large clitoris that resembles a penis.

Addison's disease

This disease is a result of failure of the adrenal gland to secrete hormones, and in particular cortisol and aldosterone. The major cause of adrenal failure is an autoimmune process whereby the patient's immune system 'attacks' the adrenal glands, gradually destroying the adrenal cortex. In the past, tuberculosis was a common cause of such disease.

The clinical features of Addison's disease include weakness, fatigue, weight loss, low blood pressure, nausea and vomiting, low body temperature, and hyperpigmentation (areas of skin become darker than normal, especially around the nipples and skin creases). Moreover, there is an increased risk of dying from an injury or an acute illness because cortisol normally enables the body to cope with such states.

The treatment of Addison's disease involves the administration of cortisol and aldosterone for the patient's entire life. If the patient develops an acute illness or undergoes an operation, the dosage of cortisol must then be increased.

Adrenalin

The inner portion of the adrenal gland, the medulla, secretes a hormone called **adrenalin** (or **epinephrine**). This hormone is secreted at times of physical or emotional stress and prepares the body to deal more effectively with the stress. Adrenalin secretion works in parallel with the sympathetic autonomic nervous system, and the two systems have similar bodily effects.

Adrenalin increases the output of the heart and lungs, dilates the airways, decreases blood flow to the skin (hence the skin becomes pale and cold), causes sweating (a 'cold' sweat), increases blood flow to the muscles, causes the pupils to widen and has many other effects. When a stressful event occurs suddenly, one can sense that the pulse rate increases, the breathing becomes more rapid, and the skin becomes cold and clammy.

Pheochromocytoma

This is a tumor of the adrenal gland that secretes excessive adrenalin and related substances into the bloodstream. Patients with this disease therefore suffer episodes, of fast heart rate, sweating and so on, in the absence of a stressful stimulus.

THE PANCREAS

The pancreas is both an exocrine and an endocrine gland. An **exocrine gland** is one that secretes its product into a duct, which then drains into the digestive system or onto the skin or mucous membranes. An **endocrine gland** is one that secretes its product directly into the bloodstream. In the case of the pancreas, its exocrine portion secretes digestive enzymes into the pancreatic duct, which drains into the duodenum (see the description of the structure and anatomic location of the pancreas on pp. 90–92).

The endocrine cells in the pancreas are found in structures called the **islets of Langerhans**. These are groups of cells (like islands) scattered throughout the exocrine tissue of the pancreas. The endocrine portion of the pancreas mainly secretes two hormones – **insulin** (produced by β cells within the islets) and **glucagon** (produced by the α cells).

Insulin is secreted in response to a rise in the level of blood glucose (a monosaccharide sugar that serves as the major fuel for the body), which happens after a normal meal. Its effect is to cause glucose to leave the bloodstream and enter the cells of the body, which lowers the level of glucose in the blood and provides the cells with their energy source.

Apart from regulating the blood sugar level, insulin has other functions in the body. One is the provision of the **satiety signal** for the body. Satiety is physiologically defined as the state when the level of sugar and other food products rise following a meal. In a satiated state, the body stores foodstuffs that it can later utilize in case of hunger.

Insulin also promotes the storage of excess foods in the body, and stimulates the utilization of glucose for various purposes. Food is stored by the:

- conversion of glucose (a monosaccharide) to **glycogen** (a polysaccharide) in the liver
- conversion of glucose to fat in the fatty (adipose) tissue
- conversion of amino acids to protein, mainly in muscle tissue.

In the hunger state, the external supply of food ceases and the body has to subsist on its stores. As a result, the blood level of glucose falls as glucose is depleted for energy. The fall in blood glucose level (**hypoglycemia**) inhibits the secretion of insulin by the pancreas and stimulates the production of other hormones, which constitute the **hunger signal**.

Glucagon, also secreted by the pancreas, is one of the important hormones involved in the **hunger signal**. A fall in insulin levels and a rise in glucagon levels act to maintain the blood glucose at a constant level in the face of varying utilization of glucose by body tissues. The level of blood glucose must remain constant because there are tissues, especially the brain, that depend on a steady supply of glucose.

The source of the glucose in a hunger state depends on the duration of the food deficit. During a short deficit (e.g. overnight), the **glycogen** stores (the polysaccharide stored in the liver) are broken down and release glucose into the bloodstream. During a prolonged deficit (more than 24 h), the muscle proteins break down into amino acids, which are converted into glucose in the liver. However, the liver is unable to convert fatty acids to sugar and thus the production of glucose from protein involves the breakdown of muscle tissue.

During starvation, fatty (adipose) tissue breaks down into fatty acids, which enter the bloodstream. The fatty acids supply most of the body's tissues (those that are not dependent solely on glucose) with their energy needs during the starvation state.

In summary, during a state of satiety, when the blood glucose level rises after a meal, the insulin level (satiety signal) rises and the glucagon level (hunger signal) falls. These hormonal changes promote utilization of glucose by the body tissues as well as the storage of fuel (food). In a state of starvation (when the blood glucose level falls), the level of insulin in the blood falls and the glucagon level rises. These hormonal changes reduce the utilization of glucose by the body's tissues, and stimulate the breakdown of food reserves and the production of glucose from protein in the liver.

DIABETES MELLITUS

Diabetes is the most common endocrine disease and is due to a disturbance of the hormonal control of the hunger and satiety systems. There are two main types of diabetes – juvenile onset diabetes and adult onset diabetes.

Juvenile onset diabetes – diabetes mellitus type 1 (insulin-dependent diabetes)

This disease usually has its onset during childhood, but can occasionally appear at later ages.

It is an autoimmune disease in which the patient's own immune system destroys the insulin-producing cells in the pancreas (the β cells). The destruction of these cells is gradual, over a period of years, and only when approximately 90% of the cells have been destroyed does the disease manifest itself.

Juvenile diabetes is the result of lack of insulin production, with abnormally high blood glucose levels – a state called **hyperglycemia**. Following a meal, the glucose level normally rises and, because no insulin is secreted (which would normally promote entry of glucose into cells), it remains high. Despite high blood glucose levels, the tissues are actually deprived of glucose and function as if in a state of starvation because the satiety signal (insulin) is missing. In an effort to provide an alternate energy source for the body, adipose tissue breaks down into fatty acids, which enter the bloodstream, and the protein in muscle tissue breaks down into amino acids, which reach the liver via the blood. The liver then converts the amino acids to glucose, which is released into the bloodstream, thereby helping to raise the blood glucose concentration further.

The high level of glucose in the blood causes the diabetic patient to excrete large volumes of urine (**polyuria**), which results in drinking large amounts of water (**polydipsia**). The literal meaning of the term diabetes mellitus is 'sweetened siphon' (Latin). The urine of diabetic patients contains large amounts of glucose, and actually has a sweet taste. (In the past doctors used to diagnosis diabetes by tasting the urine!) Because of the breakdown of the fat and protein tissues in the body, the patient loses weight, despite a constant feeling of hunger and eating large amounts. There is a characteristic smell (acetone) on the breath of these patients.

If not treated with insulin, the patient will ultimately die. In the past, insulin was derived from cows or pigs but sophisticated genetic engineering processes are now used to produce human insulin from bacteria. It is administered by injections into the subcutaneous (beneath the skin) tissues two to four times a day.

Despite treatment with insulin, it is not easy to control blood sugar levels. Poor control of blood sugar will, in the long term (over a period of more than 10 years), cause damage to many body tissues and organs, including the heart, kidneys, eyes and limbs. These effects are basically related to damage of the blood vessels and nerves.

Diabetic foot

Some diabetic patients develop necrosis (gangrene) of the foot. Because the nerves leading to the foot (as other nerves) are damaged by the abnormal sugar control, the patient might not feel much pain from a foot injury. Because the blood vessels are also affected, there is poor blood flow to the injured area in the foot, the injury does not heal and necrosis may develop. On occasion, this necessitates amputating part or all of the affected foot or leg.

It is therefore very important that diabetic patients take great care to ensure that their limbs remain clean and free of infection.

Other important complications of diabetes include damage to the kidneys, the eyes and the coronary arteries of the heart, as well as impotence in the male due to poor penile erection. Some of these complications can be prevented or lessened, and thus it is important that a person with diabetes obtains regular medical checkups.

Hypoglycemia

An important and life-threatening complication of juvenile diabetes is **hypoglycemia**, a state in which the level of glucose in the blood falls below normal. Hypoglycemia can be caused by injection of too much insulin, or by eating too little after an insulin injection. The clinical features of hypoglycemia include pallor, sweating, weakness, rapid pulse, dizziness, confusion, loss of consciousness, convulsions and even death. Most of these are the result of the brain not receiving enough glucose for proper function. The treatment of hypoglycemia is to give glucose either by mouth (if the patient is conscious and able to swallow) or by intravenous infusion if the level of consciousness is impaired.

Adult onset diabetes – diabetes mellitus type 2 (non-insulin-dependent diabetes)

This type of diabetes usually appears at a later age. It is often associated with obesity and usually runs in families (the risk of developing type 2 diabetes is higher if a first-degree relative has the disease).

In this disease, the problem is not a lack of insulin, but rather an inadequate response to insulin (**insulin resistance**). In other words, the problem is not in the pancreas but in the body tissues that insulin affects. Adult onset diabetes is often diagnosed incidentally during a routine blood test that shows abnormally high levels of glucose. Over a period of years, the high glucose levels cause damage to many organs in the body, similar to that in juvenile diabetes. In many cases, type 2 diabetes can be treated by non-medicinal means, including weight reduction, dietary changes and alterations in lifestyle.

The medications used in adult onset diabetes increase the production of insulin by the pancreas or increase the sensitivity of tissues to insulin, and thereby help to overcome the insulin resistance.

16

The female reproductive system and its diseases

There are several basic differences between the male and female reproductive systems. The male system starts functioning at puberty and remains functional throughout life, with sperm being produced continuously. The female system, on the other hand, although it also starts functioning at puberty, remains functional only until the menopause (average age 50 years). Ova ('eggs') are produced in the female only during the fetal period (which occurs *in utero*), and the female infant is born with her full complement of ova (singular = ovum). After birth, the number of ova in the body steadily diminishes.

The male reproductive system completes its reproductive role during intercourse, when semen is ejaculated into the vagina. At that moment, the female reproductive system begins its reproductive role, which ends epproximetly 38 weeks later with childbirth.

The female reproductive system (Figs 16.1 and 16.2) consists of the external genitalia called the **vulva**, a short tubular organ that opens out onto the vulva (the **vagina**), the **uterus** ('womb'), two tubes connected to the uterus, called the **uterine** or **fallopian tubes**, and the two **ovaries**. Throughout the fertile period, the reproductive system functions in a

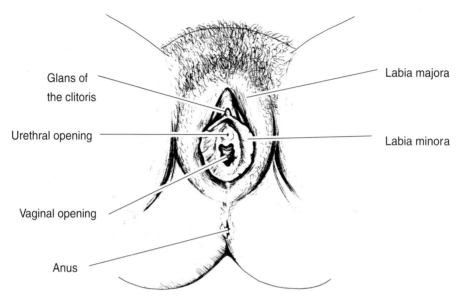

Figure 16.1   The vulva.

cyclical manner; this cycle temporarily stops during pregnancy.

During each cycle, one of the ovaries releases an ovum (a process called **ovulation**) into the fallopian tube. The ovum starts moving down the tube towards the uterus. If sperm reach the fallopian tube at that time, the egg can be fertilized by one of the sperm and the process of development into an embryo begins. The fertilized egg continues its journey down the tube and reaches the uterus, where it embeds into the wall of the uterus (a process called **implantation**), and the development of the embryo into a mature baby continues, ending in birth.

During the menstrual cycle the ovary secretes sex hormones that prepare the lining of the uterus for implantation of a fertilized ovum. If fertilization has not taken place, this lining separates from the wall and is shed; this is the process of **menstruation**. Following menstruation, the cycle starts again and the lining of the uterus builds up again to await a fertilized ovum.

VULVA

The **labia majora** (in Latin: *large lips*) are thick folds of skin, covered with hair, which form the outer border of the vulva (Fig. 16.1). The **labia minora** (in Latin: *small lips*) are thin folds of hairless skin on the inner side of the labia majora. The upper ends of the labia minora partly surround an elongated organ called the **clitoris**, which consists of erectile tissue (i.e. tissue that is capable of being distended with blood and becoming rigid). The body of the clitoris ends in a 'head' called the **glans**, covered by a fold of skin called the **prepuce** (foreskin). The structure of the clitoris is similar to that of the penis. During sexual arousal, the clitoris fills with blood and swells up. There is a network of sensory nerves in the glans of the clitoris and stimulation of it plays an important role in the female orgasm.

Below the clitoris, between the folds of the labia, is the opening of the urinary tract, the **urethra**. Below the urethra is the opening of

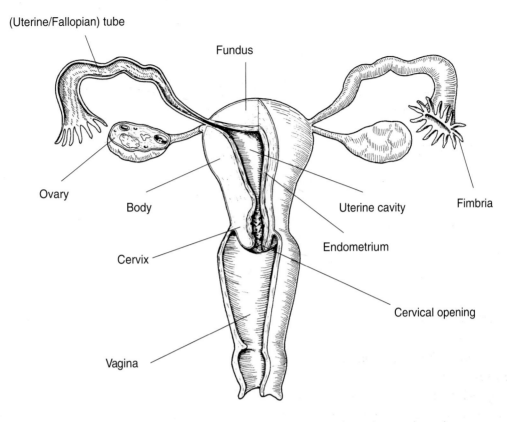

Figure 16.2   The female reproductive tract – the vagina, uterus, uterine tubes and ovaries.

the vagina, which is closed off in the virginal state by a thin membrane of skin called the **hymen**. The hymen has an opening in its center to enable the menstrual blood to drain out of the vagina at the time of menstruation. Below the lower end of the labia majora are two glands called the **vestibular glands** or **Bartholin's glands**. At times of sexual arousal, these glands secrete an oily secretion, which lubricates the vaginal opening.

VAGINA

The vagina is a canal approximately 8 cm long. Its external opening lies in the vulva, and its other end ends at the cervix (the neck of the uterus) (see Fig. 16.2). In front of (anterior to)

the vagina lie the urinary bladder and the urethra, and behind (posterior to) it lies the rectum (see Fig. 16.5).

Within the mucosal lining of the vagina are special bacteria that secrete a mild acid, which acts to protect the vagina from invasion by harmful microorganisms. At times of sexual arousal, the walls of the vagina become lubricated with an oily secretion to aid penetration by the penis. As the penis enters the vagina, the vaginal walls also stretch and elongate.

UTERUS

The uterus (see Fig. 16.2) is a hollow structure with muscle walls. In a non-pregnant woman it is approximately 8 cm long and 4 cm wide. The uterus can be divided into three parts: the **fundus**, which is the portion above the point of entry of the fallopian tubes; the **body**, which is the portion between the fundus and the **cervix**, the neck. The cervix is cylindrically shaped and its lower end connects with the upper part of the vagina. The walls of the cervix are composed mainly of connective tissue, rather than muscle as is the rest of the uterus.

The walls of the uterus comprise three layers. The outermost layer is the **peritoneum**, which is the thin membrane that envelops the abdominal organs. Next is the thick muscular middle layer and finally the innermost layer, which is composed of the mucosal lining of the uterus.

The cavity of the uterus is approximately 10 cm^3 in volume, and is T-shaped. Its lower portion continues into the cavity of the cervix – the **cervical canal**. (Note that the cervical canal is not defined as part of the uterine cavity). The upper part of the uterine cavity (the arms of the T) is continuous on each side with the cavity within the fallopian tubes.

During pregnancy, the uterus undergoes profound changes. Its volume increases from 10 milliliters to over 10 liters. The muscle of the pregnant uterus grows and stretches, while the cervix remains closed. During childbirth, the uterus contracts strongly and the cervix opens, expelling the fetus from the uterus and propelling it through the cervical canal and vagina.

Endometrium

This is the mucosal lining of the uterus, which undergoes marked cyclical changes due to the effect of the sex hormones.

The endometrium is composed of two layers. The outer layer (nearest the cavity of the uterus) is shed during **menstruation** and then regrows, whereas the deeper inner layer is not shed at all but serves as a basis for regrowth of the outer layer. The regrowth of the outer layer of the endometrium is due to the action of the hormone **estrogen**, which is secreted by the ovaries until the mid-point of the menstrual cycle (usually 14 days). At the mid-point of the cycle, due to the action of a hormone called **progesterone**, the endometrium starts to accumulate nutritional substances in preparation for possible pregnancy. If fertilization does not take place, this outer layer of the endometrium separates from the underlying inner layer and is passed out through the cervix and vagina. This process is known as menstruation. Following menstruation, a new menstrual cycle begins.

FALLOPIAN (UTERINE) TUBES

The fallopian tubes (see Fig. 16.2) are thin, muscle-walled tubes approximately 12 cm long. They are sometimes called the uterine tubes. One end of the tube opens into the uterine cavity and the other end is open to the abdominal cavity, close to the ovary. This open end of the fallopian tube ends in a wider, funnel-shaped structure with finger-like fringes (called **fimbria**) at its free end. The fallopian tube plays a crucial role in 'capturing' the ovum released from the ovary during ovulation and 'delivering' it to the uterus. During ovulation, the end of the tube moves towards the ovary and the fimbria move in a beating motion and 'suck' the ovum into the open end of the tube. Within the mucosal lining of the fallopian tube are tiny moving hairs (cilia),

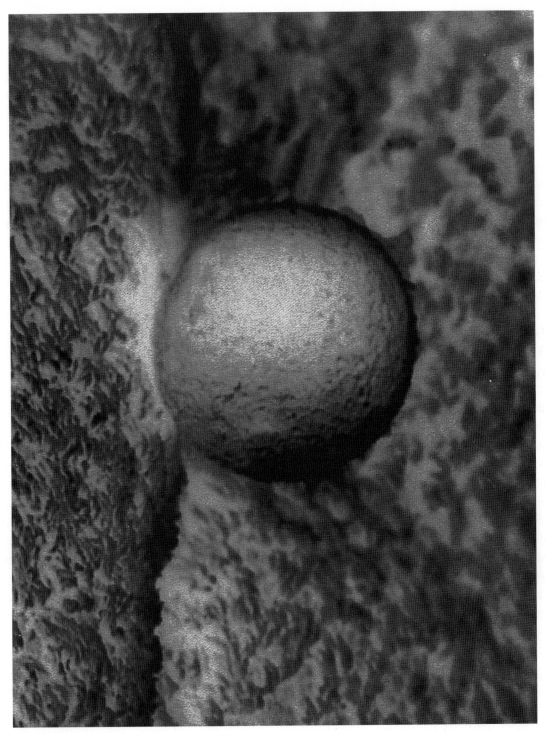

Micrograph of an ovum in a fallopian tube.

similar to those lining the respiratory tract, which sweep the ovum towards the uterus. Fertilization of the ovum by the sperm takes place within the fallopian tube, usually within the one-third that is farthest from the uterus.

OVARIES

The ovaries are two small, elliptical organs (3×1.5 cm) within the pelvic cavity, one on each side of the uterus, near the ends of the fallopian tubes (see Fig. 16.2). They have two functions: storage of ova, with the release of one mature ovum into the fallopian tube each month, and the production of female sex hormones.

The female sex cells are formed within the ovaries of the developing fetus between the first and fifth months of fetal life. By the end of the fifth month, the number of sex cells (oocytes) within the fetal ovary has reached its maximum (approximately 3 million oocytes in each ovary). Shortly before birth the fetal sex cells begin to degenerate and, by the age of puberty only approximately 400 000 oocytes remain. Of these, only about 450 will mature and will be eventually released at ovulation; most of the remaining ova degenerate.

Hence, when an ovum is fertilized, it is roughly as old as the woman herself. For this reason, the number of abnormalities in fetuses seen in women over the age of 40 is relatively high, because they are derived from 'old' ova.

Within the ovary, the ova are surrounded by a layer of cells called **granulosa cells**. The entire structure of the ovum and the surrounding cells is called a **follicle**. At the beginning of every cycle, a group of follicles starts to undergo a maturation process during which the cells surrounding the ovum divide and the follicle grows (Fig. 16.3). This growth of the follicle is stimulated by a hormone called **follicle stimulating hormone (FSH)** secreted by the pituitary gland. As the follicle matures and grows, the cells surrounding the ovum secrete the sex hormone **estrogen**, which stimulates the endometrium (lining of the uterus) to grow following menstruation. At the middle of the cycle one large follicle (approximately 2 cm in diameter) is produced, and the other follicles degenerate.

Ovulation takes place in the middle of the cycle (in a 28-day cycle), or about 14 days before the onset of menstruation in a cycle that is not 28 days long.

A pituitary hormone called **luteinizing hormone (LH)**, stimulates the process of ovulation. As the level of LH in the blood rises, the large follicle bursts open and releases the ovum from the ovary. The ovum enters the open end of the fallopian tube. The follicle undergoes a series of changes to become a **corpus luteum** (Latin = *yellow body*), which itself secretes the sex hormone **progesterone** to prepare the endometrium for possible pregnancy. If fertilization does not take place, the corpus luteum degenerates towards the 28th day of the cycle and the levels of progesterone fall, causing the thickened outer layer of the endometrium to degenerate and be shed during menstruation.

THE MENSTRUAL CYCLE

The menstrual cycle lasts an average of 28 days, although it is shorter in some women and longer in others. The cycle is controlled by the brain, via hormones secreted by the hypothalamus and the pituitary glands (Fig. 16.4).

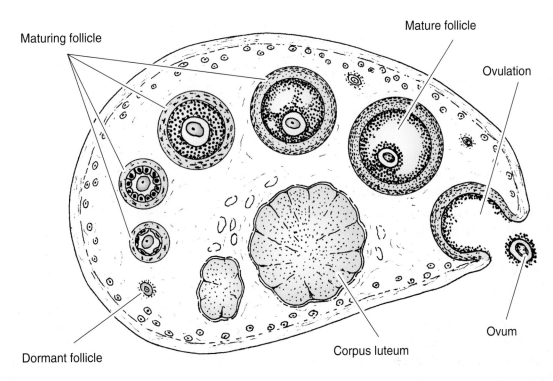

Figure 16.3   Maturation of follicles. In the ovary, one follicle is shown maturing from the initial stage until maturity and ovulation. Following ovulation the follicle becomes a corpus luteum.

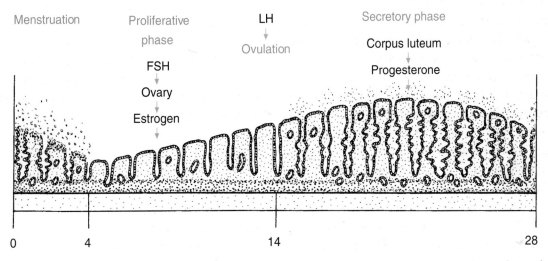

Figure 16.4   The female menstrual cycle. This diagram shows the changes occurring in the endometrium at the various stages of the cycle, which lasts 28 days.

The cycle can be divided into three phases:

1. menstruation
2. the proliferative (follicular) phase
3. the secretory (luteal) phase.

The first phase of the cycle starts with the first day of the menstrual bleed and lasts, on average, 4 days. The second phase starts when the bleeding stops, and lasts until day 14, when ovulation occurs. During this stage, the pituitary gland secretes the follicle stimulating hormone, which acts on the follicles within the ovary, causing them to grow and secrete the hormone **estrogen**. Estrogen stimulates the endometrium following menstruation to grow (hence this stage is called the **proliferative phase**).

On day 14 of the cycle, the pituitary gland secretes luteinizing hormone, which causes the largest and most mature follicle to burst and release the ovum. The residue of the follicle becomes the **corpus luteum**, which in turn secretes the hormone **progesterone**. The rest of the follicles that developed during that cycle degenerate. The progesterone acts on the endometrium and promotes the storage of 'food' and energy supplies to await the arrival of a fertilized ovum.

If fertilization does not take place, the corpus luteum degenerates, the level of progesterone falls and the thickened endometrium is shed as the menstrual bleed.

FERTILIZATION AND PREGNANCY

Fertilization occurs when a single sperm penetrates an ovum, producing the first cell of the embryo, known as a **zygote**.

During a normal single ejaculation by the male, approximately 250 million sperm are discharged into the female's vagina. The high acidity of the vagina makes it a hostile environment for sperm and only some manage to penetrate the mucus that coats the cervix of the uterus and actually enter the uterine cavity. Even fewer sperm manage to reach the fallopian tubes. Once in the tubes, the sperm must 'swim' against the current created by the tiny hairs lining the fallopian tubes. The task of the sperm is to come into contact with the ovum – this usually happens in the outer third of the fallopian tube. Of the original 250 million sperm ejaculated into the vagina only about 200 get close to the ovum, and only one actually penetrates the ovum and fertilizes it. The purpose of this extreme selection process is to ensure that only the strongest, healthiest sperm survive to fertilize the ovum.

An ovum can only be fertilized within 24 hours of ovulation: sperm can survive in the woman's body for only 72 hours. Before fertilization takes place, the sperm undergo changes to enable them to penetrate the cell wall of the ovum, and begin to secrete 'dissolving' enzymes that aid in the penetration of the ovum wall. Immediately after being penetrated, the ovum undergoes changes that make it impenetrable to any other sperm.

Each sperm contains within its nucleus 23 chromosome, which carry the genes contributed to the fetus by the father. Of the 23, 22 are single 'ordinary' chromosomes, or **autosomes**, and one is a **sex chromosome** – either an X chromosome or a Y chromosome. The sex of the fetus is determined by the sex chromosome from the sperm: if the sperm contains an X chromosome, the fetus will be a female; if it contains a Y chromosome, the fetus will be male. The ovum also contains 23 single chromosomes – 22 autosomes and one sex chromosome (always an X chromosome), which represent the genetic contribution from the mother. The zygote formed as the result of fertilization therefore contains 23 pairs of chromosomes (44 autosomes and 2 sex chromosomes).

Once the ovum has been fertilized, it starts to divide, even as it is travelling down the fallopian tube towards the uterus. The initial single cell divides in two to give 2 cells, both of which divide in two to produce 4 cells, which divide to produce 8 cells, which form 16 cells, then 32 cells, and so on. Within 3 days of fertilization, the embryo consists of several tens of cells. Five days after fertilization, when it consists of about 128 cells, it reaches the uterus and 'burrows' (implants) into the thick endometrium that has been prepared to receive it. Some of the embryo cells then develop into fetal tissues, others develop into membranes that surround the fetus, some become the placenta and still others become the umbilical cord.

The developing fetus produces a hormone called **hCG (human chorionic gonadotrophin)**, which is necessary for the maintenance of the corpus luteum. (It is the increasing level of this hormone – hCG – that forms the basis of pregnancy tests). The corpus luteum produces progesterone, which is essential for the continuation of the pregnancy. If the ovum is not fertilized, the corpus luteum degenerates (because there is no hCG to maintain it); the progesterone level then falls, resulting in degeneration of the endometrium and its shedding during menstruation.

The **placenta** (Fig. 16.5) is formed within the uterine endometrium from cells derived both from the embryo and from the mother. Maternal blood, which contains oxygen and nutrients, reaches the uterus and flows into large lake-like spaces in the placenta. Blood vessels from the fetus reach the placenta via the umbilical cord, and there they pass through these spaces filled with maternal blood. Oxygen and nutrients from the maternal blood permeate through the walls of the fetal blood vessels and carbon dioxide and waste products in the fetal blood pass out of the blood vessels into the maternal blood around them. In this way, while the fetal and maternal bloods do not actually mix, exchange of various substances does take place between them. The **umbilical cord** contains two arteries, which carry blood from the fetus to the placenta, and one vein that brings blood from the placenta to the fetus.

The fetus lies in a fluid-filled sac called the **amniotic sac**; the fluid is called **amniotic fluid**. This fills the fetal lungs, ensuring that they develop normally in preparation for breathing air at birth.

During the course of a pregnancy, a woman's body undergoes many changes. For example, the blood volume increases by 50%, cardiac output increases, the kidney and lung functions increase and changes appear in the skin, such as increasing pigmentation (becoming darker) of the areolae of the breasts (the area around the nipple). On average, a pregnant woman gains approximately 12 kg in weight.

BIRTH (LABOR)

Birth normally takes place 40 weeks after the date of the last normal period. During this process, the cervix gradually opens (this is measured to monitor the progress of the birth). The uterine muscle starts to contract with increasing frequency (**contractions** or 'labor pains') in response to the secretion of the hormone **oxytocin** by the pituitary gland. Each time a contraction occurs, the muscle fibers shorten and the infant is slowly expelled

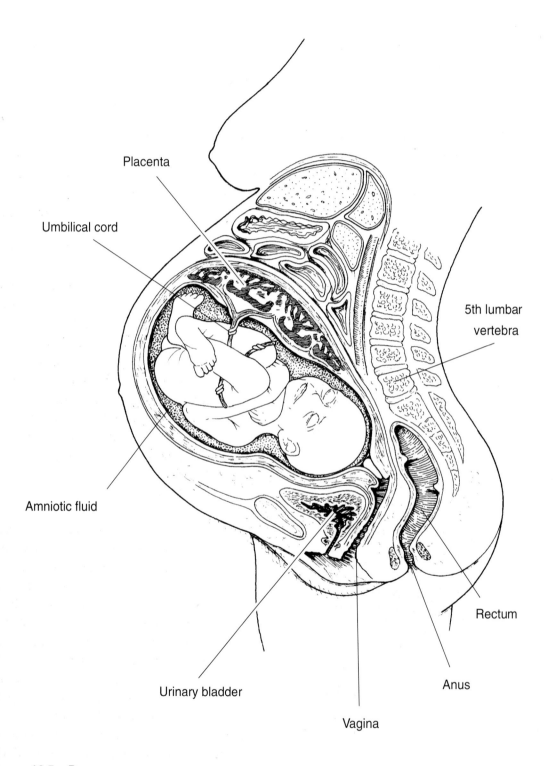

Placenta

Umbilical cord

Amniotic fluid

5th lumbar vertebra

Rectum

Anus

Vagina

Urinary bladder

Figure 16.5 Pregnancy.

further from the uterus. At some stage during the labor, the bag of membranes ruptures (**'the waters break'**) and the infant, who usually lies in a 'cephalic presentation' (head down), passes through the birth canal and into the outside world. The sudden transition to the new 'air' environment stimulates the baby to start breathing and, a short time later, the amniotic fluid in the lungs is fully absorbed and disappears.

BREAST

The breast is a gland that secretes milk to feed the infant (Fig. 16.6).

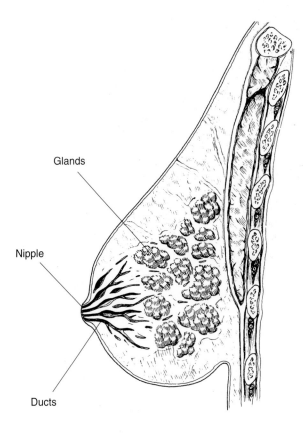

Figure 16.6   The breast: shown in sagittal section.

Until puberty, the female breast is not fully developed. As a result of the secretion of the hormone estrogen by the ovaries, the breast starts to enlarge and develop.

In a mature woman, each breast contains approximately 15–20 lobes. Each lobe contains a main duct, which opens out into the **nipple** at its outer end and branches out into a network of small tubules within the lobe of the breast at its other end. At the end of each tubule is a tiny gland that is normally dormant. Between the tubules there is abundant fatty tissue.

During pregnancy, as a result of the secretion of various hormones, such as estrogen, progesterone and prolactin, the 'dormant' glands at the ends of the tubules 'come to life', and increase in both number and size.

Stimulation of the nipple by the infant during breast feeding produces hormonal changes that cause the production and secretion of milk. If breast feeding stops, the breast returns to its pre-pregnancy state.

FEMALE INFERTILITY

Infertility is defined as the inability to become pregnant after a year of sexual intercourse during which no contraception was used.

Approximately 15% of couples have problems of infertility – in some 40% the problem lies with the male partner; in about 50% the problem is with the female and in about 10% the cause of the problem is unknown.

Infertile women can be classified into two main categories: those who are unable to ovulate and those who do ovulate but in whom fertilization does not occur (e.g. in the case of disease or abnormalities of the fallopian tubes).

Non-ovulation is the result of a problem in the function of the hypothalamus (that part of the brain that secretes GNRH), the pituitary gland (which secretes FSH and LH) or the ovaries.

There are several ways to determine whether ovulation has occurred:

- **Temperature changes**: the body temperature rises by about 0.5°C following ovulation.
- **Hormone levels:** the level of progesterone (the hormone secreted by the corpus luteum) on the 21st day of the cycle can be measured. If ovulation has not occurred (and there is no corpus luteum), the level of progesterone will be low.
- **Ultrasound**: the ultrasound machine is an imaging device that provides an image of the ovaries and the follicles within them. If follicles do not mature, ovulation cannot take place.

The fallopian tubes could be damaged following infection in the tubes themselves or elsewhere in the abdomen. As a result, adhesions that interfere with the free passage of the ovum down the tube can develop and affect fertility. This problem can be diagnosed by injecting contrast medium (a substance that is visible on X-ray) into the uterus and tubes and photographing them with X-ray.

The management of infertility involves hormonal or surgical treatment, depending on the nature of the underlying problem.

In vitro fertilization (IVF)

In vitro (from the Latin = *in glass*) fertilization (IVF) refers to fertilization of an ovum outside the woman's body. The reasons for performing IVF include abnormalities of the fallopian tubes (inoperable blockage of the tubes), infertility from unknown causes and abnormalities of the sperm.

In IVF, the woman is first injected with GNRH, which suppresses the natural secretion of the sex hormones and, in effect, stops the menstrual cycle. Next, a series of injections of follicle stimulating hormone (FSH) is given. As a result, the follicles in the ovary start to mature but, unlike the natural process in which only one follicle matures, in this case several follicles mature. The size of the follicles is monitored by ultrasound examinations and blood levels of the sex hormones are measured repeatedly.

When the follicles have reached a certain size (approximately 2 cm) and the hormone levels are appropriate, an injection of the hormone **chorionic gonadotrophin** is given, which produces ovulation. Just before ovulation, the mature ova are 'sucked' out of the ovary through a fine needle. The ova are placed in a small laboratory dish together with approximately 200 000 sperm. If fertilization takes place, the embryo begins to divide and, when it has reached the stage of 4–8 cells (usually 48 hours after fertilization), it is inserted into the woman's uterus.

Usually, several embryos are inserted, in the hope that one of them will implant in the endometrium and continue to develop. It is possible that several embryos will develop in the dish and they cannot all be transferred to the uterus. The excess embryos are frozen (for many years, if necessary) and transferred to the patient when another pregnancy is desired.

Another development that has now become routine is **intracytoplasmic sperm injection (ICSI)**. In cases where the male partner has very few sperm, or where the sperm are not very active or able to penetrate the ovum, a single sperm can be selected and inserted into the ovum.

The success rate (number of births achieved) of IVF is currently approximately 18%. This is a rapidly advancing area of medicine and new techniques are being introduced all the time.

DISORDERS ASSOCIATED WITH PREGNANCY AND CHILDBIRTH

Abruption of the placenta

Sometimes the placenta separates from the uterus too early; this is known as placental abruption and the reason for it is generally unknown.

There are various degrees of placental abruption, ranging from only a few millimeters to complete separation of the placenta from the uterine wall. In the latter case, the fetus will die because its oxygen supply is cut off.

Clinically, placental abruption is manifested by vaginal bleeding and tenderness over the uterus. If abruption is diagnosed in time, an emergency cesarean section must be performed in an attempt to save the baby's life.

Cesarean section

A cesarean section is an operation performed to deliver an infant by cutting into the uterus and removing it through the incision. In Western countries, about 20% of all births are by cesarean section.

The indications for performing a cesarean section include both emergency and non-emergency situations. Emergencies include situations in which rapid action is necessary to save the infant or the mother, such as placental abruption, fetal distress (where the baby shows signs of lack of oxygen) and labor that is obstructed and cannot progress. Non-emergency indications include situations such as an infant with an overly large head that cannot readily pass through the mother's pelvis (e.g. in infants of diabetic mothers), an infant lying in an abnormal position within the uterus such that vaginal birth is problematic, and triplets.

DISORDERS ASSOCIATED WITH MENOPAUSE

Menopause is defined as the permanent cessation of a woman's menstrual cycle. On average, the menstrual cycle stops at the age of 50 and thus more than one-third of a woman's life is after the menopause.

Menopause occurs because the follicles in the ovary gradually stop functioning and no longer produce estrogen. During this 'winding down' period (known as the **climacteric**), the woman can experience irregular menstruation, hot flashes (or flushes), night sweats, sleeplessness, mood swings, anxiety, irritability, poor concentration and memory lapses. These features can be severe enough to interfere with day-to-day function but, once the menstrual cycle has ceased completely, the symptoms will also disappear.

After the menopause, certain diseases become more common. The process of thinning of the bones **(osteoporosis)** accelerates after the menopause. Hence, it is not uncommon for postmenopausal women to suffer bone fractures.

The incidence of heart disease also increases significantly after the menopause (estrogen protects against heart disease, which may explain why heart disease is much more common in men than in women prior to menopause but its incidence rises in post-menopausal women).

Apart from these illnesses, lower levels of estrogen cause the mucosal lining of the genital passages to become thinner and dryer, which can result in pain during intercourse, and avoidance of intercourse altogether.

The symptoms are all amenable to treatment consisting of sex hormones (**hormone replacement therapy**). The hormones replaced are estrogen and progesterone, thereby continuing the sequence of the menstrual cycle artificially. A disadvantage of this treatment is that hormones given after the menopause appear to increase the incidence of breast cancer, although the decrease in heart disease, strokes and osteoporotic fractures is much greater.

BREAST CANCER

Cancer of the breast is the most common form of cancer in women, and rarely occurs in males. The chances of a woman developing breast cancer during her lifetime are more than 12%. With increasing age, the risk also increases.

Some of the factors associated with an increased risk of developing breast cancer include early age of first menstrual period, menopause at a later age, not having had any pregnancies, genetic factors (the risk of breast cancer is higher in women who have had a first degree relative with the disease) and possibly a diet rich in saturated fat.

Cancer of the breast is more common in Western countries than in the Far East and Asia.

It usually presents as a hard, irregular lump. The mass grows over time and can infiltrate the muscle tissue deep to (under) the breast and the skin overlying the breast. It might also send metastases (particles of cancer tissue that separate off the main mass and lodge elsewhere in the body) to the lymph glands in the axillae (armpits), the liver, brain, bones, skin and other organs.

The likelihood of being cured of breast cancer depends on the characteristics and extent of spread of the tumor. If the disease is diagnosed at an early stage, the prospect of cure is in the order of 90%; if the tumor has invaded the lymph glands in the axilla, the likelihood of cure is 40%.

The type of treatment also depends on the extent of spread of the cancer. A tumor that does not involve the axillary lymph glands is treated either by removing the entire breast or, more commonly by excising the mass itself, with subsequent radiotherapy to the breast. If the lymph glands are involved or if there is distant spread of metastases, treatment involves chemotherapy in addition to surgical management. It is essential to diagnose breast cancer early. Every woman over the age of 50 should undergo an annual mammography (a special radiologic examination of the breasts).

BENIGN CONDITIONS OF THE BREAST

Not every lump in the breast is a cancer. In fact, most are non-cancerous.

Fibrocystic disease. This is a very common condition in which the breasts contain many vaguely defined lumps. When examining the breasts with the hands the breast tissue does not feel 'smooth' but is rather 'lumpy'. Sometimes, the breasts become painful at certain stages of the menstrual cycle and occasionally there is a discharge from the nipple. Fibrocystic disease of the breast is a benign (non-malignant) condition that does not require any specific treatment.

Fibroadenoma. This is a benign growth that appears in young women as a firm, mobile lump in the breast. The differentiation between fibroadenoma and a carcinoma can only be made definitively after removing the lump and examining it under the microscope.

CARCINOMA OF THE UTERUS

Carcinoma of the uterus is the most common malignancy of the female genitalia (not including the breast). This tumor usually appears at around the age of 60.

The factors related to the onset of carcinoma of the uterus include obesity, few or no pregnancies, early onset of menstruation and late menopause, diabetes, cancer of the breast and estrogen medication.

The tumor arises from the endometrium, fills the uterine cavity and spreads into the muscle of the uterine wall, the cervix, the fallopian tubes and other pelvic organs. Metastases can appear in the lymph nodes of the pelvis and, at a more advanced stage of the disease, in the liver and lungs.

The most common sign of uterine cancer is vaginal bleeding in women who have already undergone menopause ('postmenopausal bleeding'). Sometimes there is abdominal pain or a foul smelling vaginal discharge.

The treatment of uterine cancer depends on the extent of tumor spread and includes hysterectomy (removal of the uterus) and removal of the uterine tubes and ovaries, combined with radiotherapy and/or chemotherapy. If the cancer is confined to the uterus, there is a 70% chance of survival.

The male reproductive system and its diseases

The male reproductive system completes its 'reproductive' function as soon as sexual intercourse has taken place and fertilization of the female's ovum has occurred. This is in contrast to the female reproductive system, which completes its task only 9 months later, at childbirth. Furthermore, unlike the female reproductive system, the male reproductive system retains its ability to fertilize ova throughout life.

The male reproductive system has two main functions:

1. Production of sperm and semen, and their delivery to the female reproductive system.
2. Production of the male sex hormone – **testosterone**.

THE TESTES

The testes produce sperm and testosterone. Within the developing fetus, the testes are in the abdomen until the 28th week of gestation. At this stage, they start to move downwards until they eventually enter the scrotum in the 32nd week of gestation.

The **scrotum** (Fig. 17.1) is a sac of skin that contains the testes, the epididymis and part of the spermatic cord. The reason that the testes

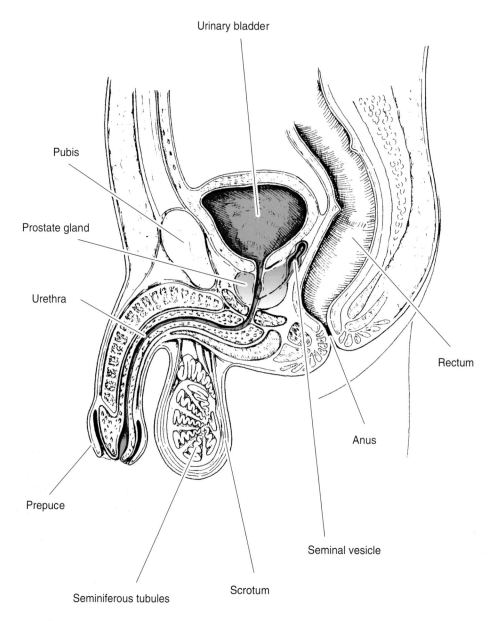

Urinary bladder

Pubis

Prostate gland

Urethra

Rectum

Anus

Prepuce

Seminal vesicle

Seminiferous tubules

Scrotum

Figure 17.1   The male reproductive system: a sagittal section through the pelvis.

are situated in the scrotum and not in the abdomen (which would afford them more protection), is that the production of sperm requires a temperature about 2°C below normal body temperature.

The testis is surrounded by a layer of tough connective tissue, which divides it up into lobules. Each lobule contains between one and four tiny tubules, each of approximately 0.2 mm diameter and 30–70 cm in length. The total length of these tubules is approximately 250 m. These tubules, called the **seminiferous tubules**, are the site where the sperm are formed. In the walls of the seminiferous tubules are cells that produce the sperm, as well as supporting cells.

The process of sperm production is called **spermatogenesis**, and takes approximately 72 days.

Spermatogenesis starts at puberty, when the male reproductive system becomes mature, and it continues throughout life. It is important to note that the quality of the sperm does not diminish with increasing age. Sperm are produced by the division and differentiation of primordial sex cells ('germ cells') in the walls of the seminiferous tubules. The outermost part of the wall of the seminiferous tubules contains the primordial cells, which bear no resemblance to mature sperm. These cells divide and form other cells with a slightly different appearance; these cells in turn divide, and their shape continues to change until finally they reach the form of the mature sperm, which are released into the cavity of the tubule. These sperm cells are still not ready to fertilize ova, but must undergo further maturation outside the testis.

In the course of spematogenesis (the production of sperm cells from primordial germ cells), the number of chromosomes in each cell is halved, from 46 chromosomes (23 pairs) in the primordial cell to 23 single chromosomes in the mature sperm. There are two types of mature sperm – those that contain a male sex chromosome (Y) and those that contain a female sex chromosome (X) – however, their external appearance is identical.

The **sperm cells**, which are approximately 65 thousandths of a millimeter long, comprise a head, a mid-piece and a tail (Fig. 17.2). The

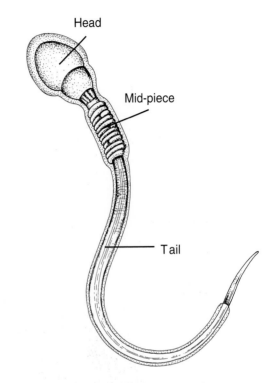

Figure 17.2   Structure of a sperm cell.

head, which contains the chromosomes (the genetic material), is covered by a cap containing digestive enzymes that enable the sperm cell to penetrate the wall of the ovum.

The mid-piece of the sperm cell is like a 'motor', which makes the tail spin like a propeller and propels the sperm cell forward.

Apart from the production of sperm, the testis has another important function, the secretion of the male sex hormone, **testosterone**. Special cells situated between the seminiferous tubules produce this hormone, which is important in stimulating the formation of the external male sex organs in the developing fetus, in producing the secondary sexual characteristics in the adult male at puberty, and in spermatogenesis.

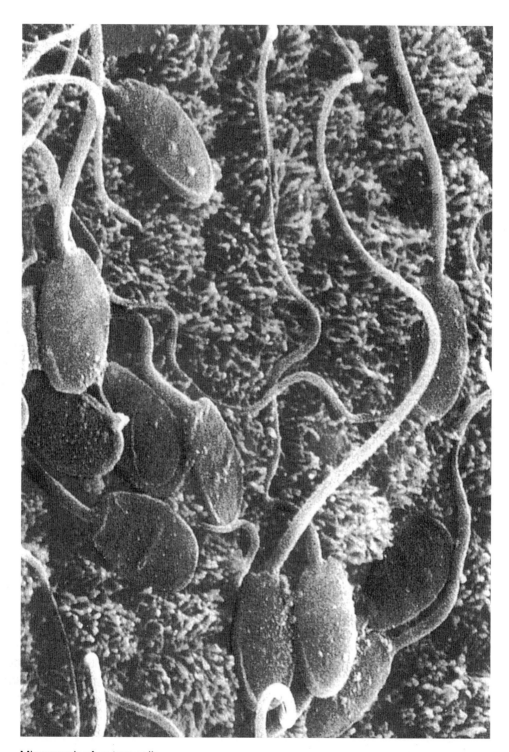

Micrograph of sperm cells.

Testosterone is produced in the testes and secreted into the bloodstream; hence the testes function as endocrine glands. The secretion of testosterone is controlled by the sex hormones secreted by the pituitary gland. The secondary sexual characteristics include the appearance and distribution of body hair (including pubic hair), increase in muscle mass, deepening of the voice and enlargement of the penis and testes. After puberty, testosterone plays an important role in spermatogenesis, in the production of semen and in penile erection during sexual arousal.

EPIDIDYMIS

The sperm cells that are released into the seminiferous tubules are collected in a convoluted tube outside the testis, the **epididymis** (Fig. 17.3). The epididymis is an elongated structure that sits on top of the testis (within the scrotum), and can actually be felt through the scrotum. In the epididymis, the sperm undergo a further maturation process, which takes 2 weeks and during which the sperm acquire the ability to move.

SPERMATIC CORD

From the epididymis the sperm move into the spermatic cord (**vas deferens**), which starts at the lower end of the epididymis, heads upwards and enters the abdominal cavity through the inguinal (groin) canal. From there, the spermatic cords (there are two – one from each testis) pass above the urinary bladder. Behind the lower part of the bladder, the spermatic cords enter the prostate gland, where they join the urethra. The wall of the spermatic cord contains a thick layer of smooth muscle to

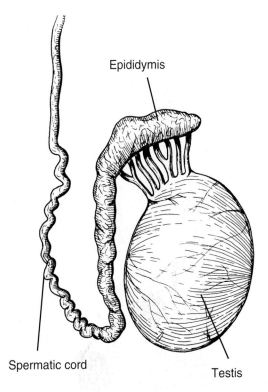

Figure 17.3   The testis, epididymis, and spermatic cord.

propel the sperm and the seminal fluid (semen) into the urethra during ejaculation.

THE GLANDS THAT PRODUCE THE SEMINAL FLUID

Seminal fluid is produced by two types of glands. The **seminal vesicles** are two elongated glands, approximately 5 cm long, situated on the posterior (back) wall of the urinary bladder (Fig. 17.4). A duct emerges from each gland. This enters the spermatic cord, which becomes the **ejaculatory duct**. The ejaculatory duct enters the prostate gland, within which it joins the urethra. The fluid produced by the seminal vesicles contains glucose to nourish the sperm, as well as certain vitamins and

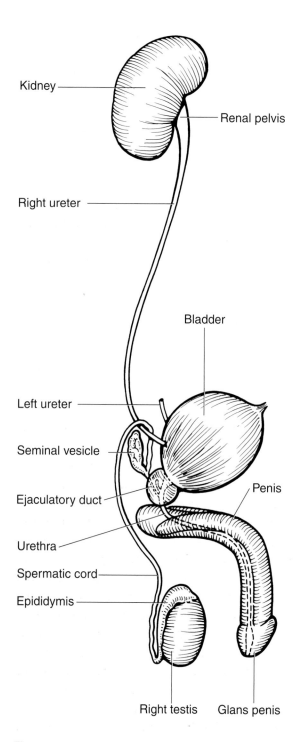

Kidney

Renal pelvis

Right ureter

Bladder

Left ureter

Seminal vesicle

Ejaculatory duct

Penis

Urethra

Spermatic cord

Epididymis

Right testis   Glans penis

Figure 17.4 The male reproductive system: showing the position of the different glands.

other nourishing substances. Most of the volume of the seminal fluid is derived from the seminal vesicles.

The **prostate gland** is situated immediately below the bladder (see Figs 17.1 and 17.4) and is shaped like an inverted pyramid approximately 3 cm high. Within the prostate gland, the spermatic cord (at this stage called the ejaculatory duct) joins the urethra. The prostate gland contributes an alkaline fluid to the semen, whose function is to neutralize the acidity of the vagina. The prostatic secretion also contains other substances, such as zinc, which are needed by the sperm. This secretion is discharged into the urethra via a short duct.

Cowper's glands are a pair of small glands that produce a small amount of a fatty fluid that lubricates the tip of the penis during sexual stimulation.

THE PENIS

The penis is composed of three cylinders of tissue (Fig. 17.5). The two upper cylinders contain erectile tissue (this brings about an erection), while the lower cylinder contains the urethra. One half of the length of the cylinders is actually within the pelvis, that portion of the penis being called the **root of the penis**. The tip of the penis is called the **glans**, and it is continuous with the lower cylinder. The **prepuce** (or foreskin) is an extension of the skin of the penis that extends over the glans.

Erectile tissue is connective tissue (not muscle) that contains many spaces filled with blood. During an **erection**, the arteries supplying blood to the penis dilate and more blood flows into the spaces within the erectile tissue. The veins that drain blood away from the penis constrict, so less blood can flow out

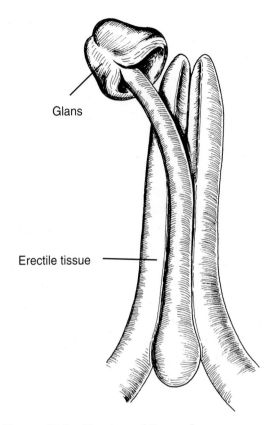

Glans

Erectile tissue

Figure 17.5 Structure of the penis.

through them. As a result, blood is 'trapped' within the erectile tissue cylinders, the pressure within them rises and the penis becomes rigid and elongated, producing an erection.

The constriction of the veins and dilatation of the arteries is under the control of the autonomic nervous system. An erection results from sexual stimulation of the nervous system, either by direct physical stimulation of the penis or by a sexually arousing situation.

SEMEN AND EJACULATION

The **ejaculate (semen)** contains sperm and seminal fluid, most of the ejaculate being the seminal fluid that is derived from the various glands as outlined above.

Ejaculation is the process of discharging semen from the penis during orgasm. During ejaculation, the smooth muscle in the semen-producing glands and in the spermatic cord contracts rhythmically and the semen is discharged out of the opening of the penis. The volume of ejaculate varies between 1 and 5 cm^3. Each cubic centimeter of ejaculate contains about 50 million sperm, hence the number of sperm in one ejaculation is approximately a quarter of a billion.

If ejaculation takes place repeatedly within a relatively short time, the volume of the ejaculate does not decrease significantly but the number of sperm per cubic centimeter of ejaculate does diminish.

BENIGN PROSTATIC HYPERTROPHY (BPH)

This condition appears in men over the age of 50; its incidence increases with age. It is an extremely common condition in which the tissue of the prostate gland enlarges. The prostate is an organ that continues to grow throughout life, under the influence of testosterone, and, in some men, this growth is excessive. The enlarging prostate presses on the urethra, which runs through its center, and causes obstruction to urine flow (sometimes this gets to the stage of complete obstruction).

The symptoms include difficulty in starting to urinate ('hesitancy'), a weak stream that stops before the bladder is empty, dribbling after urination and frequent urination.

The muscle of the bladder wall, which must work harder to push the urine past the obstruction, becomes enlarged and thickened. The increased pressure within the bladder can cause urine to 'leak' back, upwards into the ureters and even up to the kidneys (urinary reflux), which can cause kidney infection and damage. The treatment of BPH is either with medication or by surgical treatment, depending on the severity of the situation.

CANCER OF THE PROSTATE

Cancer of the prostate gland is the most common cancer in males, although it is not the most common cause of death from cancer in males (lung cancer is); its incidence increases with age.

Cancer of the prostate gland tends to produce metastases (cancer cells that spread to areas distant from the original tumor) in bones and other organs in the pelvis.

The initial clinical symptoms are obstructive, similar to those of benign prostatic hypertrophy. In the early stages of the disease, it can be treated by surgical removal of the prostate gland. However, if the cancer has spread to other organs, it is incurable. Some prostatic cancers can be detected at an early stage by rectal examination, which is recommended for all men over the age of 40 annually.

UNDESCENDED TESTIS

The testes in the fetus are located in the abdomen but, from the 28th week of gestation they start to move downwards, and normally reach the scrotum by the 32nd gestational week. If something goes wrong with this descent, a situation arises where at birth one or both testes still remain in the abdomen, not in the scrotum. This is called **cryptorchidism**, or undescended testis.

A testis that remains within the abdomen is liable to degenerate and cease to function and, furthermore, has an increased likelihood of developing cancer. It is therefore important that surgery is performed to 'bring down' an undescended testis into the scrotum as early as possible – usually before the age of 2 years.

TORSION OF THE TESTIS

The testis receives its blood supply via blood vessels that come from the abdomen and reach the testis with the spermatic cord. If the testis twists within the scrotal sac, these blood vessels can also become twisted and obstructed, depriving the testis of its blood supply. If the blood supply is not restored within 6 h, the testis undergoes necrosis (tissue death).

Torsion of the testis often occurs following physical exertion. Its symptoms are severe pain and extreme tenderness to touch.

The treatment is immediate surgery, with untwisting of the testis and tieing it so that it cannot twist again.

MALE INFERTILITY

Most cases of male infertility are due to poor quality of sperm. This can be related to low numbers of sperm, to decreased motility (ability to move) of the sperm, to distortion of the shape of the sperm and other factors. These factors can be evaluated quite easily in the laboratory.

There are many causes for poor quality sperm, including some congenital (= from birth) diseases, abnormalities of the veins draining blood from the testes, infections that damage the testis (e.g. the mumps virus) and exposure to irradiation.

Today, various techniques are used to improve the quality of the sperm, by separating the defective sperm from the normal ones. It is important to stress that infertility can also be the result of the interaction of male and female factors. It is possible that a man with poor quality sperm is unable to fertilize one woman but is able to fertilize another.

We now know that many cases of infertility are related to male factors, particularly sperm quality, whereas in the past it was generally assumed that infertility was due to the female.

IMPOTENCE

The definition of impotence is the inability to achieve and/or maintain an erection.

The most common cause of impotence is psychological. Other causes include disease of the blood vessels or nerves leading to the penis, diabetes (which affects both the blood vessels and the nerves) and sex hormone abnormalities.

The treatment of impotence can involve psychologic therapy, the injection of a substance into the penis that causes an erection, implanting a prosthesis into the penis or, most recently, drugs that increase blood in the penis, causing it to become erect.

18 The immune system

The immune system is made up of many different components present in almost every part of the body. In addition to those organs that are specifically related to the immune system, components of the system are also present in other body systems.

The immune system plays a crucial role in protecting the body from 'foreign' invaders; however there are a number of diseases in which the immune system attacks its own body and causes disease. Such diseases are called **autoimmune diseases**.

The study of AIDS, a disease caused by a virus that attacks the immune system, has resulted in massive research into the immune system and, as a result, much new information has become available recently.

FUNCTIONS OF THE IMMUNE SYSTEM

Defense against foreign invaders

There are microorganisms that are capable of entering the body and causing various diseases.

Viruses.   These are extremely small particles (there is some dispute as to whether they should be classified as living organisms) made up of some genetic material within a lipid and protein envelope. The virus can invade cells of the body and make them produce more viruses of its own kind. Eventually the cell bursts and releases many new virus copies, which proceed to invade other cells. There are many different types of virus, each attacking specific cells in the body and causing specific diseases. Rubella, measles, influenza, polio and AIDS are some examples of the many diseases caused by viruses.

Bacteria (singular = bacterium).   These are living organisms whose structure is similar to that of a body cell. They can invade the body and remain either within its cells or between them. Some bacteria secrete a **toxin** that can damage body tissues. As opposed to viruses, which cannot replicate by themselves but only within some other cell, bacteria replicate in a similar manner to body cells (cell division). Two well known species of bacteria that can cause disease are *Streptococcus* and *Staphylococcus*.

Fungi.   These are living organisms that grow either in colonies or as single units. They have certain characteristics that distinguish them from bacteria. One fungus that causes disease is called *Candida*.

Protozoa.   These unicellular organisms can cause serious diseases. They have certain features (that will not be discussed here) which distinguish them from bacteria and fungi. One well known such protozoa is called **ameba**.

There are also multicellular organisms (i.e. whose body is made of many cells), such as **worms**, that can cause various diseases. Unlike viruses, bacteria, fungi and protozoa, these are not microscopic in size.

It is important to emphasize that there are many types of viruses, bacteria and fungi that do not cause any disease, in fact, these represent the majority of the microorganisms.

Millions of microorganisms are constantly attempting to invade the body but the immune system prevents their entry into the body or destroys them upon entry. If an infectious agent does manage to enter the body and multiply, it can cause disease, the nature of which depends on the type of invader. The infectious agent is usually destroyed by the immune system, which protects the body against disease.

Removal of damaged body tissues

Following an injury or disease, some destruction of body tissues may occur. These damaged or dead tissues must be removed before the repair process begins. Cells of the immune system act as 'cleaners' and remove such tissue efficiently.

Destruction of cancerous cells

The immune system has an important task in destroying cancerous cells as they arise. In patients with abnormal immune function (e.g. AIDS patients), various types of cancer appear more frequently.

The immune system can be divided into two major divisions. One part acts to prevent the entry of foreign invaders into the body, and the other part deals with foreign invaders once they have entered the body.

ANATOMIC BARRIERS

The mechanisms and systems that prevent the entry of foreign substances or organisms into the body include the skin, the mucosa of the respiratory and reproductive systems, 'good' bacteria within the digestive system and the flow of liquid or air.

The skin

The skin is an important barrier against invasion of the body. The outer layer of the skin is called the **epidermis** and is made of several layers of epithelial cells. The outermost layer comprises dead skin cells that are constantly being shed, with new cells coming up from the deeper layers to take their place. Under the thin epidermis is a thicker layer called the **dermis**, composed of strong connective tissue. The dermis contains the blood vessels that nourish the skin, as well as the hair follicles, sweat glands and sebaceous glands. Under this connective tissue layer is a layer of fat. Healthy skin provides a formidable barrier to invasion by microorganisms. Injury to the skin, such as an extensive burn, allows millions of bacteria to enter the body through the damaged area. In fact, patients with very severe or extensive burns usually die of infection. A further problem is severe loss of body fluids by evaporation, leading to serious dehydration.

The respiratory mucosa

The respiratory mucosa tissue contains ciliary cells and mucus cells that trap invading microorganisms and other particles and remove them from the airways before they can reach the lungs. The mucus glands produce a sticky layer, which coats the lining of the respiratory passages and traps particles and microorganisms. The ciliary cells have tiny microscopic hairs (cilia) on them that beat rhythmically and sweep the mucus layer (together with any particles trapped in it) out

of the respiratory tract to the exterior. Any disease or injury to this system may result in recurrent lung infections.

The vaginal mucosa

The vaginal mucosa contains special acid-producing bacteria. The acidity prevents microorganisms from entering the body via the vagina. This is an example of 'good' bacteria present in the body protecting against the entry of 'bad', disease-causing bacteria.

The digestive system

The digestive system contains a large number of bacteria in the mouth and in the large bowel. Such 'good' bacteria make up the **normal flora** and play an important role in preventing the entry of harmful bacteria.

The urinary tract

The urinary tract system prevents the entry of foreign invaders by the principle of liquid flow: a foreign invader entering the urinary system is swept out of the body by a flow of urine. A disease that interferes with the normal flow of urine, such as kidney stones or prostatic hypertrophy, increases the risk of infection in the urinary tract and elsewhere.

INTERNAL IMMUNE MECHANISMS

The body's internal immune mechanisms include specific organs of the immune system, such as the spleen and lymph nodes, as well as immunologically active cells and proteins. Most of such cells and proteins are found in the blood, although they are also present to some extent in all body tissues.

Cells of the immune system

The body contains many types of immunologically active cells, all of which are various types of **leukocyte (white cell)**. Leukocytes are formed in the bone marrow and released into the bloodstream, where between 5000 and 10 000 leukocytes per cubic millimeter are found.

Neutrophils

These make up approximately 70% of the white cells in the blood. They are constantly being produced in the bone marrow and then enter the bloodstream, in which they circulate throughout the body. They have a lifespan of 6–8 hours.

Their task is to engulf and destroy foreign invaders and they are the first line of defense against invaders (especially bacteria). Neutrophils move towards the foreign substance, become attached to it and then surround and engulf it so that the invader is contained inside the neutrophil within a 'bubble' (vesicle) formed by a portion of the neutrophil cell wall. The next stage is the union of this 'bubble' containing the foreign invader with other vesicles within the neutrophil that contain digestive enzymes. In this way the foreign invader is destroyed.

During an infectious illness, the number of neutrophils produced by the bone marrow increases significantly, which is reflected by an increased number of neutrophils in the blood (**neutrophilia**). An increase in the number of white blood cells is called **leukocytosis**.

A significant decrease in the number of neutrophils is called **neutropenia**. This is a serious situation, which could result in fatal infection. Neutropenia usually occurs as the result of disease of the bone marrow, where the neutrophils are normally produced.

Macrophages

These make up approximately 10% of the white cells of the blood; those that are actually circulating within the blood are called **monocytes**. Macrophages are also found within various body tissues, such as the subdermis (the layer immediately beneath the skin), liver, lungs, spleen and lymph nodes. Unlike neutrophils, which live for a very short time, macrophages can live for years. Macrophages also engulf and digest foreign invaders and damaged body tissues and, importantly, they secrete substances that regulate the activity of the entire immune system.

Lymphocytes

These constitute approximately 20% of the white blood cells. There are two main types of lymphocyte – type B and type T. **Type B lymphocytes** are the cells that produce proteins called **antibodies**. **Type T lymphocytes** are further divided into several subtypes, of which the two main ones are **cytotoxic** (or 'killer') **T cells** and **helper T cells**. A cytotoxic T cell is a T cell that is able to destroy body cells infected by viruses. A helper T cell is a T cell that secretes substances needed by the type B lymphocytes to produce antibodies.

The AIDS virus attacks helper T cells, so there are less of them in the body. As a result, the whole immune system is affected and the patient becomes very susceptible to infections.

Antibodies

Antibodies are proteins produced by the B lymphocytes. An antibody molecule has a central body with two arms; different types of antibody differ in the structure of the ends of the arms. The arms bind specifically to various foreign substances, depending on the physical and chemical structure of the arm and the foreign substance (like a key that fits a specific lock) (Fig. 18.1).

Each particular type of antibody is produced by a specific type of B cell. Under normal circumstances (even without prior exposure to foreign invaders), the B cells in the blood are capable of producing antibodies against virtually any foreign substance (there are many millions of different subtypes of B cell).

Following entry of a foreign substance into the body (for example, a bacterium), the B cells that produce the antibody against that particular substance multiply and produce the specific antibodies. This process takes several weeks.

The action of antibodies

Antibodies bind to a protein in the foreign substance called an **antigen**.

A single bacterium contains many such proteins, so there will be many different types of antibody directed against various antigens on the bacterium. Each antibody attaches only to its specific antigen. When an antibody becomes attached to a foreign substance, it neutralizes the substance in several different ways.

Occasionally, the very act of the antibody attaching to the invader prevents the foreign substance from affecting the body (for example, when an antibody attaches to a toxin or poison).

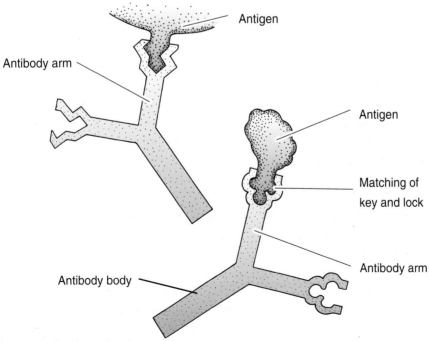

Figure 18.1   Antibody and antigen.

The attachment of an antibody to an antigen makes the foreign substance appear much more 'palatable' to the white cells, enabling them to engulf it much more readily. This is because the white cells themselves contain receptors that are attracted to the antibody, which is, in turn, attached to the (foreign) antigen.

When an antibody binds to an antigen, changes also take place in the antibody that significantly strengthen its binding to white cells.

The attachment of an antibody to an antigen stimulates and activates another part of the immune system – the **complement system**. This is a system of proteins that helps to eliminate foreign substances from the body. Complement is attracted to the antigen–antibody complex and is able to destroy the invader. It also improves the ability of the white cells to engulf whatever substance the complement has attached to.

The first time that the body is exposed to a specific invader an **immunologic memory** for that substance is triggered. The number of specific B cells that produce antibody against that invader increases significantly. Moreover, the amount of circulating antibody against that particular substance also increases. If the invader enters the body again, it does not cause disease because it is met with large amounts of antibody: immunity has been produced.

The principle behind **immunization** (vaccination) is the creation of such an immunologic memory. By deliberately injecting a dead or weakened bacterium or virus (which cannot cause disease) into the body, the immune system is 'tricked' into producing antibodies and immunologic memory against it. This type of immunization is known as **active immunization**, because the immune system is stimulated to actively produce the antibodies required.

In contrast, **passive immunization** is the injection of preformed antibodies into the body. This is usually done in urgent situations where there is no time to wait for the body to produce its own antibodies, as for example, in the case of a snakebite.

Where do these preformed antibodies against the snake venom come from? They are derived from an animal (e.g. a horse) into which a small amount of the snake venom was injected. The animal produces antibodies against the snake venom and these antibodies are harvested and injected into a human patient when needed. The (horse-derived) anti-snake venom antibodies become attached to the snake venom antigen in the patient and neutralize it, enabling recovery. However, the structure of the antibodies produced by the animal differs slightly from human antibodies, so they themselves now constitute a foreign protein in the patient. Therefore, within a few weeks of having received the horse antibodies, the body produces its own antibodies against the horse antibodies. Should that patient then be given an injection of horse-derived antibodies for a second time, these will now be immediately destroyed by the patient's immune system. Furthermore, serum obtained from animals might contain other antigens that are 'foreign' to the patient, and which might result in a severe allergic reaction.

Organs of the immune system

Lymphatic tissue

This tissue comprises a variety of cells belonging to the immune system (mainly lymphocytes and monocytes) that are found in various organs of the body. For example, there are large numbers of such cells in the wall of the digestive tract. Their task is to prevent unwanted foreign matter from entering the body via the digestive system.

Within the mouth and throat are several groups of lymphatic tissue. The **palatine tonsils** (generally referred to as just 'tonsils') are found at the back of the mouth cavity and, in effect, are a part of the lymphatic tissue guarding the entrance to the digestive tract. Other groups of lymphatic tissue are present on the rear third of the tongue, as well as the upper part of the back wall of the pharynx (the **adenoids**).

If some infectious agent (e.g. streptococcal bacteria) enters the pharynx and causes an infection (called **pharyngitis**), the lymphatic tissue (mainly the tonsils) swells and appears red and 'inflamed', while the immunologically active cells within it are mobilized to fight off the invader.

Lymph nodes

These are structures situated lying along the lymphatic vessels at many sites in the body (Fig. 18.2). They act as filters for the immune system, and trap foreign substances. Lymphocytes within the lymph nodes then produce antibodies against the foreign substance. All lymph nodes are connected to **lymphatic vessels**, which bring lymphatic fluid to them and to other vessels draining the lymphatic fluid away (Fig. 18.3).

Because the lymphatic system drains excess fluid from virtually every tissue in the body (except the brain, where the system is absent), virtually all foreign matter that gets into the body ultimately finds its way into the lymphatic system and passes through lymph nodes at some point in the body.

There are many white blood cells in lymph nodes – mainly lymphocytes and macrophages. The lymphatic fluid from the tissues comes into contact with these white blood cells in the lymph nodes. Any foreign matter present in the fluid is trapped by the white cells and antibodies are produced against it. This is why, during an infection, the lymph nodes often become swollen – the immunologically active cells within them multiply rapidly.

It is sometimes convenient to think of the lymph nodes as belonging to two different groups. There are the 'external' lymph nodes, which can be felt on physical examination, the main ones being in the neck and under the jaw, the axillae (armpits) and groin. The other group of lymph nodes are 'internal' and cannot be felt. These are present within the various body cavities – the chest cavity, the abdominal cavity and the pelvis. This differentiation into 'external' and 'internal' lymph nodes is based purely on their location – structurally and functionally, they are the same.

The spleen

This is a flat, elongated organ composed of friable (crumbly) blood-containing tissue. It is located in the upper left of the abdomen, against the upper left side of the stomach and adjacent to the 10th and 11th ribs. The ribs protect this fragile organ from external trauma (Fig. 18.4).

The spleen is the largest mass of lymphatic tissue in the body. It contains various types of white blood cell, which trap and destroy foreign invaders carried to it by the blood. It also produces antibodies against these invaders. The spleen has a very rich blood

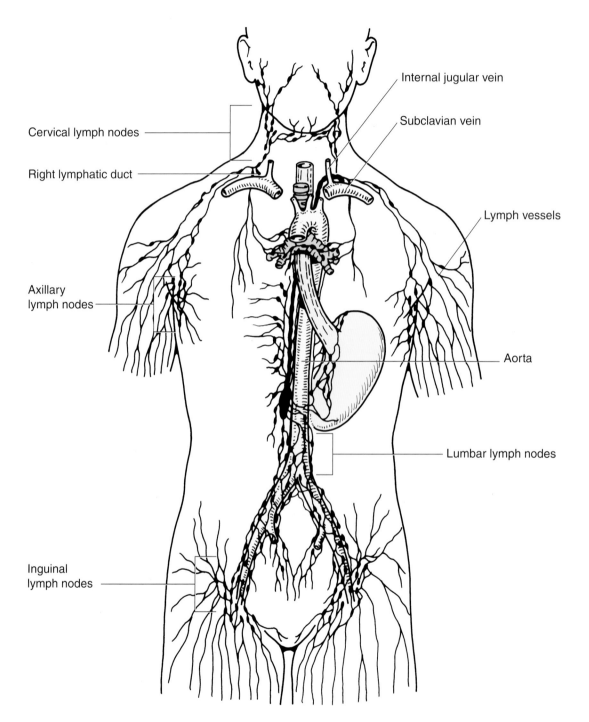

Figure 18.2 Lymph nodes and lymph vessels. The lymph vessels drain lymphatic fluid from the upper and lower extremities and from the abdomen and chest back to the blood circulation via the subclavian vein.

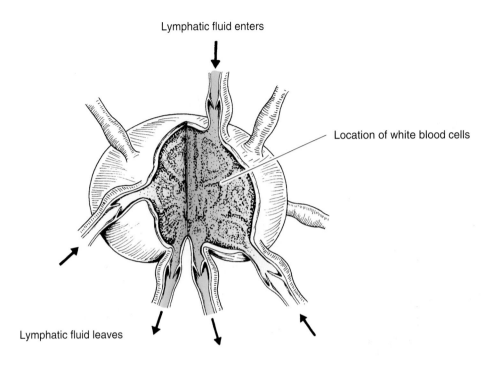

Figure 18.3 A lymph node.

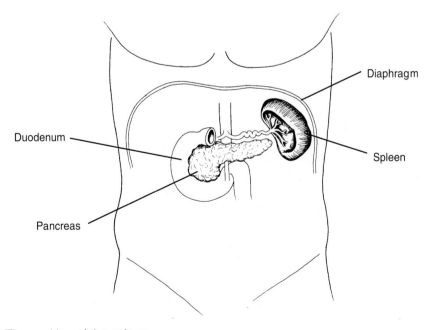

Figure 18.4 The position of the spleen.

supply and thus serves as the main blood filtering unit of the immune system.

Apart from its central role in the immune system, the spleen also acts as the 'graveyard' for worn-out red blood cells (the lifespan of a red blood cell is about 120 days). These are engulfed by macrophages, and their components (iron, hemoglobin, etc.) are recycled. The spleen can also produce new red blood cells when necessary (e.g. following massive blood loss, when the bone marrow is unable to meet the demand for new red cells).

The thymus

This organ is often called the 'thymus gland', although it does not actually secrete anything. The thymus is a flat organ with two lobes. It is situated in the upper anterior chest cavity, between the sternum (breastbone) and the pericardium (covering of the heart). In the infant, the thymus is at its largest relative to the size of the body. At adolescence, the thymus becomes smaller and in the adult it is very small relative to the body.

The thymus is composed of lymphatic tissue (mainly lymphocytes), and plays a crucial role in the development and maturation of the immune system. The T lymphocytes undergo a 'learning' process within the thymus. (They are, in fact, called T cells because they 'come from' the thymus.) Once the immune system has matured, the thymus has no further function and can be removed without compromising the patient's immune function.

19 Diseases of the immune system

IMMUNE DEFICIENCY DISEASES

Disease or malfunction of the immune system results in various infections and cancers. Diseases that affect specific parts of the immune system result in the appearance of different infections. This is because different components of the immune system deal with different infectious agents – some deal with viruses, some with fungi, some with bacteria, and so on.

Immune deficiency diseases can be divided into two main groups – congenital (= from birth) and acquired diseases.

Severe combined immune deficiency

Severe combined immune deficiency (SCID) is a very rare but well-known congenital disease. Children with this disease have virtually no lymphocytes – neither T cells nor B cells – and consequently suffer from repeated severe infections. Very few patients survive beyond 1 year of age. In an effort to protect them from infections, such patients often have to spend their lives isolated from the outside world, within a protective 'bubble'. The only form of treatment that offers some hope is bone marrow transplantation.

Acquired immunodeficiencies are usually the result of one of two causes. The most common cause is some disease or abnormality of the bone marrow, which affects the production of white cells. The second major cause of acquired immune deficiency is AIDS, due to the HIV virus.

Bone marrow disease

Neutrophils, which make up 70% of the white blood cells, are constantly being produced in the bone marrow. These cells, which live only for 6-8 hours, constitute the body's first line of defense against bacterial infection. Because neutrophils have a short life span, anything that affects the bone marrow can very quickly result in a decrease in the number of neutrophils in the blood (**neutropenia**). When the number of neutrophils in the blood falls below 200 per cubic millimeter, there is a real danger to life because of overwhelming bacterial infection.

Most cases of bone marrow depression are related to treatments for cancer, such as chemotherapy or irradiation. Those treatments attack all rapidly dividing cells in the body, including cancer cells, but unfortunately bone marrow cells are also rapidly dividing and are therefore also affected. The effect on the bone marrow is usually only temporary, and it recovers. During the period that the white blood cell count is low, the patient is susceptible to infections and must be treated promptly with antibiotic therapy. There are also other reasons for bone marrow depression, including certain medications and diseases.

Acquired immune deficiency syndrome (AIDS)

AIDS is probably the most talked about disease in the world today. It is caused by a virus called HIV (human immunodeficiency virus). This virus attacks a type of T lymphocyte, the **helper cells**, and decreases its numbers significantly. As long as the number of T lymphocytes in the body exceeds a certain minimum, the immune system can function normally. However, as soon as the number of T cells falls below that minimum, the patient succumbs to infections that can be ultimately fatal.

AIDS is transmitted by sexual intercourse, by infected blood and blood products, via infected needles and from an infected mother to her unborn child. Ordinarily, it is not possible to be infected from a patient's saliva or from mere physical contact with an AIDS patient.

In Western countries, the majority of AIDS patients are males who became infected following homosexual intercourse, or from using infected needles to inject drugs.

In developing countries (Africa, India, Thailand, etc.), the incidence of AIDS is similar for men and women (in fact, women are slightly more frequently affected than men), and most patients are infected following heterosexual intercourse. The number of AIDS patients and HIV carriers in the world (a carrier is someone who has been infected with the HIV virus but does not show any symptoms of the disease) in 1997 was approximately 22 million, with the majority of patients being in Africa. While the number of new cases of AIDS in Western countries appears to be declining, in the developing countries the incidence is rising steadily.

Clinical features of AIDS

There are several stages of the disease.

Acute phase. Some 3–6 weeks after being infected with HIV, about one-half of the patients experience an acute flu-like illness: headache, fever, sore throat, muscle pains, lack of appetite, nausea and vomiting, enlargement of lymph nodes and a rash. This stage lasts 1–2 weeks and then resolves.

Asymptomatic phase. At this stage, the patient has no symptoms of the disease. The asymptomatic phase lasts on average 10 years, but there are cases in which it has been as short as 1 year or as long as 15 years. During this phase, the patient is called a carrier, and not an AIDS patient. However, the disease is still active during the carrier stage and the number of helper T cells steadily decreases.

Early symptoms. At this stage, generalized enlargement of the lymph nodes appears, there may be fungal infection of the mouth, low-grade fever and weight loss.

Late symptoms. This is the final stage of AIDS, and ends with the patient's death. This stage is characterized by the appearance of a variety of infections and cancers. It is usually a lung infection that ultimately kills the patient. The infections are referred to as 'opportunistic infections' because they do not normally occur in someone with an intact immune system. They 'seize the opportunity' of attacking AIDS patients because their immune systems are weakened.

In addition to infections, the AIDS patient might show evidence of neurologic damage resulting from infections, brain tumors and direct damage to brain cells by the HIV virus. The symptoms can include personality changes, a general decline in intellectual capacity, unstable gait or seizures.

At present, combinations of drugs given simultaneously (a 'cocktail') can significantly increase life expectancy but does not irradicate the virus entirely. It is possible, however, that the disease is no longer fatal and AIDS patients can live for a long time.

LYMPHADENOPATHY

There are several areas in the body in which lymph glands are present under the skin, such as in the groin, the axillae and the neck. When these nodes become enlarged they can be quite easily felt under the skin. However, the 'internal' lymph nodes, within the chest, abdomen or pelvis cannot be felt. There are two main reasons why lymph nodes become swollen:

Infection or some inflammatory process. In this case, the lymph nodes become swollen because of the increased activity of the lymphatic tissue within them. A localized infection, for example in the throat, will cause the nodes in the neck to swell, while an infection localized to the foot will result in swelling of the lymph nodes in the groin. Generalized swelling of lymph nodes usually indicates some generalized infectious process throughout the body (e.g. infectious mononucleosis).

Malignancy. Lymph nodes can be the site of a primary lymphatic malignancy, when the white blood cells within the node become cancerous. Alternatively, they can be the site of secondary malignancy, in which metastases from a tumor elsewhere in the body spread via the lymphatic vessels, reach the lymph node and grow there into a malignancy, causing the node to enlarge.

A primary cancer of the lymph nodes is called **lymphoma**. There are different types of lymphomas, depending on which particular type of cell becomes cancerous. Some types are more common in children and other types more common in adults. Some types are very aggressive and develop rapidly (over weeks), while others develop very slowly (over years).

Some of the symptoms of lymphoma include enlargement of the lymph nodes (often noticed first in the neck), fever, night sweats, loss of weight and generalized itching. Enlargement of lymph nodes within the chest, for example, could cause pressure on important structures such as the trachea (windpipe) and result in breathing difficulties.

The treatment of lymphoma includes radiotherapy and chemotherapy (depending on the particular type of lymphoma) and, in some cases, there is a very good cure rate (90%).

AUTOIMMUNE DISEASES (RHEUMATIC DISEASES)

Autoimmune diseases are diseases in which the immune system attacks its own body tissues. The immune system does not normally attack its own body tissues because these are not recognized as foreign. (We still do not fully understand how the immune system recognizes and differentiates between self and non-self).

If tissues from another person are transplanted into the patient, the immune system will attack those tissues. Thus, in organ transplantation, medications have to be given to suppress the immune system and prevent rejection of the transplant.

In autoimmune diseases, the immune system, for some unknown reason, mistakenly identifies some body tissue as being 'foreign' and attacks it. Such patients have 'autoantibodies' (antibodies that attach to specific cells in the patient's body).

The joints are commonly involved in this autoimmune process, although any organ in the body can be affected, giving rise to many different diseases.

Treatment of these diseases involves suppression of the immune system using medication, such as steroids and chemotherapy.

Systemic lupus erythematosus (SLE)

SLE is an autoimmune disease which occurs mainly in women and is sometimes called the 'disease of a thousand faces' because of the wide range of clinical manifestations that can occur.

In SLE, antibodies appear that are directed against the genetic material in the nuclei of the cells, such that the immune system attacks many different tissues within the body.

The symptoms of SLE reflect disease of the nervous system, the skin, the kidneys, the joints and others. The disease is called 'lupus erythematosus' because of a reddish rash that appears over the bridge of the nose and the cheeks, giving the patient a wolf-like facial appearance (from the Latin *lupus* = wolf and the Greek *erythema* = flush).

Rheumatoid arthritis

In this autoimmune disease, antibodies are formed against certain components of the joints, destroying them. The small joints of the hand are particularly involved in rheumatoid arthritis, although other joints are also commonly affected. This is a common chronic disease, which requires long-term immunosuppressive drug therapy and usually results in joint deformities and disability.

20

Sight and hearing

SIGHT

The sense of sight supplies the brain with an enormous amount of very precise information about the external environment. Loss of sight is a very severe impairment in comparison with the loss of the other senses.

The energy source that stimulates vision is light. Light stimulates special receptors in the eye, called **photoreceptors**, which convert the light stimulus into an electrical signal, which is transmitted via nerves to the visual center in the brain.

The visual system can be divided into an optical portion (including the lens of the eye), which conducts the light rays from the external environment to the photoreceptors, and a neurologic portion, which includes the photoreceptors and all the neurons related to the visual system. Today, most diseases of the optical system can be managed quite successfully, but it is more difficult, and sometimes impossible, to treat disease or injury of the neurologic portion.

The eye

The **orbit** of the eye is a conical bony depression in the skull containing the globe of the eye (eyeball) and the muscles that move it. The walls of the orbit are made up of several skull bones. There are six **extraocular muscles** (Fig. 20.1), which move the globe. All but one have their origin at the back of the orbit and all are inserted into the eyeball. These muscles can cause extremely precise movements of the eyeball.

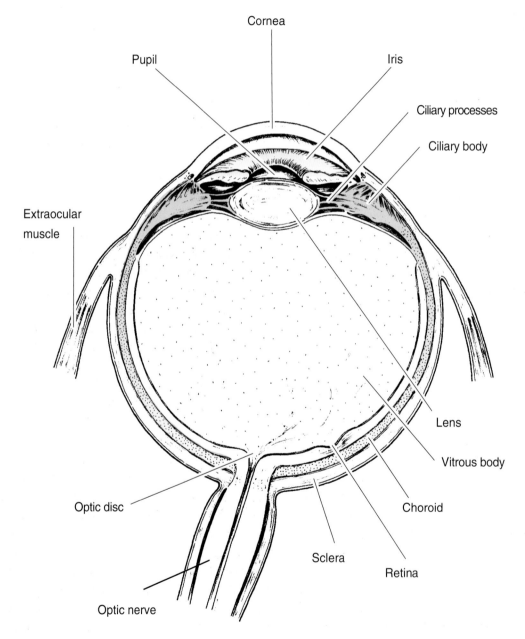

Figure 20.1   Structure of the eye.

The wall of the eyeball is made of three layers.

The outermost layer of the eye. This is composed of tough connective tissue, and is called the **sclera** (from the Greek *scleros* = hard). This is the white of the eye. The sclera is present all around the globe, except for the anterior part, where it becomes a transparent layer called the **cornea**.

The cornea is continuous with the sclera but, because it is transparent, it is not easily seen. Its task is to refract the light rays that reach the eye to produce an image on the retina at the back of the eye. The cornea does not contain any blood vessels (which is why it is transparent) but it does, contain many nerves, which transmit pain and touch sensations. The slightest touch on the cornea, even a puff of air, causes an instant blink reflex, with the eye closing to protect the cornea. A scratch or other injury to the cornea causes intense, prolonged pain.

The second layer of the eye. This is made up of three parts: the **choroid**, the **ciliary body** and the **iris**.

The choroid is a vascular layer that nourishes the retina. Near the front of the eye, the choroid (which lies underneath the sclera) forms a thickened ring-shaped structure, the ciliary body. The ciliary body holds the **lens** in place and controls the shape of the lens. The lens is a transparent structure that refracts the light rays reaching the eyes and focuses them onto the retina. Although most of the refraction occurs at the cornea, the lens can also affect the path of the light rays by changing its shape. The purpose of this mechanism is to ensure that a sharp image is produced on the retina.

The ciliary body has small finger-like processes coming out of it, the **ciliary processes**, which hold the lens by means of tiny filaments attached tightly to the edge of the lens. Inside the ciliary body are involuntary smooth muscles that pull the ciliary body forward when they contract.

When one looks at an object nearby, the eye performs a process called **accommodation**. The muscles in the ciliary body contract, the tension on the ligaments holding the lens decreases and the lens springs into a more convex shape (becomes thicker). This increases the refraction of the light rays, allowing to focus the image of the near object onto the retina. The reverse process occurs when looking at a distant object. The muscles in the ciliary body relax, the edges of the ciliary body move further away from each other, applying tension to the ciliary processes and the filaments attached to the lens, which is 'pulled out' to become flatter. This focuses the image of the distant object on the retina. The alteration in the shape of the lens acts as a focusing mechanism, as in a camera.

Accommodation is an active process requiring muscular effort, and can therefore be tiring. Indeed, the ciliary muscle is one of the most frequently used muscles in the body. Trying to focus on near objects for prolonged periods tires the ciliary muscles, which might be unable to maintain the effort, and the image becomes blurred as it slips out of focus. This does not occur when looking at distant objects, because in this situation the muscle is relaxed.

The opaque iris is the colored portion of the eye and is situated immediately in front of the lens. It is a dome-shaped structure with a central hole – the **pupil** of the eye – through which light enters. Its periphery is connected to the front of the ciliary body. The iris contains two smooth muscles, a circular muscle and a longitudinal muscle. The pupil looks black because there is no light source inside the eye (as in the opening to a cave). The two pupils are normally equal in size. When the longitudinal muscle fibers in the iris contract, the opening in the center enlarges and the pupil dilates; when the circular muscle contracts, the pupil constricts. The change in the size of the pupil controls the amount of light that enters the eye, in exactly the same way as the diaphragm of a camera controls the amount of light reaching the film.

The strength of the light determines the size of the pupil: in bright light, the pupil constricts and in poor light it dilates. The muscles of the iris are innervated by the autonomic nervous system and are not under voluntary control. Various diseases can affect the size of the pupils.

The reason that the iris is colored is that it contains pigment to prevent light from getting through. The color of a person's eyes is determined by the amount of pigment in the iris. A large amount results in a black iris, and little pigment results in a light blue iris. (An albino individual has no pigment and has serious visual problems.) Between the iris and the cornea is a space (the **anterior chamber**) filled with a clear fluid that is constantly being produced and reabsorbed. If the amount of this fluid becomes excessive (e.g. by interference with its absorption), the pressure in the anterior chamber rises, giving rise to a disease called **glaucoma**. This disease can destroy nerves in the retina, leading to blindness, and must be treated promptly.

The innermost layer of the eye. This is called the **retina**. The retina contains photoreceptor cells and nerve cells with many synapses (connections between two nerve cells) among them.

Some of the nerve cells in the retina have long axons, which converge from all over the retina into a small area called the **optic disc**, to form the **optic nerve**. The optic nerve passes through the choroid and the sclera at the back of the orbit, and enters the skull.

Photoreceptors are elongated cells that convert light impulses to electrical charges, which are then conducted along the nerves. There are two kinds of photoreceptors – **rods** and **cones**. The rods are extremely sensitive to light and are used for night vision. They are scattered all over the retina (it is estimated that there are some 120 million rods in each eye). The cones, of which there are some 6 million in each eye, are responsible for color vision. They are concentrated in an area of the retina called the **fovea**. This is also the most important area for visual acuity and, when focusing on an object, the eyes normally move to make the light rays from the center of the object fall on the fovea. Injury or illness of the fovea in effect results in blindness.

The retina contains millions of nerve cells that process the information arriving from the photoreceptors and transmit it to the brain via the optic nerve. The visual pathway ends in the visual center in the brain, located in the occipital lobe at the back of the brain.

Most of the volume of the eyeball is filled with a clear gelatinous substance called the **vitreous body**. This substance fills all of the space behind the lens, up to the retina. A light ray passing through the eye on its way to the retina passes through the following structures: the cornea, the clear liquid between the cornea and the lens, the pupil (not an actual structure but a hole in the center of the iris), the lens and the vitreous body. All these structures normally are completely transparent.

The conjunctiva and the lacrimal system

The **conjunctiva** is a thin, vascular membrane that covers the internal surface of the eyelids and part of the sclera of the eye up to the edge of the cornea. It forms a sac that prevents foreign matter from entering the eyeball.

Tears are formed in the **lacrimal glands** (Latin *lacrima* = tear), which are situated in the upper outer part of the orbit (Fig. 20.2). The tears sweep across the eye and are then drained away into the lacrimal drainage system through two tiny holes in the edge of each eyelid, towards the medial (nasal) side. From there they are drained into the **lacrimal sac**, which is situated at the medial wall of the orbit, and finally into the nasal cavity. (this is why one needs to blow one's nose if crying). The tears rinse out the conjunctival sac and the cornea and clear away any foreign matter. In addition, the tears keep the cornea moist and prevent it from drying out.

Diseases of the eye

Hyperopia. Also called **hypermetropia**, hyperopia is long-sightedness and is the most common abnormality of sight. It results from abnormal refraction of light rays from distant objects, such that they do not focus on the retina but a little behind it, causing a blurred image.

Myopia. This is near sightedness and occurs when light rays from a near object are focused in front of the retina, again resulting in a blurred image.

These problems are very easy to correct by placing a lens (spectacle or contact lens) in front

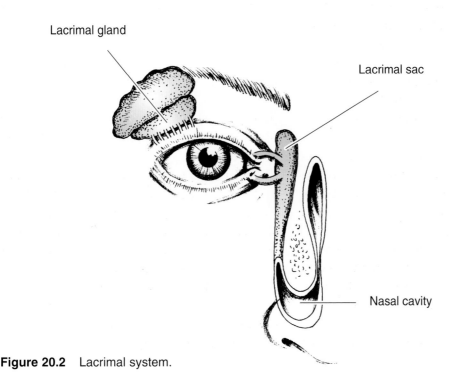

Figure 20.2   Lacrimal system.

of the eye to correct the refractive error and cause the light rays to focus on the retina itself.

Diseases of the cornea

A scratch on the cornea is extremely painful. The cornea usually heals completely but sometimes a scar remains, which can interfere with sight. A common cause of corneal injury is exposure to very bright light without protective goggles (e.g. when welding) or exposure to prolonged ultraviolet light (the discotheque syndrome), resulting in corneal burns. This causes considerable pain but, in most cases, the cornea recovers completely.

Various infectious agents (e.g. the Herpes virus) can damage the cornea and cause it to become opaque, which interferes seriously with vision. In many cases, the only treatment is a corneal transplant, a commonly performed procedure.

Diseases of the lens – cataract

The cataract is a clouding (opacification) of the lens. It usually appears in older persons as a result of age-related degenerative changes in the lens. It can also result from certain diseases (e.g. diabetes), injury to the lens or some medications (e.g. corticosteroids). The opacification of the lens leads to progressive loss of vision in the affected eye. Treatment consists of removing and replacing the lens with an artificial lens, the most common eye surgery performed today.

From the age of approximately 50, the lens progressively loses its elasticity, causing increasing difficulty to focus on nearby objects (reading). This problem is called **presbyopia**, and requires the use of reading glasses, which aid in nearby focusing.

Glaucoma

Glaucoma results from an increase of pressure in the eye, usually due to inadequate absorption of the fluid in the anterior chamber of the eye. This fluid is constantly being produced and reabsorbed and normally there is a balance between the rate of production and the rate of absorption. In most cases, the increased pressure does not cause any immediate symptoms but, with time, it causes damage to the retina and, if untreated, will eventually lead to visual disturbance and blindness. The initial treatment is by means of medications and, if this proves unsuccessful, several operations can be carried out to lower the pressure within the eye.

Conjunctivitis

Conjunctivitis is an inflammation of the conjunctiva, usually caused by a virus or bacteria. As a result of the infection, the blood vessels in the conjunctiva dilate and become engorged with blood and the eye looks red (the so-called 'red eye'). In most cases, the infection can resolve without treatment, although topical antibiotic drops are often used to speed healing.

THE HEARING AND BALANCE SYSTEM

The ear

The ear can be divided into three divisions: the external ear, the middle ear and the inner ear (Fig. 20.3)

The external ear

This comprises the **auricle** and the **external auditory meatus**.

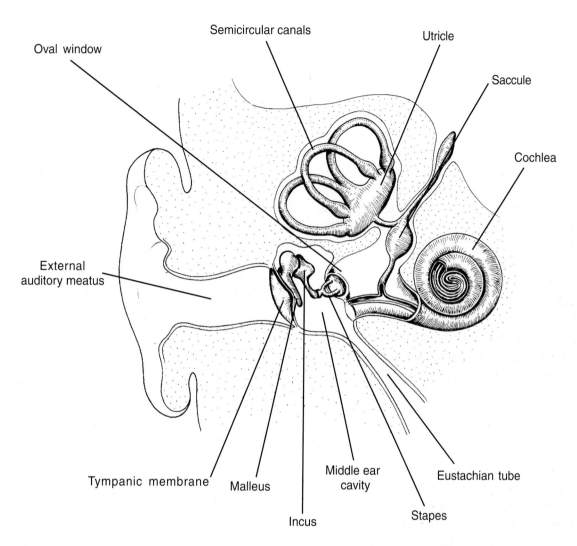

Figure 20.3   The ear.

The auricle consists of elastic cartilage covered with skin. Its function is to 'gather' the sound into the external auditory (hearing) meatus. The cartilage of the ear continues to grow throughout life, and in the elderly the ear is relatively large.

The sound waves pass along the external auditory meatus until they reach the **tympanic membrane** (the eardrum). The external auditory meatus is a canal approximately 2.5 cm long; its outer two-thirds is made of cartilage and the inner one-third of bone. The skin lining of the auditory canal contains glands, which secrete a fatty substance called **cerumen** (wax). At the (inner) end of the auditory canal is the tympanic membrane. This is a thin, round sheet, approximately 1 cm in diameter, that vibrates when sound waves reach it and transmits the sound waves into the middle ear.

The middle ear

The middle ear is an air-filled space situated within the temporal bone in the skull. Within the middle ear are three tiny bones called the **auditory ossicles**, which transmit and magnify the vibrations of the eardrum. These ossicles are called the **malleus**, the **incus** and the **stapes**.

The vibrations of the tympanic membrane are transferred via the auditory ossicles to the inner ear. Two tiny muscles are attached to the auditory ossicles, which involuntarily contract in case of a very loud noise. This dampens the transmission of the vibrations to the middle ear and protects the neurologic system in the middle ear from damage. The **auditory tube** (or **Eustachian tube**) is a thin tube that connects the middle ear with the pharyngeal cavity. This tube ensures that the air pressure in the middle ear is the same as that in the external environment. If the auditory tube becomes blocked (e.g. in case of a respiratory infection), changes in the external pressure (as can occur when diving or flying) result in pressure differences on either side of the eardrum, which cause pain.

The inner ear

The inner ear is situated within the temporal bone and contains the **cochlea**, which contains the hearing receptors, as well as the **vestibular** (balance) **system**.

The cochlea is a fluid-filled tube, with a central partition along its length on which the hearing receptors rest. It is curled in a way that resembles a snail's shell, hence its name (Latin *cochlea* = snail shell). Between the middle ear and the inner ear are two small 'windows' covered by a thin membrane. One of the three auditory ossicles in the middle ear, the malleus, is attached to the inner side of the tympanic membrane, and the base of the third ossicle (the stapes) is connected to one of those windows, called the **oval window**. This arrangement forms a continuous 'chain', which transmits vibrations. Sound waves cause the tympanic membrane to vibrate; these vibrations are transmitted by the auditory ossicles to the oval window, which vibrates in turn and causes movement of the fluid in the cochlea. The membrane partition along the length of the cochlea is of variable thickness and different areas of this partition respond to different frequencies of vibration. High frequency sounds cause the thicker part of the membrane to respond and lower-frequency waves stimulate the thinner part of the membrane.

The vibrations of the membrane partition cause the receptor cells along its length to vibrate and these, in turn, transmit an electrical charge to the nerve ends that connect to them. The sound receptors are mechanoreceptors, because they respond to vibration.

The axons of these sound receptors form part of the eighth cranial nerve, the vestibulocochlear nerve. This transmits the information from the ear to the hearing center in the brain, in the temporal lobe.

Balance

The organ involved in maintaining balance is also found in the inner ear and is separate from the auditory system. This organ comprises two structures, the **utricle** and the **saccule**, which respond to linear acceleration forces, as well as three **semicircular canals**. The three semicircular canals are arranged perpendicular to each other and are oriented in the three planes of space. They respond to acceleration in non-linear directions.

Each of the above organs contains balance receptors. The balance receptors are connected to nerve endings that transmit the impulses via the eighth cranial nerve to the balance center in the brain.

The balance center in the brain receives information from three sources:

1. balance organs in each ear
2. the eyes
3. special receptors in the muscles and joints that transmit information regarding the position and degree of tension of the muscles and joints at any given moment.

If the information from these sources is not fully correlated, this causes nausea. For example, reading while travelling sends 'conflicting' signals to the brain because the information arriving from the balance organs in the ears indicates movement of the body, while the information arriving from the eyes (looking at a book or newspaper) indicates absence of movement between the body and the environment.

Vertigo is a sensation that the world is rotating or spinning and occurs in case of damage or disease involving the balance system. Persistent vertigo can be a very debilitating condition, which must be treated by drugs or even surgery.

Hearing loss

Hearing loss can be conductive, sensory or neural in nature.

Conductive hearing loss. This involves a disruption in the conduction of sound waves from the outer or middle ear and is caused by dysfunction of the external ear or middle ear. The former commonly results from obstruction of the external auditory meatus by cerumen, debris or foreign bodies, or from perforations of the tympanic membrane. The latter results from diseases of the auditory ossicles, dysfunction of the auditory tube, fluid in the middle ear, infection and tumors of the middle ear.

The most common cause of conductive hearing loss is **cerumen impaction**. Cerumen is a fatty protective substance secreted in the external auditory meatus. In most individuals the ear canal is self-cleaning. Recommended hygiene consists of cleaning the external opening with a washcloth over the index finger, but without entering the canal itself. Daily cleaning of the actual canal (e.g. with cotton swabs) produces irritation of its skin and increases cerumen production, which can result in build-up and impaction. Treatment of impaction includes detergent ear drops, mechanical removal, suction or irrigation.

The auditory (Eustachian) tube connects the middle ear to the pharynx and provides ventilation and drainage of the middle ear. It is normally closed, opening only during swallowing or yawning. Upper respiratory tract infection or allergy can cause edema of the tubal lining and block the passage of air through the tube. Air trapped within the middle ear is absorbed, producing negative pressure. The patient usually reports a sense of fullness in the ear and mild to moderate hearing loss. In children, the auditory tube is narrower and more easily blocked. The negative pressure leads to filling of the middle ear with fluid, a condition known as **serous otitis media**. If prolonged medication fails to relieve this condition, a ventilation tube placed through the tympanic membrane can often restore hearing.

Sensory hearing loss.   This is caused by damage to the central sensory organ of hearing, the cochlea. Aging, noise trauma, viral infections, ototoxic drugs and fracture of the temporal bone can produce sensory hearing loss. The damage is usually irreversible and the primary goals of treatment are prevention of further loss, improvement of function with amplification devices ('hearing aids') and auditory rehabilitation.

The most common cause of sensory hearing loss is normal aging, called presbyacusis, and involves a progressive, predominantly high-frequency and symmetric hearing loss. Approximately 50% of people over 75 years of age experience hearing difficulties, usually a loss of speech discrimination that is especially pronounced in a noisy environment.

Noise trauma is the second most common cause of sensory hearing loss. Loud sounds (exceeding 85 dB) are potentially injurious to the cochlea, especially with prolonged exposure, and include industrial machinery, explosives and loud music. Using protection devices can prevent the injury.

Neural hearing loss.   This results from lesions involving the eighth cranial nerve or the hearing center of the brain. It is relatively uncommon and can be a sign of brain disease.

The skin

The **skin** forms the outermost covering of the body. The hair, nails, sweat glands, and sebaceous glands are all parts of the skin (Fig. 21.1).

FUNCTIONS OF THE SKIN

- Protection against physical and chemical damage.
- Prevention of fluid loss by surface evaporation.
- Location for the receptors for touch, pain and temperature.
- Location for the first stage in vitamin D production.
- Body temperature regulation by changes in the blood flow to the skin and via sweating.

STRUCTURE OF THE SKIN

The skin is composed of three layers: the **epidermis**, the **dermis** and the **subcutaneous tissue**.

Epidermis

The epidermis consists of multiple layers of epithelial cells. The cells at the bottom of the epidermis (furthest from the surface of the skin) are cuboid in shape and divide continuously. As

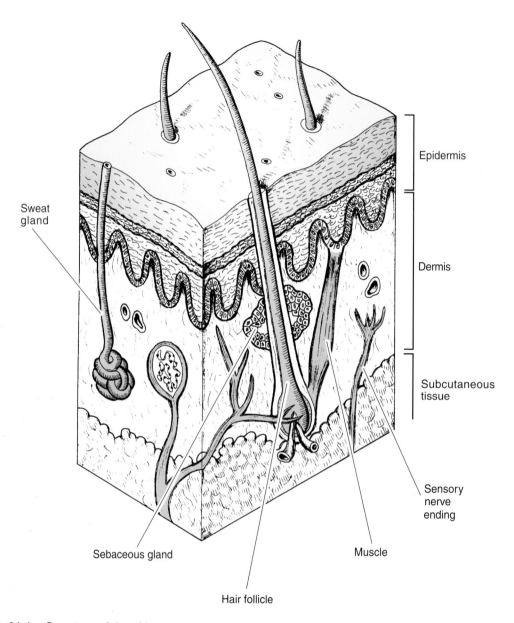

Sweat
gland

Epidermis

Dermis

Subcutaneous
tissue

Sensory
nerve
ending

Sebaceous gland

Muscle

Hair follicle

Figure 21.1   Structure of the skin.

thay divide, the cells are pushed towards the surface of the skin by the newly formed cells beneath them and, as they migrate upwards, they die and become flatter and flatter in shape. When the cells reach the surface of the skin, they are shed. This process of replication and

shedding of dead cells proceeds continuously throughout life.

Melanocytes are round cells with elongated processes. They are found in the basal (innermost) layers of the epidermis. They produce a substance called **melanin**, a black pigment, which passes through the processes of the melanocytes to the superficial layers of the epidermis and gives the skin its color. Exposure to the sun increases the production of melanin, causing the skin to become darker.

Dermis

The dermis is a thick, tough connective tissue layer beneath the epidermis, which provides the skin with its strength. The dermis contains cells called fibroblasts, as well as an intercellular substance that contains **collagen** (a protein fiber). Both fibroblasts and collagen are embedded in a gelatinous material.

Subcutaneous tissue

This layer is composed mainly of fat and its thickness varies considerably between thin and fat individuals and according to the area of the body. The subcutaneous tissue functions as an energy store and also provides an insulating layer to maintain body temperature.

Sebaceous glands

These are present in the dermis and are connected to the hair follicles. They secrete a fatty substance, which coats the hair and the outer surface of the skin.

Sweat glands

These are present in the dermis and the subcutaneous layer and secrete sweat onto the surface of the skin. Apart from the lips and the genitalia, virtually all of the skin contains sweat glands.

Sweat comprises mainly water and salts, as well as a small amount of uric acid, urea and ammonia. It plays a very important role in regulating body temperature. If the body temperature rises, the blood-flow to the skin increases (the skin becomes flushed) and more sweat is secreted. As the sweat evaporates from the body surface, it cools the skin, thereby cooling the blood flowing through it.

Hair

Hair is made of a tough substance called **keratin** and grows out of a structure called a **hair follicle**.

The hair follicle is formed from epidermal cells that have moved down into the dermis. The hair is formed by the division of cells at the base of the follicle. The new cells push the older cells up along the follicle towards the surface of the skin. In a process similar to that occurring in the cells of the epidermis, the cells die as they move up the hair follicle and the hair at the surface is composed of dead cells and keratin. Each hair follicle goes through cycles of growth and resting phases.

A sebaceous gland is attached to each hair follicle and sebum produced by the gland is secreted onto the surface of the growing hair. Each hair follicle also has a tiny muscle attached to it. When this muscle contracts, it causes the hair to stand on end.

Hair growth is influenced by the secretion of the male sex hormone, testosterone, which is responsible for the growth of tough, dark hairs in specific areas such as the face, chest and buttocks.

AGING OF THE SKIN

With aging, normal skin undergoes atrophic changes that make it thinner, wrinkled and dry. Solar ultraviolet radiation accelerates this process. The aging process involves both the epidermis and dermis layers of the skin.

The division of cells at the bottom of the epidermis, which produces new epidermal cells, is slowed down. The number of melanocytes in the epidermis is reduced and the dark pigment produced by these cells is no longer distributed equally in the upper layers of the epidermis, so that dark spots (lentigo) and bright spots appear. The dermis layer also undergoes degenerative changes: the number of fibroblasts declines, the intracellular matrix is damaged and the strength and elasticity of the skin diminishes, making it vulnerable to trauma. The growth rate of hair and nails diminishes by 30%; the hair becomes gray, and later white, as the result of a reduction in the number of the melanocytes in the hair follicles. The production of sebaceous glands is also decreased and the skin becomes dry.

PATHOLOGY OF THE SKIN

Skin lesions have many forms and can appear as a symptom of acute illness or as part of a chronic, either systemic or localized, disease.

Skin rash

This can develop in many infectious diseases. For example, the viral disease **Rubella** (German measles) is accompanied by a discrete erythematous rash. The rash begins on the face and spreads to the body, lasting for about 3 days.

The viral disease **varicella** (chickenpox) is accompanied by a rash that appears initially as red papules, which rapidly progress to oval vesicles on an erythematous base. The vesicles ulcerate, crust and then heal.

Skin rash often develops as part of an allergic reaction. **Urticaria** (hives) comprises transient lesions composed of a central blanched wheal surrounded by an erythematous halo. The lesions are round or oval in shape and are often pruritic. Urticaria develops within minutes of contact with the allergen, and eventually disappear completely.

Skin rash can also be a manifestation of systemic disease. For example, the autoimmune disease systemic lupus erythematosus is accompanied by a reddish rash on the cheeks and the bridge of the nose, giving the patient a wolf-like facial appearance.

Acne vulgaris

This is the most common skin disease among young people in the second and third decades of life, and up to 85% of adolescents have some degree of acne. It is distributed equally between males and females, although males tend to have a more severe form. Acne is caused by chronic inflammation of the sebaceous glands. The sebaceous glands normally secrete a fatty substance, which drains to the hair follicles and to the outer surface of the skin. Hyperproliferation of epithelial cells in the hair follicle can block the drainage process and lead to the formation of a **comedone**, a plug of keratin and fat which blocks the opening of the sebaceous gland on the surface of the skin. Subsequent bacterial infection of the comedone leads to the formation of erythematous papules and pustules. Acne appears mainly on the face, upper chest, back and arms. The eventual healing of the lesions can result in the formation of scars. The treatment of acne includes local drugs (antibiotics and retinoids), and so prevent the formation of comedones which prevent the formation of acne.

Malignent melanoma

This highly malignant skin tumor accounts for the majority of deaths due to skin disease, although many are preventable by early diagnosis and excision. Melanoma originates from melanocytes normally present in the epidermis and often appears in sun-exposed areas. The tumor penetrates the skin and sends metastases to lymph nodes, liver, lung, bone and brain. Once metastatic disease is established, the likelihood of cure is very low.

Benign mole

This is a small, well-circumscribed lesion with well-defined border and a single shade of pigment from beige or pink to dark brown. In the first decade of life, moles often appear as small, flat, brown lesions. Over the next 2 decades moles increase in size and often become raised. Suspicious moles that may be melanomas are usually more than 6 mm in diameter, have an irregular and asymmetrical border and irregular topography, which can be partly raised and partly flat. The color is variable mixtures of tan brown, black and pink. A patient with a large number of moles is statistically at increased risk for melanoma and should undergo careful periodic examination. Suspicious moles are usually excised and examined for pathology.

22

Cancer

Cancer refers to a large group of different diseases, all of which are caused by the uncontrolled multiplication of cells and the formation of a mass of tumor cells. (Note: the word **tumor** means swelling or lump, it is not the name of a disease.)

The human body, which contains billions of different cells, begins as a single cell following the union of the sperm and the ovum. The body which contains billions of cells of different types, develops from one single cell. This cell divides exponentially, and the new cells that are formed undergo a process of **differentiation**. During differentiation, the newly formed cells undergo various changes, which ultimately produce mature cells of different types. These cells must also migrate to different sites to form the various tissues of the body. The processes of cell division and differentiation are controlled and coordinated in a very complex manner to produce an organized, functioning body.

In the human body, there are three types of cells:

1. **Cells that are unable to divide**: these are cells that were able to divide when the body was developing but, once that process ended, lost their ability to replicate themselves.

Nerve cells (neurons) and muscle cells are examples of cells that are unable to divide. Their numbers diminish progressively throughout life.

2. **Cells that can divide under certain circumstances**: these are cells that do not divide normally but, under special circumstances will start doing so. Liver cells, for example, do not usually divide in adults. However, if there is damage or injury to the liver, with destruction of a large number of liver cells, the remaining cells start to divide and produce new liver tissue to replace the loss. Once the regeneration of the liver tissue is complete, the replication of the cells stops.

3. **Cells that are dividing continuously throughout life:** these are cells that have a short lifespan: dead cells are constantly being replaced by new cells. Red blood cells live for an average of 120 days, and then die in the 'red cell graveyard' – the spleen. To compensate for this loss, the bone marrow is constantly producing new red blood cells. White blood cells of the neutrophil type are also constantly being produced in the bone marrow, released into the bloodstream, and die after 8 hours. Both red and white blood cells are formed from a common stem cell present in the bone marrow. This stem cell divides and then undergoes differentiation to one of the types of blood cell. Some of the cells become red blood cells, some become white blood cells. This process is very precisely regulated to meet the requirement at any given time. Other cells that are dividing constantly are skin cells and the mucosal cells of the digestive system.

A **tumor** is formed when the control system that regulates cell division and differentiation becomes abnormal: a single cell might fail to respond to the control system, it starts dividing uncontrollably, producing more cells, which also divide uncontrollably, eventually producing a mass of cells, or tumor. (Note: cancer of the blood cells, is an exception to this because it does not produce a tumor mass but rather an excess of cells within the vascular system.)

The tumor might interfere with body functions by compressing and destroying healthy tissue around it, or by secreting substances that compromise normal tissue functions.

The type of tumor is determined by the type of cell from which it originated, as well as the organ in which it appeared. Tumors derived from epithelial cells are referred to by the general term **carcinoma**, and tumors derived from connective tissue or muscle tissue are called **sarcoma**. **Gastric carcinoma** is a tumor that originates in the mucosa of the stomach (epithelial cells); **gastric sarcoma** is a tumor that arises from the smooth muscle cells in the wall of the stomach.

Within a tumor are subtypes of cells, depending on the particular cell type in the tumor. If the tumor cells resemble the normal cells within which the growth appeared, the tumor is called **well differentiated**. If the tumor cells do not resemble the cells from which they arose, the tumor is called **poorly differentiated**.

FACTORS RELATED TO THE DEVELOPMENT OF TUMORS

A cancer develops when a single normal cell undergoes some change in its genetic material. This change makes the cell uncontrollable, eventually producing the tumor.

Both external and internal factors are involved in the formation of cancerous cells.

Age. For each type of cancer there is a typical age group when it tends to occur. There are some cancers that occur in childhood but most occur in adults. The precise reason why a certain cancer appears at certain ages is not known.

Gender. Certain cancers appear more frequently in males and others in females. This difference is obviously related not only to anatomic differences (men cannot develop cancer of the uterus and women cannot develop prostate cancer) but probably also to differences in hormonal factors, and possibly differences in lifestyle.

Heredity. It is well known that some types of cancer are influenced by hereditary factors. For example, the daughter of a woman who had breast cancer has a higher risk of herself developing breast cancer than a woman whose mother did not have cancer of the breast. Apparently, the tendency for the cells in the breast to become malignant is transmitted genetically.

In those types of cancer with a strong hereditary influence, it is recommended that close relatives of the patient undergo appropriate screening tests to detect the disease as early as possible. For example, first-degree relatives of someone who has carcinoma of the colon should have an annual colon examination to detect the development of a colon cancer at an early stage, when it can be more successfully treated.

Geographic location. There are marked differences in the incidence of certain cancers in different parts of the world; these differences are probably related to environmental factors. For example, cancer of the stomach is very common in Japan but quite uncommon in the United States and Europe; breast cancer is very common in the United States and in Europe, but uncommon in China. Interestingly, among Chinese women who emigrate to the United States and adopt an American lifestyle, the incidence of breast cancer is similar to that in the United States.

Diet. There is an association between the type of diet and the incidence of certain types of cancer. For example, pickled, cured and smoked food is associated with the occurrence of stomach cancer. A diet rich in saturated fats and low in fiber is associated with an increased tendency to develop cancer of the colon.

Infection. Certain infections increase the risk of developing some types of cancer. For example, infection of the cervix of the uterus by human papilloma virus increases the incidence of cancer of the cervix. Chronic infection with hepatitis B or C virus is associated with the development of cancer of the liver.

Radiation. Exposure to solar rays increases the incidence of skin cancer. Exposure to ionizing radiation (such as from the atom bomb), increases the incidence of a variety of cancers. It is known that ionizing radiation directly damages the genetic material within cells, and in this way can turn them into malignant or cancerous cells.

Smoking and air pollution. Cigarette smoke and air pollution contain substances that affect the incidence of certain cancers. There is a clear association between smoking and cancers of the lung, larynx and throat, and even cancer of the urinary bladder.

Carcinogens. These are substances that result in an increased incidence of certain cancers. For example, asbestos dust is associated with the development of a lethal type of lung cancer.

BENIGN TUMORS

A benign tumor is one that does not invade healthy tissues around it and does not produce metastases (see below). The tumor usually presses on surrounding tissues as it grows and a border of connective tissue generally forms around it.

Benign tumor cells are usually **well differentiated**, that is, they resemble the normal cells from which the initial tumor cell developed. For example, a **leiomyoma** (often called a 'fibroid') is a tumor made up of muscle cells derived from the smooth muscle in the wall of the uterus (Fig. 22.1). It is a very common tumor, occuring in one in four women. It grows slowly and is usually asymptomatic. If it becomes very large (leiomyoma can reach more than 20 cm in diameter), it can cause clinical problems because of pressure on surrounding structures.

It is usually quite easy to remove a benign tumor, because the growth is surrounded by a capsule and can therefore be readily separated from the surrounding tissues. On occasion, however, a benign tumor can endanger the patient's life if it occurs in certain critical anatomic locations. For example, a benign tumor in the brain stem can press on vital structures in the brain, yet, because of its location, cannot be removed without causing damage to surrounding healthy brain tissue.

MALIGNANT TUMORS

Certain characteristics differentiate malignant from benign tumors.

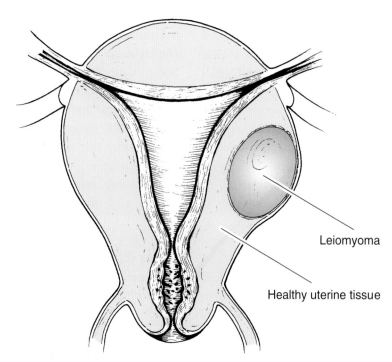

Leiomyoma

Healthy uterine tissue

Figure 22.1   Leiomyoma (fibroid) – a benign tumor of the uterus.

Invasion of healthy tissue. Malignant cells invade and damage the surrounding healthy tissue (Fig. 22.2). A cancerous mass with tentacle-like extensions that spread out into the surrounding tissue resembles the shape of a crab, from which the term **cancer** is derived (the Latin word *cancer* = crab).

Seeding metastases. A **metastasis** is a 'daughter colony' of a primary cancerous growth. The cells within a metastasis are identical to the tumor cells in the primary tumor but are situated at some distance from it. Metastases occur when cells break off the primary tumor and move to another area in the body, where they develop into a secondary tumor. There are several ways by which metastatic cells spread:

- **Lymphatic spread**: cells break off from the primary tumor, enter the lymphatic vessels, and finally reach the lymph nodes, where they develop into a secondary tumor. The development of a tumor mass within lymph nodes results in enlargement of the lymph nodes, known as **lymphadenopathy**. For example, cancer of the breast tends to spread to the axillary (armpit) lymph nodes, which then become enlarged.

- **via the blood**: tumor cells break away from the primary growth, enter the vascular system and move in the bloodstream to distant areas, where they develop into a secondary tumor. Common sites for such metastases are the lungs, liver, bones and brain.

- **Spread within cavities:** tumor cells within the thoracic or the abdominal cavity can break away from the primary tumor, move around within the cavity and then develop into a secondary tumor in another part of the cavity.

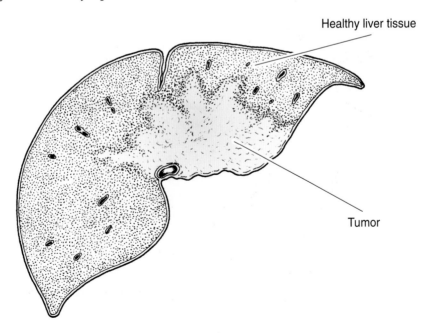

Healthy liver tissue

Tumor

Figure 22.2 Malignant tumor of the liver. Tumor cells are shown invading the healthy surrounding tissue. There is no clear-cut border between the tumor tissue and the healthy tissue.

Rate of growth. A malignant tumor often grows rapidly, spreads through the body and kills the patient if left untreated.

Type of cells. Malignant tumors contain cells of different degrees of differentiation, from highly to poorly differentiated.

CLINICAL FEATURES OF CANCER

The clinical features of cancer can be divided into localized features, resulting from their direct effects on surrounding tissues, and multisystem features caused by harmful substances in the bloodstream secreted from the tumor cells.

Localized features

A cancerous growth might produce a mass that can be felt. For example, cancers in the breast produce lumps that can be felt when they are only 0.5 cm in diameter.

Tumors can press on nearby tissues and organs and cause malfunction. For example, a cancer of the esophagus causes difficulty in swallowing because it blocks the passage of food. Cancer of the rectum can result in changes in bowel movements (often alternating constipation and diarrhea), changes in the size or shape of the stool or the appearance of blood in the stool. Cancer of the pancreas can block the bile duct and cause jaundice. A cancer developing in an organ can affect the function of that organ. For example, a brain tumor could cause neurologic signs, such as paralysis.

Multisystem features

These are the result of the effects of substances secreted into the bloodstream by the cancer cells. Loss of appetite, weight loss and general emaciation, weakness, pain, depression, anemia, and neurologic signs can appear with various cancers.

In most types of cancer, the local phenomena usually appear first, although sometimes the general, multisystem phenomena appear before the localized ones.

TREATMENT OF CANCER

The aim of treatment is to achieve a **cure**, namely to destroy all of the cancerous cells while causing minimal damage to normal body tissues. In some cases this cannot be achieved, and then the aim of treatment is to minimize the patient's suffering (**palliation**).

There are basically three forms of treatment for cancer: surgery to remove the tumor, chemotherapy and radiation.

Surgery. This is carried out either to produce a cure or palliation. In the case of benign tumors, surgery is an effective and relatively straightforward form of treatment. In the case of malignant tumors, the fact that the tumor invades healthy tissues often makes it hard to remove without damaging normal tissue around it. In cases where the cancer has already seeded distant metastases to other places in the body, surgery cannot cure it. In such cases, the aim of surgery is to relieve the patient's discomfort, for example by removing a tumor of the colon in order to relieve bowel obstruction.

Chemotherapy. This is treatment using medications (usually intravenous) that kill tumor cells. Because the medication is injected into the bloodstream, it can reach the tumor cells throughout the body. Chemotherapeutic drugs attack rapidly dividing cells, and so destroy cancer cells. The problem with chemotherapy is that normal rapidly dividing cells in the body will also be attacked. This is the reason for some of the severe side-effects of chemotherapy, such as hair loss, nausea and vomiting (due to damage to the rapidly dividing cells in the gastrointestinal mucosa) and suppression of the production of all blood cells, including red and white blood cells and thrombocytes. The damage to the white blood cells is the most significant because it compromises the body's defense system and predisposes to various infections. The use of chemotherapeutic drugs is therefore limited by their side-effects, which can themselves be lethal.

Radiotherapy. This also destroys rapidly dividing cells and, like chemotherapy, also destroys healthy dividing cells. However, unlike chemotherapy, which affects the entire body, radiotherapy is usually aimed at the tumor site(s) only.

In many cases, combinations of surgery, chemotherapy and radiation are used. The particular type of treatment depends on the nature of the cancer, its location, the degree of spread and the patient's wishes and general state of health.

The specific type of cancer is diagnosed by pathologic examination of a sample of the tumor under the microscope (biopsy), as well as by various biochemical and immunologic tests. Different cancers react differently to different forms of treatment. For example, certain types of lymphoma (a cancer originating in the lymph nodes) are very sensitive to chemotherapy but cannot be treated surgically. On the other hand, carcinoma of the esophagus responds poorly (if at all) to chemotherapy and radiation but, in its early stages, is amenable to surgical removal. Breast cancer is commonly treated by a combination of surgery, radiotherapy and chemotherapy.

The extent of spread of a cancer is diagnosed on the basis of the physical examination of the patient, various imaging investigations and the results of laboratory tests. It is accepted practice to classify the spread of a malignant tumor by **staging**. A growth that is confined to one area of the body is an early-stage tumor. A growth that has spread to the regional lymph nodes (those close to the primary tumor) is of an intermediate stage. A tumor that has seeded metastases to distant areas of the body is of an advanced stage.

Other factors taken into account when deciding upon treatment include the patient's wishes, age and other illnesses that may be present. In general, a more aggressive approach is taken with a young cancer patient and less aggressive treatment is given to a debilitated older patient unlikely to survive aggressive treatment for long.

PROGNOSIS

The prospect of recovering from cancer depends on the type of tumor, the degree of its spread (its stage) and the type of treatment. The likelihood of cure is calculated statistically on the basis of data gathered from many patients and is used in deciding which treatment to offer.

For any given stage of spread of a tumor, there are data providing the likelihood of cure, or survival for 5 or 10 years from the time of diagnosis (referred to as **5-year** or **10-year survival rates**).

For example, the 5-year survival rate following diagnosis of breast cancer at an early stage is between 80 and 90%. If the tumor has spread to the axillary lymph nodes, the 5-year survival drops to between 40 and 60%. If bone metastases are present at the time of diagnosis, the 5-year survival is only 10%.

It is important to note that the prognosis statistics do not predict the course for any given individual but denote a statistical risk for an entire patient population. Because of the way in which prognosis statistics are derived, they cannot be used for a completely accurate prediction in any given case and treatment is still influenced by the clinical experience of the physician and the wishes of the patient. This is the art of medicine.

PREVENTION

A healthy lifestyle significantly lessens the risk of developing cancer. The concept of a 'healthy lifestyle' includes proper nutrition and avoidance of exposure to carcinogens (e.g., cigarette smoke). Early detection is also critical in improving the prognosis in most types of cancer, highlighting the need for routine regular medical check-ups. In other words, prevention depends as much on the patient as on the physician.

Index